AN INTRODUCTION TO CARDIAC
ELECTROPHYSIOLOGY

AN INTRODUCTION TO CARDIAC ELECTROPHYSIOLOGY

Edited by

Antonio Zaza

*Dipartimento di Fisiologia e Biochimica Generali
Università di Milano, Milano, Italy*

and

Michael R. Rosen

*Department of Pharmacology
College of Physicians and Surgeons
Columbia University, New York, USA*

 harwood academic publishers
Australia • Canada • France • Germany • India • Japan • Luxembourg
Malaysia • The Netherlands • Russia • Singapore • Switzerland

Amsteldijk 166
1st Floor
1079 LH Amsterdam
The Netherlands

British Library Cataloguing in Publication Data

An introduction to cardiac electrophysiology
  1. Heart – Electric properties 2. Heart cells – Electric properties
  I. Zaza, Antonio II. Rosen, Michael R. (Michael Robert), 1938–
  612.1'71

ISBN   90-5702-457-8

Contents

Contributors

Paul B. Bennett
Senior Director, Ion Channel Research
MRL, Pharmacology WP26 – 265
Merck & Co.
770 Sumneytown Pike
West Point, PA 19486
USA

Ofer Binah
Rappaport Family Institute for Research
  in the Medical Sciences
Faculty of Medicine – Technion
PO Box 9697, Haifa IL 31096
Israel

Penelope A. Boyden
Department of Pharmacology
College of Physicians and Surgeons
Columbia University
630W 168th Street
New York, NY 10032
USA

Chris Clausen
Department of Physiology and
  Biophysics
Health Science Center of the State
  University of New York
Stoney Brook, NY 11794-8661
USA

Ira S. Cohen
Department of Physiology and
  Biophysics
Health Science Center of the State
  University of New York
Stoney Brook, NY 11794-8661
USA

Mario Delmar
Department of Pharmacology
SUNY Health Science Center
  at Syracuse
766 Irving Avenue
Syracuse, NY 13210
USA

José Jalife
Department of Pharmacology
SUNY Health Science Center
  at Syracuse
766 Irving Avenue
Syracuse, NY 13210
USA

J.P. Johnson
Department of Medicine
560 MRB II
Vanderbilt University School of
  Medicine
Nashville, TN 37232-6602
USA

Judith M.B. Pinto
Department of Pharmacology
College of Physicians and Surgeons
Columbia University
630W 168th Street
New York, NY 10032
USA

Michael R. Rosen
Department of Pharmacology
College of Physicians and Surgeons
Columbia University
630W 168th Street, New York, NY 10032
USA

Contributors

Walter Spinelli
Cardiovascular and Metabolic
  Diseases
Wyeth – Ayerst Research
CN 8000
Princeton, NJ 08543-8000
USA

Antonio Zaza
Dipartimento di Fisiologia e Biochimica
  Generali
Università di Milano
Via Celoria 26
20133 Milano
Italy

Introduction

This book is intended for students interested in the biological and physical bases for the electrical activity of the heart. Our goal in preparing the volume was to tie together basic concepts of electricity and of the structure and function of the cell membrane in explaining the mechanisms that determine the generation of the cardiac action potential and its propagation from cell to cell. The book is not intended to be a compendium, but a primer. It is by design incomplete, but we trust it will provide some of the tools needed for the informed student of electrophysiology and its diverse literature.

The foci of the first four chapters, respectively, are electricity, the molecular biology of the channels that permit ions to flow across the cell membrane, the generation of the cardiac action potential and its subsequent propagation. The next three chapters provide specific examples of the modulation of electrical activity: by the autonomic nervous system, by pharmacological agents, and by disease. In these chapters the intent is not to be all-encompassing, but rather to provide mechanistic examples of how the function of the cardiac myocyte and the heart are altered by commonly occurring intercurrent factors. Finally, to provide the reader with a dynamic representation of the contribution of ionic currents to the action potential, Chapter 8 includes a diskette with a computer model of the Purkinje-fiber action potential for interactive study.

There are many people we wish to thank for their efforts: first, our students, whose frequent requests for a brief, fundamental approach to electrophysiology provided the impetus for taking on this project; second, the authors, who have worked exceptionally hard to write and rewrite such that the information they provided could be integrated into a cohesive whole; and third, Eileen Franey, who contributed considerable time and effort towards the preparation of the volume.

Antonio Zaza
Michael R. Rosen

1 Electricity and Electrophysiology

Ofer Binah

INTRODUCTION

This chapter illustrates the physical interpretation of processes involved in the genesis and propagation of the cardiac impulse. Mathematical descriptions have been provided to help in the understanding and practical application of physical relationships. Analytical derivation of these equations is not an essential component of this chapter, and has been largely omitted.

Most of the concepts introduced here will be referred to in subsequent chapters. Although some of them might appear complex at first reading, they will become more obvious as their practical implications are described. The reader is encouraged to use this chapter as a basic reference to help understand the central role of physics in cardiac electrophysiology.

BASIC CONCEPTS IN ELECTRICITY

A Brief History of the "Electricity" Concept

It has been known since ancient times that when amber is rubbed, it can attract light objects such as small pieces of paper. In 1600, Sir William Gilbert (1544–1603) coined the term *electrics*, from the Greek word for amber (*elektron*) to describe substances that acquire the capacity to attract (Laider and Meiser, 1982). It was later discovered that materials such as glass, when rubbed with silk, exert forces opposed to those of amber. These findings led to the distinction between two types of electricity: *resinus* (from substances like amber) and *vitreous* (from substances like glass). Later, Benjamin Franklin (1706–1790) established the convention used today that the type of electricity produced by rubbing silk on glass is positive, while the resinous type of electricity is negative. "Bioelectricity" was first demonstrated in 1791 by Luigi Galvani (1737–1798), who brought a nerve of a frog's leg in contact with an electrostatic machine, causing a contraction of the leg muscles. In 1800 Alessandro Volta (1745–1827) developed the "Voltaic pile" allowing him to produce shocks and sparks, that previously had been observed with friction machines. In subsequent years, William Nicholson (1753–1815) and Sir Anthony Carlisle (1791–1842) were the first to decompose water by electric current, and subsequently Michael Faraday (1791–1867) introduced the important concepts of electrolysis, cathode and anode.

The Electric Force, the Electric Field and Coulomb's Law

Electrical phenomena can arise whenever electrical charges of opposite sign are separated. Electrical charges exert an electrostatic force on other charges: opposite charges attract and like charges repel. All matters are composed of charged particles, when normally the number of positive charges is equal to the number of negative charges, thus causing bodies to be electrically neutral. A mole of any atom or molecule contains **Avogadro's number** ($N = 6.02 \cdot 10^{23}$) of protons and the same number of electrons. The quantity of charge is measured in coulombs (C) (after Augustin de Coulombs, 1736–1806), and the charge of a proton is $e = 1.6 \cdot 10^{-19}$ C. Avogadro's number of elementary charges is called the **Faraday Constant** (F) and is equal to: $6.02 \cdot 10^{23} \cdot 1.6 \cdot 10^{-19} \sim 10^5$ C $\cdot$ mol^{-1}. This is the charge on a mole of Na$^+$ or K$^+$ or on 0.5 mol of Ca^{2+}.

The electrical force as it implies to biological systems is the force generated between 2 electrical charges (Figure 1). As the distance between the charges increases, the force that is exerted decreases. When two charges (q and q_1) are separated by a distance R, the electrical force between them is given by Coulomb's law:

$$F = K(qq_1/R^2) \tag{1}$$

The charge q is measured in coloumbs (C), and K is the electrical force constant determined experimentally, $9 \cdot 10^9$ N $\cdot$ m^2 $\cdot$ C^{-2}. One coulomb is defined as the electrical charge that will cause two equally charged balls, separated by 1 meter, to be repelled by $9 \cdot 10^9$ newton (N). One coulomb is an enormous amount of charge, and is much larger than any electric force encountered in the laboratory (Sanny and Moebs, 1996). In electrostatic experiments, objects typically acquire a charge of 10^{-6} C. In SI units the constant K is usually written not as K, but as $1/(4\pi\varepsilon_0)$. The constant ε_0 is the **permittivity of free space**. Its numerical value is: $\varepsilon_0 = 1/(4\pi k) = 8.85418 \cdot 10^{-12}$ C^2 $\cdot$ N^{-1} $\cdot$ m^2. When K is substituted with $1/(4\pi\varepsilon_0)$ Coulomb's law becomes:

$$F = 1/(4\pi\varepsilon_0) \cdot (qq_1/R^2) \tag{2}$$

The electric interaction between two charges is described using the concept of the electric field. When the charge q_1 (Figure 1) is replaced with another charge q_2 (placed at the same distance R from q), the fixed factor $1/(4\pi\varepsilon_0) \cdot q/R^2$ is then multiplied by q_2 instead by q_1. This prior "information" $1/(4\pi\varepsilon_0) \cdot q/R^2$ that was present before q_1 was added, is the **electric field** (E) created by the charge q. The

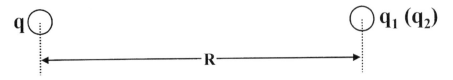

Figure 1 The electrical force between two charges is proportional to the size of the charges and the distance separating them.

electric field is determined only by the charge q generating the electric field and by the distance from it. This information determines the force "felt" by a single unit charge (1 C) placed at a distance R from q. The electric field E operating on a charge $q_1 = 1\,\text{C}$, is therefore: $E = 1/(4\pi\varepsilon_0) \cdot q/R^2$, and is constant at a distance R from the charge q. Importantly, the electric field has a direction, and it is the direction towards which a positive charge will move. A negative charge will therefore move in the opposite direction of the electric field. The relationships between the electric field (E) and the electric force (F) is:

$$F = qE \tag{3}$$

Potential Difference and Electrical Work

As electrical charges exert an electrostatic force on other charges (opposite charges attract and alike charges repel), **work** (W, force · distance) must be performed in order to bring a charge q_1 (or q_2) to a certain point in an electric field (Figure 2):

$$W = 1/(4\pi\varepsilon_0) \cdot (qq_1/R) \tag{4}$$

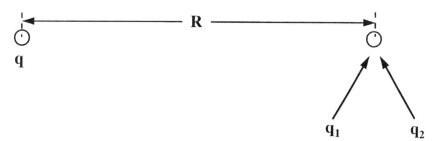

Figure 2 Work is required to bring a charge q_1 (or q_2) from infinity to a point separated by the distance R from a charge q.

Work per unit charge, referred to as **electrical potential** and designated by V, can be obtained by dividing equation 4 by q_1:

$$V = 1/(4\pi\varepsilon_0) \cdot (q/R) \tag{5}$$

The potential difference between two points is the work that must be done to move a unit of positive charge (1 C) from one point to the other, i.e., it corresponds to the **potential energy** of the charge. One volt (V) is defined as the potential energy required to move 1 C of charge along a distance of 1 meter against a force of 1 N.

Conductors and Insulators

Any matter is composed of a positive nucleus and circulating negative electrons. The electrons which do not circle a specific nucleus are called free electrons, and are the charge carriers. When a voltage difference (ΔV) is induced across two sides of a substance containing free electrons, it will cause free charges to move from the low potential (V_2) to the high potential (V_1), so that free electrons will move from V_2 to V_1, thereby generating an electric current (Figure 3).

Therefore, the net movement of charges through a conductor is represented by the electric current. A matter containing a large number of free electrons is called a **conductor** (e.g., copper, silver, iron), and a matter which has few or no free electrons is called an **insulator** (e.g., wood, plastic, rubber). Since electrons are always the free charges, charge movement in a conductor will be carried out by negative charges.

A convention establishes that the direction of current is defined by movement of positive charges, irrespective of the sign of the particles (electrons, anions, cations) that physically carry the current. Thus, current flows from the high positive potential (i.e., the $+$ pole) to the low positive potential (i.e., the $-$ pole). The larger the charge movement within a conductor in a unit time, the larger the current in the conductor. The **electric current** (I) is defined as the quantity of charge (dq) passing during time (dt):

$$I = dq/dt \tag{6}$$

Current is measured in amperes (A), so that movement of $1\,C$ through a conductor during a second causes a current of $1\,A$. In electrolyte solutions, current is transported by the movement of charged ions within the aqueous environment. Thus, in contrast to solid conductors in which only electrons move, current in electrolyte solutions corresponds to the movement of molecules. The currents measured in biological systems are small, ranging in magnitude from picoamperes (pA, $10^{-12}\,A$) to microamperes (μA, $10^{-6}\,A$). Typically, when a Na^+ channel is open, 10^4 ions cross the membrane each millisecond. This current equals to $1.6\,pA$

Direction of electrons movement

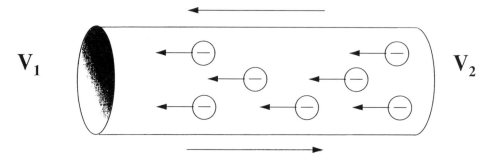

Direction of electrical current

$$\mathbf{V_1 > V_2}$$

Figure 3 A voltage difference (ΔV) across two sides of a substance containing free electrons, causes free charges (electrons) to move from the low potential (V_2) to the high potential (V_1).

$(1.6 \cdot 10^{-19}\,\text{C/ion} \cdot 10^4\,\text{ions} \cdot \text{ms}^{-1} \cdot 10^3\,\text{ms} \cdot \text{s}^{-1})$. The **current density** J_e, is the electric current per unit cross-sectional area:

$$J_e = I/A \tag{7}$$

Conductance and Resistance

The current (I) that flows when a potential difference (V) is applied to the ends of a conductor is defined by **Ohm's law** (Figure 4): $I = V/R$, or $V = IR$, that is, the potential energy (voltage) across a conductor is directly proportional to the current that moves through it. The larger the resistance (R), the larger the voltage generated by a given current. As shown in the top panel of Figure 4, according to Ohm's law the dependency of I on V is linear; the slope of the relation between I and V is referred to as conductance ($G = I/V = 1/R$).

In an **ohmic conductor** such as that depicted in the upper panel of Figure 4, G is a constant, i.e., it is independent of V. In some conductors (including most ion channels) G is a function of V; thus the relation between I and V diverges from linearity. Such non-linear conductors are often defined as **non-ohmic conductors** (Figure 4 bottom panels). The current (I) is measured in amperes (A); V, voltage

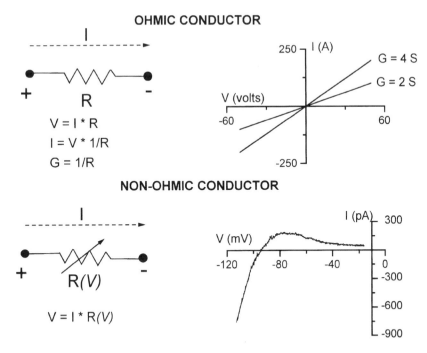

Figure 4 Ohmic and non-ohmic conductors. Upper panels: in conductors behaving according to Ohm's law (ohmic conductors), conductance (G) is a constant at all potentials and the current-voltage (I–V) relationship is linear (right panel). The right panel shows that a higher conductance corresponds to a steeper I–V relationship. Bottom panels: in a non-ohmic conductor, resistance is a function of potential (the arrow across the resistor means that resistance is variable). The right lower panel shows the I–V relation for a non-linear conductor such as a potassium channel.

difference measured in volts (V); G, conductance measured in siemens (S); R, measured in ohms (Ω): $1 \text{ ohm} = (1 \text{ siemens})^{-1}$. The resistance ($R$) of a conductor is determined by its cross sectional area (A), by its length (l) and by its resistivity (ρ), an intrinsic property of the conductive material:

$$R = \rho \cdot 1/A \tag{8}$$

Resistivities ($\Omega \cdot \text{cm}$) of common conductors are: aluminum $2.6 \cdot 10^{-8}$, copper $49 \cdot 10^{-8}$ and silver $1.6 \cdot 10^{-8}$. For the particular case of an electrolyte solution, ρ is termed the **electrolyte resistivity**, and κ ($1/\rho$) is called the **electrolyte conductivity**. Metallic conductors (having many free electrons) have low resistivity, while lipids (e.g., biological membranes) have high resistivity. The resistivity of electrolyte solutions is much higher than that of metallic conductors and depends on the ionized salt concentrations. Several resistivities of biological significance are (at 20°C): frog Ringer's solution $80\,\Omega \cdot \text{cm}$, mammalian saline $60\,\Omega \cdot \text{cm}$ and seawater $20\,\Omega \cdot \text{cm}$ (Hille, 1984).

Parallel vs. Series Circuits

The left panels of Figure 5 illustrate resistors connected **in series**. In a series circuit,

- the current is the same at all points in the circuit
- total resistance is the sum of individual resistances: $R_{tot} = R_1 + R_2 + \cdots R_n$; thus total resistance is larger than any of the individual resistances;

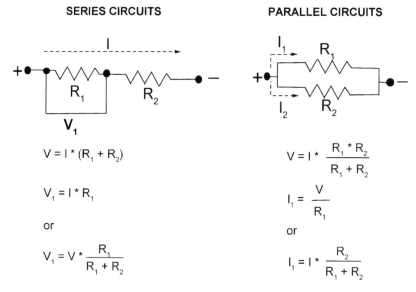

Figure 5   Series vs. parallel circuits. In the series circuit, current (I) is the same in all circuit points and total voltage (V) is the sum of voltage drops across resistances R_1 and R_2; thus series resistances act as a "voltage divider". Total resistance is the sum of partial resistances. In the parallel circuit current splits among the branches ("current divider") in a way proportional to the ratio between branch resistances. Total conductance ($1/R$) is the sum of branch conductances.

The right panels show resistors connected **in parallel**. In a parallel circuit:

- Total current splits among the branches of the circuit ($I = I_1 + I_2$). The proportion of total current flowing in each branch depends on the proportion of total circuit resistance contained in that branch vs. other branches
- Total resistance is given by: $R_{\text{tot}} = (R_1 \cdot R_2 \cdots \cdot R_n)/(R_1 + R_2 + \cdots R_n)$; thus total resistance is inversely proportional to the number of parallel resistors.

Two examples, relating to bioelectrical phenomena highlight the consequences of series vs. parallel configurations. In cell membranes individual ionic channels are connected in parallel; thus as the number of open channels increases the membrane resistance decreases and conductance increases. In contrast, within a bundle of myocardium, cells are connected to one another as series elements, with resistance being partly accounted for by cell membranes. The larger the number of cell borders (membranes) crossed by the conductive path, the larger the electrical resistance of the path.

Voltage Source

A voltage "source" or "generator" is a device generating and maintaining an electrical potential difference (a form of energy). If the poles of a voltage source are connected by a conductor, current flows through the conductor, thus dissipating the potential difference. According to Ohm's law, the lower the resistance of the circuit, the larger the current generated. Thus, to maintain a potential difference across a low resistance conductor, a voltage source must be able to provide a large amount of charge. The "ideal" voltage source is the one able to maintain a constant potential difference irrespective of the circuit resistance; the latter represents the electrical "**load**" imposed to the voltage source. Any real voltage source deviates from ideality whenever the load becomes large relative to the energy stored in the source. This is well illustrated by the common experience that a battery can light the high resistance filament of a bulb (small load) for many hours, but it is quickly exhausted if its poles are short-circuited by a low resistance wire (large load).

Capacitors

A capacitor (or condenser) is a device able to accumulate charge (capacitors can actually be used as voltage sources). A capacitor (Figure 6) consists of two conductive plates facing one another, separated by a small layer of non conductive substance (dielectric).

When the two plates are respectively connected to the poles of a voltage source (Figure 6 middle panel), positive charge starts to accumulate on one plate and negative charge on the other. This is possible because, as reaching the plate, each positive charge is electrostatically attracted by the negative charge residing on the opposite plate. The energy absorbed by such an electrostatic interaction subtracts from the potential field generated by the charge; this allows many charges to be attracted and stored on the plates. The ability to store charge is referred to as

Ofer Binah

OPEN CIRCUIT

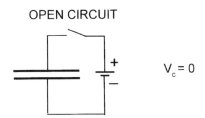

$V_c = 0$

CAPACITOR CHARGING

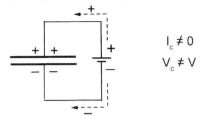

$I_c \neq 0$

$V_c \neq V$

CAPACITOR CHARGED

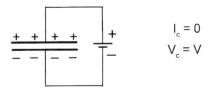

$I_c = 0$

$V_c = V$

Figure 6 Charging a capacitor with a voltage source (battery). Closure of the circuit (middle panel) is followed by capacitative current (I_c) flow. Capacitative current persists as long as the voltage across the capacitor plates (V_c) is different from that of the voltage source (V). When $V_c = V$ (the capacitor is fully charged), I_c ceases (bottom panel). Opening of the switch at this time would be followed by persistence of charge on the capacitor's plates (not shown).

capacitance, which is defined as the amount of charge (Q) that can be stored when the potential difference V is applied to the plates of a capacitor:

$$C = Q/V \qquad (9)$$

As distance between the plates decreases the electrostatic interaction is enhanced, thereby increasing capacitance. Larger plates can store more charge. Thus, the potential difference that exists between the capacitor plates when the capacitor is fully charged is given by:

$$V = 1/\varepsilon \cdot Q \cdot d/A \qquad (10)$$

Where d is the distance between plates, A is the area of the plates and ε is the **dielectric constant**, a measure of how the medium interposed between the two plates is effective in reducing the electric field between the plates. Another important feature of the dielectric medium, defining its insulator properties, is **dielectric strength**. A large dielectric strength allows a strong potential difference to build up across the plates before charge starts to flow across the plates (short-circuiting of the capacitor). The capacitance of a parallel-plate capacitor can be calculated from:

$$C = Q/V = \varepsilon \cdot A/d \qquad (11)$$

In SI units, A is expressed in square meters, d in meters, and C in farads. One farad (F) is the capacitance required to store 1 Coulomb of charge by applying a potential difference of 1 Volt; this represents a huge capacitance.

Until the plates are fully charged, positive charge moves from the positive battery pole to the positive plate and negative charge moves from the negative pole to the negative plate (Figure 6 middle panel). Thus, during charging of the capacitor, a current is generated in the two branches of the circuit, even if no charge actually moves through the dielectric separating the plates. This current is referred to as **capacitive current** (I_c). Capacitive current flows in the circuit until the voltage across the capacitor plates equals the voltage source (Figure 6 bottom panel), implying that capacitive current will flow only during charging or discharging of the capacitor plates. If a charged capacitor is disconnected from the voltage source (open circuit), the charge will remain on its plates; if the plates are then connected, the charge flows through the conductor from the positive plate to the negative one (capacitor discharge), producing a capacitive current that is the mirror image of the one occurring during the charging process.

ELECTRICITY IN BIOLOGICAL SYSTEMS

"Linear" Electrical Properties of Biological Membranes: Parallel RC Circuit Model

Cell membranes are very efficient capacitors: two conductive elements (intra and extracellular environments) are separated by a very thin dielectric medium (the phospholipid bilayer); this results in a specific capacitance (capacity per unit area) of near $1.0\,\mu F \cdot cm^{-2}$, slightly higher than that of a pure lipid bilayer ($0.8\,\mu F \cdot cm^{-2}$). Since this value of specific capacitance is remarkably constant among all biological membranes, a reasonable estimate of the cell surface area can be obtained experimentally by measurement of electrical capacitance of the cell. The capacitance of a typical ventricular myocytes is about $10^{-10}\,F$ (100 pF), that leads to an estimated membrane surface area of about $10{,}000\,\mu^2$.

Cell membranes are crossed by ion channels that can be viewed as conductors (or resistors). As will be detailed in the following chapters, under particular conditions ion channels behave as ohmic resistors. Thus, according to the simplest model, biological membranes can be represented by a capacitor (the phospholipid bilayer) connected in parallel with a linear resistor (parallel RC circuit) (Figure 7).

The properties of this simple circuit are very important in explaining the response of membrane potential to current flow through ionic channels. Such properties may be examined by analyzing the time course of potential and current changes occurring when a square current pulse is applied across the ends of a parallel RC circuit via a current generator (Figure 7). When the generator circuit is open (Figure 7A) no current flows through it, the potential across the resistor R is null and the capacitor C is uncharged. After the switch is closed (Figure 7B), current starts to flow in the

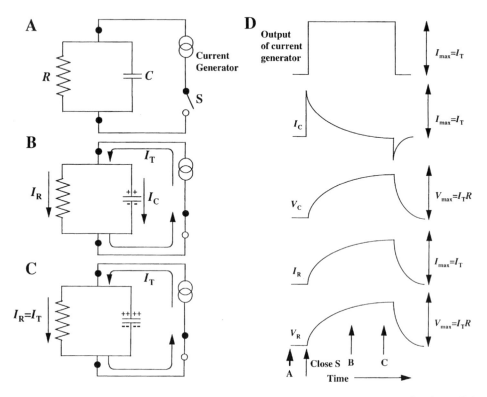

Figure 7 Electrical responses to a square current pulse, in a circuit composed of a capacitor in parallel with a resistor. [A] The circuit before switch S is closed. [B] Shortly after the switch S is closed. [C] The charge on the capacitor has reached its steady state value. [D] Time course of the changes in I_C, V_C, I_R, and V_R in response to closing the switch. In the lower trace of panel D, "A" "B" and "C" represent the corresponding panels on the left side of the Figure.

circuit, via its resistive and capacitive branches. At any instant, total current (I_T) equals capacitive current (I_C) plus the current through the resistor (resistive current, I_R). At the very first instant, the capacitor is not yet saturated and absorbs all the charge available. Thus, for an instant after circuit closure, I_C is equal to I_T. At this time I_R, and the resulting potential (V_R), remain null. As charge accumulates on the capacitor, a potential difference V_C builds up across its plates, and opposes further charge accumulation. Thus, the proportion of I_T flowing through the resistive branch increases progressively, producing a growing voltage across the resistor R (Ohm's law); I_C decreases correspondingly. As less and less current flows into the capacitor, its rate of charging will be slowed, accounting for the exponential shape of the curve of V_C (and V_R) vs. time. When the capacitor is fully charged, all the current flows through the resistive branch and $V_R = I_T R$. The value of V_R at any instant t during the current pulse can be computed as follows:

$$V_R(t) = I_T R(1 - e^{t/\tau}) \tag{12}$$

The term τ that represents the time constant of the exponential charging and discharging of the capacitor, is equal to the product $R \cdot C$ and has the dimension of time. When $t = \tau$, $(1 - e^{t/\tau}) = 0.63$, and $V_R = 0.63 \, I_T R$; therefore, at a time equal to τ, V_R is 63% of its steady state value; approximately 5 τ are required before the charge process is almost completed.

An important consequence of the properties of the parallel RC circuit is that, upon a change in transmembrane current, the potential across the membrane resistive component changes with a delay, determined by a charge (or discharge) of membrane capacitance. Whereas the final magnitude of membrane potential (V) depends only on a current (I) flowing through the resistive component ($V = IR$), the rate of potential change (dV/dt) is determined entirely by charge (or discharge) of the capacitative component:

$$dV/dt = -I_c/C_m \qquad (13)$$

where C_m is membrane capacitance. In this setting a larger current is required to produce the same rate of depolarization in a larger cell (large C_m) than in a smaller one. The negative sign simply reflects the convention that a current with a negative sign produces a positive change in membrane potential (and vice-versa).

Since the values of C_m and dV/dt can be measured during the excitation cycle, equation 13 allows estimation of the magnitude of the net instantaneous current underlying each phase of the action potential in a single myocyte. On the other hand, membrane resistance (or conductance) can be estimated (Ohm's law) by measuring the voltage change occurring during sustained injection of small transmembrane currents of known amplitude.

IONIC (ELECTROLYTE) SOLUTIONS AS CONDUCTORS

Hydration of the ion

An electrolyte is a substance that yields ions ("charged chemical species") to solution, as evidenced by the solution's showing electrical **conductivity**. Substances, such as NaCl, KCl and HCl, occur almost entirely as ions when they are in aqueous solutions, and are known as strong electrolytes, as compared to the weak electrolytes (CH_3COOH) which are present only partially as ions. A crystal (e.g., NaCl, $CaCl_2$) consists of positive and negative ions in the pure state. When an ionic crystal (NaCl) is dissolved in a polar solvent such as water, the ions break off from the crystal and enter the solution as solvated ions. This process is called **solvation**, or in water, **hydration**. The term "hydrated" (or "solvated") means that each ion in aqueous solution is surrounded by a relatively bulky shell of water molecules (**hydration shell**) attracted to the ion by electrostatic forces, and travelling through the solution with the ion. Despite its non-covalent nature, the interaction between the ion and the surrounding water molecules involves a remarkable change in free energy (**hydration energy**); in general, hydration energy is inversely proportional to the atomic radius of the ion. Before an ion can permeate a "narrow" channel pore, the hydration shell needs to be removed. To do so an amount of energy equal to hydration energy needs to be supplied to the hydrated ion. As will also be discussed in the following chapters, this energy may be provided by (electrostatic) interaction of the ion with a charged moiety of the channel molecule.

Activity Coefficients of and Free Concentrations of Ions in Aqueous Solutions

When an electrolyte is dissolved at a sufficiently low concentration, the distance between ion molecules within the solution is large enough to make interactions between individual molecules very unlikely. Under such conditions, the solution is defined as "ideal", and each ion behaves independently from the others. In ideal solutions, the ability of a molecule to diffuse or react with other molecules (chemical potential of the molecule) is only determined by its **concentration**. More concentrated solutions, such as those of physiological interest, are sufficiently crowded such that only a fraction of the ion concentration contributes to its chemical potential. This fraction is referred to as **activity** of the ion and is inversely proportional to the **ionic strength** of the solution, a parameter proportional to the sum of individual ionic concentrations and to their valence (the ionic strength of biological fluids is in the order of 100 mM). Thus, when calculating the chemical potential of an ion in non-ideal solutions, ion concentration is conveniently replaced by ion activity. Activity can easily be computed by multiplying the ion concentration by the **activity coefficient** of the ion in a solution of given ionic strength (tables relating activity coefficients to ionic strength are available in chemistry books). The activity coefficient for monovalent cations (e.g., Na^+, K^+, etc.) in physiological solutions is approximately 0.75 (e.g., a K^+ concentration of 10 mM corresponds to a K^+ activity of 7.5 mM) (Freedman, 1995).

In biological fluids, some ions can strongly interact with large, indiffusable molecules, such as proteins. The protein-bound and the free forms of the ion are in chemical equilibrium; in other words, the ion concentration is actually "buffered" by proteins. Under such conditions the activity of the ion, often referred to as **free ion concentration**, may be well below the one predicted by the activity coefficient. Examples of ions strongly buffered by intracellular proteins are Ca^{2+} and H^+.

Molar Conductivity

Since the number of charge carriers per unit volume usually increases with increasing electrolyte concentration, the solution's conductivity κ usually increases as the electrolyte's concentration increases. To obtain a measure of the current-carrying capacity of a given amount of electrolyte (compensated for the difference in concentration), the term **molar conductivity** Λ_m, or in case of a solution of an electrolyte, the **electrolyte conductivity** (Λ) of an electrolyte in solution has been defined as follows:

$$\Lambda = \kappa/c \tag{14}$$

where c is the solution's stoichiometric molar concentration. The importance of the molar conductivity is that it provides information on the conductivity of ions produced in a solution by 1 mole of a substance.

Independent Migration of Ions and Ionic Mobilities

An important question pertaining to an electrolyte solution is how the two ions of an electrolyte pair (e.g., Na^+ and Cl^-) contribute to the overall conductivity of the electrolyte solution. This issue was resolved by the observation made in 1875 by

Kohlrausch that, in very diluted solutions the difference that exists between the equivalent conductivities of a potassium and sodium salt of the same anion (e.g., KCl and NaCl) is independent of the nature of the anion. Thus, each member of the pair independently contributes to the molar conductivity of the solution. Kohlrausch formulated this concept as the **law of independent migration of ions**:

$$\Lambda = \lambda^+ + \lambda^- \tag{15}$$

where λ^+ and λ^- are the ion conductivities of the cation and anion, respectively, at infinite dilution.

Although, for a strong electrolyte, anion and cation independently contribute to conductivity, the proportion of total current carried by each member of the pair may be different. Indeed, since during conduction ions actually move through the solution, the ability of an ion to carry current depends on its **mobility** (u). Mobility of the ion, is defined as the speed with which the ion moves through the solution under a unitary gradient of (chemical or electrical) potential. For uncharged molecules mobility is inversely proportional to the molecular size: the larger the molecule the stronger the drag imposed by friction with the solvent. For ions in aqueous solutions, mobility also depends on the ease with which the ion is able to replace water molecules of its hydration shell. Since hydration energy is inversely proportional to molecular size, mobility is a bell-shaped function of molecular size (Hille, 1984). The SI units of mobility are $cm \cdot s^{-1}/V \cdot cm^{-1}$. Mobilities of biologically-relevant ions in water are $[10^4 \ (cm \cdot s^{-1})/(V \cdot cm^{-1})]$: Na^+, 5.19; K^+, 7.62; Ca^{2+}, 3.08; Cl^-, 7.92.

When the ion pair of an electrolyte (e.g., Na^+ and Cl^-) diffuses along a concentration gradient, the ion with higher mobility (e.g., Cl^-) moves faster than the one with lower mobility (e.g., Na^+). This results in a momentary separation of electrical charge proportional to the diffusion rate. Such a separation of charge is the basis of diffusion potentials (see below). KCl is preferred as an electrolyte conductor for electrophysiological measurements because mobilities of K^+ and Cl^- are very similar; this reduces contamination of measurement by diffusion potentials generated in the electrode.

ELECTROCHEMICAL POTENTIALS

Aqueous Diffusion of Ions due to a Chemical Gradient

Current flow (I) is the amount of material (m) passing through a cylindrical cross-sectional area, or through a membrane in a unit time (t): $I = m/t$. If the current changes with time, the differential form is used: $I = dm/dt$. Flux is current per unit area: $J = I/A$, or $1/A \cdot dm/dt$. If solutions of different concentrations ($C_1 > C_2$) are brought into contact, there is a net flow of solute from phase 1 to phase 2. The net flow continues due to the process of **diffusion** until the solute's concentration is constant throughout the solution. Diffusion results from the random thermal motion of molecules, as conceptualized by the Brownian motion of colloidal particle suspended in fluid. According to **Fick's first law of diffusion**, the flux due to diffusion is:

$$J = -D \cdot dC/dx \tag{16}$$

or the diffusion current is:

$$I = dm/dt = -DA \cdot dC/dx \qquad (17)$$

dm/dt is the net rate of flow of solute (in moles per unit time) across a plane P of area A perpendicular to the x axis; dC/dx is the value at plane P of the rate of change of the solute's molar concentration with respect to the x coordinate. As dC/dx at a given plane changes, eventually becoming zero, diffusion then stops. The SI units of the following components are: dm/dt, $mol \cdot s^{-1}$; dC/dt, $mol \cdot m^{-4}$; the **diffusion coefficient** D, $m^2 \cdot s^{-1}$; flux per unit area, $mol \cdot m^{-2} \cdot s^{-1}$. In practice, diffusion coefficients are commonly expressed as $cm^{-2} \cdot s^{-1}$. D is a function of the local state of the system (temperature, pressure) and of the composition of the solution:

$$D = RTu/N \qquad (18)$$

R, gas constant; T, absolute temperature; u, solute mobility in solution; N, Avogadro's number. The mobility of a solute in a specific solution depends on its radius and the solution viscosity.

Diffusion Across Membranes due to a Chemical Gradient

Diffusion of solutes across a membrane (in contrast to a homogeneous medium) occurs in biological systems. In the model shown in Figure 8, two solutions at different concentrations are separated by a porous membrane.

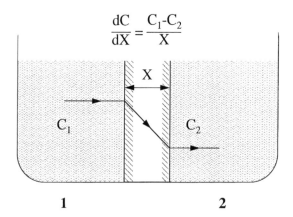

Figure 8 Two-compartment system illustrating diffusion due to a chemical potential, across a membrane with thickness $= x$.

Such a membrane contains water-filled pores, and the assumption is that diffusion through the membrane occurs at the same rate as in water. To obtain a steady state, the concentration gradient across the membrane must fall linearly (see Figure 8), as given by:

$$-dC/dx = (C_1 - C_2)/x \qquad (19)$$

Fick's law describing the rate of (current) flow through the membrane then becomes:

$$\mathrm{d}m/\mathrm{d}t = -DA \cdot (C_1 - C_2)/x = DA/x \cdot (C_2 - C_1) \qquad (20)$$

From this equation the parameter of **permeability** (P) can be defined, $P = D/x$, so Fick's law becomes:

$$\mathrm{d}m/\mathrm{d}t = PA(C_2 - C_1) \qquad (21)$$

The units of P are $\mathrm{cm} \cdot \mathrm{sec}^{-1}$, like those of velocity, and P indeed measures the velocity of substance movement through a specific membrane. Permeability is independent of the solute's concentration.

Flux of Ions Across Membranes due to an Electrical Potential Gradient

Since "bioelectricity" is generated due to movements of ions, I will expand the discussion to diffusion of ions across membranes. Interestingly, the word ION (Greek for "that which goes") was first introduced by Michael Faraday in 1834. He used the term "ions" to describe the charged components moving up to the electrodes (Hille, 1984). Firstly, I will consider ion movement due only to the electrical potential (Figure 9).

Here, the concentration of solutions on both sides of the membrane is identical ($C_1 = C_2 = C$), and the only force operating is due to the imposed electric potential: $V = \Psi_1 - \Psi_2$. The electrical force (F_Ψ) generated on one ion is:

$$F_\Psi = -ZF/N \cdot \mathrm{d}\Psi/\mathrm{d}x \qquad (22)$$

Z, ion valence (2^+ for calcium ion); F, Faraday number; N, Avogadro's number. As matter flux is: $J_m = CuF_D$, where C is the concentration; u, ion mobility and F_D the driving force, the flux therefore becomes:

$$J_m = -CuZF/N \cdot \mathrm{d}\Psi/\mathrm{d}x \qquad (23)$$

Since D (the diffusion coefficient) is: $D = RTu/N$, or $D/RT = u/N$,

$$J_m = -CD/RT \cdot ZF \cdot \mathrm{d}\Psi/\mathrm{d}x \qquad (24)$$

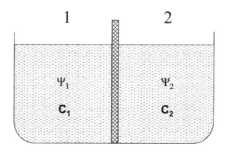

Figure 9 Two-compartment system illustrating diffusion of ions due only to the electrical potential imposed across the membrane.

For diffusion through a membrane of width $= x$, equation 24 becomes:

$$J_m = -CD/RT \cdot ZF \cdot (\Psi_1 - \Psi_2)/x = C \cdot D/x \cdot ZF/RT \cdot V = CP \cdot ZF/RT \cdot V \quad (25)$$

P, permeability (D/x); $V = \Psi_1 - \Psi_2$. From Ohm's law we know that $I = V/R = G \cdot V$, so that the electrical flux is: $J_e = G/A \cdot V$ (A, the area). Since G/A is the specific conductance g, and each mole of electrolyte contains ZF coloumbs, the matter flux is:

$$J_m = J_e/ZF = g/ZF \cdot V \quad (26)$$

If we compare in equations 25 and 26 the proportion between the flux and the voltage:

$$g/ZF = CP \cdot ZF/RT \quad (27)$$

so,

$$g = CP \cdot Z^2F^2/RT \quad (28)$$

From this equation we learn that: (1) the specific conductance is proportional to the permeability; (2) Conductance and permeability are related to each other by the constants Z, F, T and the concentration. Thus, for a membrane to conduct a specific ion, the membrane should be permeable to that ion, and a concentration gradient must exist.

Flux of Ions Across Membranes due to Chemical and Electrical Gradients

I will now consider a situation, closer to that in living cells, in which a membrane separates two solutions ($C_1 > C_2$) of the same ion, with electrical potentials Ψ_1 and Ψ_2, respectively (Figure 9). The total ion flux (J_T) is the sum of fluxes due to the chemical and electrical gradients:

$$J_T = -D(\mathrm{d}C/\mathrm{d}x + ZF/RT \cdot C \cdot \mathrm{d}\Psi/\mathrm{d}x) \quad (29)$$

or the total current (I_T) due to both fluxes is:

$$I_T = -DA(\mathrm{d}C/\mathrm{d}x + ZF/RT \cdot C \cdot \mathrm{d}\Psi/\mathrm{d}x) \quad (30)$$

For an uncharged material ($Z = 0$), $I_T = -DA \cdot \mathrm{d}C/\mathrm{d}x$, which is **Fick's first law of diffusion**. Let us examine a situation of a membrane separating two aqueous solutions in which $[\mathrm{Na^+}]_1 > [\mathrm{Na^+}]_2$. If there is no electrical potential difference between sides 1 and 2, $\mathrm{Na^+}$ will diffuse from side 1 to side 2, as if it were an uncharged molecule. If, however side 1 is electrically negative with respect to side 2, $\mathrm{Na^+}$ will still diffuse from side 1 to side 2 driven by the chemical gradient, but now $\mathrm{Na^+}$ will also tend to move in the opposite direction (from side 2 to side 1) due to the electrical potential difference across the membrane. The direction of the *net* $\mathrm{Na^+}$ movement depends on which force, the chemical or the electrical, is greater. Thus, the difference in potentials, which is the **electrochemical potential**, determines the direction and magnitude of the ion movement across the membrane.

Electrochemical Equilibrium in a System with Chemical and Electrical Gradients

When the flux due to the chemical potential balances the flux due to the electrical potential gradient, there is no net force on an ion, and the net movement of that ion will be zero; thus, the system will be in a steady state. In this situation,

$$0 = D(dC/dx + ZF/RT \cdot C \cdot d\Psi/dx) \tag{31}$$

Since $D \neq 0$, the expression within the parenthesis equals zero. Therefore,

$$d\Psi/dx = -RT/ZF \cdot 1/C \cdot dC/dx \tag{32}$$

Since the gradient for both potentials is across the same membrane, equation 32 becomes:

$$d\Psi = -RT/ZF \cdot d(\ln C) \tag{33}$$

Integrating equation 33 between Ψ_1 and Ψ_2, $(V = \Psi_1 - \Psi_2)$, and between C_1 and C_2 results in the **Nernst equation**, which is valid for ions at equilibrium:

$$V = RT/ZF \cdot \ln(C_2/C_1) \tag{34}$$

Use of Nernst equation

Equation 34 is usually converted to a form containing $\log_{10}$ (instead of the natural logarithms, $\ln x = 2.303 \log_{10} x$). Since in living cells, transmembrane potentials are measured in millivolts (mV), the units of R are selected so that at $\sim 30°C$, the quantity $2.303\, RT/F$ is equal to 60 mV. In the example shown in Figure 10, in order to maintain a tenfold concentration difference (at equilibrium) between the 2 compartments, an electrical potential difference calculated by the Nernst equation, must exist:

$$\Psi_1 - \Psi_2 = V = (-60\,\text{mV}/ + 1) \cdot \log_{10}[K^+]_1/[K^+]_2$$
$$= -60\,\text{mV} \cdot \log(10) = -60\,\text{mV} \tag{35}$$

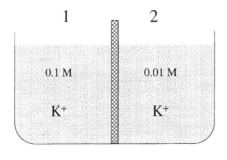

$$\Psi_1 - \Psi_2 = -60\ \text{mV}$$

Figure 10 Electrical potential difference is required to maintain a concentration difference (at equilibrium) between the 2 compartments containing 0.1 M and 0.01 M of K^+ ions, respectively. The electrical difference can be calculated by the Nernst equation.

At equilibrium, side 1 will be 60 mV negative compared to side 2. The Nernst equation thus provides the value of the electrical potential difference required to maintain a concentration difference of charged ions. This potential is also called the **equilibrium potential** or the ion's **reversal potential**. If the system shown in Figure 10 represents a living cell, than at a membrane potential (V_m) of -60 mV, the net K^+ current will be zero, in accordance with Ohm's law:

$$I_k = g(V_m - V_k) \tag{36}$$

V_k is the K^+ Nernst potential. In tissues were accurate measurements of intracellular concentrations of K^+ and Na^+ are possible, V_k and V_{Na} can be calculated. In the cat heart muscle, the values of K^+ and Na^+ concentrations are: $[K^+]_i = 151$ meq/l; $[K^+]_o = 4.8$ meq/l; $[Na^+]_o = 159$ meq/l and $[Na^+]_i = 6.6$ meq/l (Hoffman and Cranefield, 1976; Robertson and Dunihue, 1954). The corresponding Nernst potentials are: $V_k = -92.6$ mV and $V_{Na} = 84$ mV.

Diffusion Potentials

A situation resembling that in living cells occurs when a concentration gradient for a cation and an anion exists across the membrane, but the membrane permeability for the two ions differs (Figure 11).

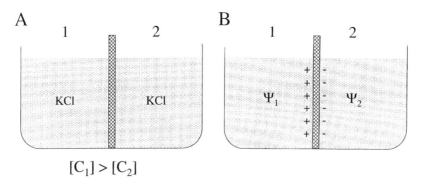

Figure 11 Two-compartment system in which a chemical gradient for a cation and an anion with different permeabilities, exists across a membrane. [A] In the initial state, a non-permeable partition separates the compartments containing different concentrations of KCl: $[C_1] > [C_2]$. [B] The partition is replaced with a membrane permeable to both ions, and diffusion is initiated. In the steady state, a diffusion potential is generated across the membrane.

In the initial state (Figure 11A), a non-permeable partition separates the compartments, which contain different concentrations of KCl : $[C_1] > [C_2]$. When the partition is replaced with a membrane permeable to both ions, diffusion along the chemical gradient will be initiated. However, since membrane permeability to Cl^- is higher than that to K^+, shortly after the beginning of the diffusion process (due to the chemical gradient), more Cl^- ions will cross the membrane than K^+ ions, thus generating an electrical potential difference across the membrane (Figure 11B). This electrical potential difference will now affect ion movement in addition to the concentration difference. The diffusion potential generated across the membrane at equilibrium, is derived from equation 29. After rearranging and integrating equation 29, the diffusion potential generated across the membrane can be calculated:

$$V = (P_k - P_{Cl})/(P_k + P_{Cl}) \cdot RT/F \cdot \ln(C_2 - C_1) \tag{37}$$

Where P_K and P_{Cl} are K^+ and Cl^- permeabilities, respectively. Clearly, if $P_K = P_{Cl}$, the diffusion potential is zero. In case either the cation or the anion permeability is zero, equation 37 becomes the Nernst equation.

The Resting Membrane Potential

When a microelectrode is inserted into a nerve fiber, cardiac muscle cell, lymphocyte, plant cell or a *paramecium*, it is seen that the inside of the cell is electrically negative compared to the outside by several tens of mV (-30 to -90 mV). This potential difference across the cell membrane has been termed the **resting potential**. As will be illustrated, the generation of the resting potential involves uneven distribution of ions across the membrane, and interaction of chemical and electrical forces.

As shown in previous sections, ion chemical gradients across a membrane can act as a battery. Intuitively, when several ions are distributed across a cell membrane, each ion tends to force the membrane potential towards its own equilibrium potential, which can be predicted from the Nernst equation. The more permeable the membrane to a certain ion, the more influence it will have on the membrane potential. For example, in a frog muscle, V_{Na} is 67 mV, V_K is -105 mV, V_{Cl} is -90 mV, and the resting potential is -90 mV. Indeed, in most cells the resting potential is slightly positive to V_k, indicating that at these range of potentials, the membrane is mostly permeable to K^+.

Quantitative analysis of the resting potential
A quantitative description of the resting potential is provided by the **Constant Field Equation**. This equation which was developed by Goldman (1943) and by Hodgkin and Katz (1949), contributed significantly to the understanding of ionic mechanisms underlying the resting potential. In developing the constant field equation, the flux of each ion is the product of its permeability coefficient and the driving force ($V_m - V_{ion}$). Several assumptions were used to develop the constant field equation: (1) The electric field across the membrane (V/x) is constant (giving the equation its name). (2) The concentration of each ion at the membrane is proportional to its concentration in the aqueous solution. (3) The partition coefficient (α) between the membrane and the aqueous solution is equal for all ions. (4) Cell membrane is homogeneous. (5) The chemical and electric energies are the only forces generating ion movement. (6) Ion currents are due only to Na^+, K^+ and Cl^- currents. Based on these assumptions and on equation 29, the calculated resting potential (under steady state conditions) is:

$$V = RT/F \cdot \ln(P_{Na}[Na]_o + P_K[K]_o + P_{Cl}[Cl]_i)/(P_{Na}[Na]_i + P_K[K]_i + P_{Cl}[Cl]_o) \tag{38}$$

If the cell membrane is permeable only to one ion, the constant field equation becomes the Nernst equation. In the resting state, as P_k is the dominant factor, the resting potential is close to V_k, but not at V_k, since the permeabilities of the other ions are not zero.

PASSIVE MEMBRANE PROPERTIES

Conduction of the action potential along a nerve, or through the cardiac electrical syncytium depends on both linear (ohmic) and non linear membrane electrical properties. Small changes in membrane potential, such as those moving membrane potential from its resting value to the activation threshold, may not affect membrane conductance (i.e., do not change the state of activation of ion channels). Under such conditions, commonly referred to as "**electrotonic**", the membrane behaves as an ohmic conductor. Since "active" membrane properties, such as voltage dependent opening of ion channels are not involved, the membrane response is said to be determined by "**passive membrane properties**".

The initial phenomena underlying propagation are determined by passive membrane properties; thus, in spite of their small magnitude, electrotonic potentials are pivotal to impulse conduction. This is well illustrated by the statement that "the main electrical characteristics of conduction are demonstrated in the passive spread of current, and it is difficult to understand conduction without an appreciation of these passive properties" (Fozzard, 1979).

The following discussion focuses on passive membrane properties, which determine the sub-threshold (electrotonic) electrical behavior of the cardiac tissue. The impact of passive membrane properties on conduction will be dealt with in chapter 4.

Electrotonic Spread of Current

Analysis of passive membrane properties was initially performed in the early forties, with measurements of membrane resistance and capacitance in nerve fibers (Hodgkin and Rushton, 1946; Davis and Lorento de Nó 1947). While working with Hodgkin and Huxley, Weidmann applied these methods to a preparation of cardiac origin, the Purkinje fibers of newborn goats, thus initiating studies on passive membrane properties in the heart (Weidmann, 1952). Weidmann's studies were performed by injecting small, "sub-threshold" currents into thin Purkinje fibers, and recording the resulting transmembrane potential changes at sites along the longitudinal axes of the fibers and at different distances from the site of current injection (Figure 12).

Weidmann demonstrated that the membrane potential decayed with distance in a way that could be fitted with a single exponential function. According to a theory based on ohmic electrical behavior (Hodgkin and Rushton, 1946), such an observation was compatible with the Purkinje fiber behaving as a uniform continuous one-dimensional cable (Jack *et al.*, 1975). Weidmann calculated that the resistivity of the internal longitudinal pathway (axial resistivity) was as low as $100–200\,\Omega \cdot cm$ (Weidmann, 1952; 1970). After comparing this value with that of Tyrode's solution ($52\,\Omega \cdot cm$), Weidmann concluded that there was very little resistance added by cell

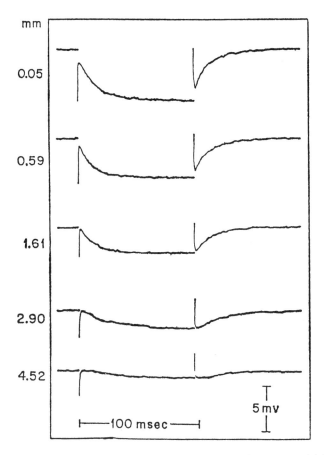

Figure 12 The electrotonic spread of subthreshold changes in membrane potential in response to a 100 msec hyperpolarizing current pulse applied to a single Purkinje strand. The membrane potential was recorded at 0.05, 0.59, 1.61, 2.90 and 4.52 mm from the current-injecting electrode (Weidmann, 1952).

boundaries, thus inferring that individual myocytes are coupled by low-resistance electrical connections (now known to be gap-junctions). A significant contribution of cell boundaries (gap-junctions) to axial resistance has been identified using a two-dimensional analysis of the effect of cellular structure on longitudinal electronic current flow (Spach and Heidlage, 1992). Although at the macroscopic level, the decay in V_m with distance was well fitted by a single exponent, discontinuities due to the contribution of gap-junctional resistance became evident at the microscopic level. Still, the uniform cable model remains a fundamental tool for the understanding of electrotonic propagation; thus, the principles of such theory will be outlined below.

Quantitative Analysis of Passive Membrane Properties

The passive membrane properties are illustrated in the simple cable model, having a smooth surface and continuous interior (Jack *et al.*, 1975). It is an accurate

Ofer Binah

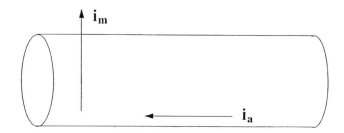

Extracellular fluid

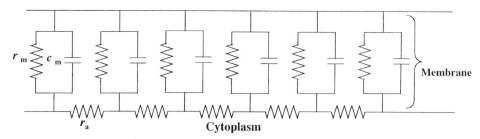

Figure 13 A one-dimensional cable model (upper panel) and its electrical analog (lower panel), divided into unit lengths. In this example, the extracellular resistance is assumed to be negligible. Each unit length of fiber is a circuit element with its own membrane resistance (r_m) and capacitance (c_m). All the circuits elements are connected by resistors (r_a) representing the axial resistance of segments of cytoplasm. Transmembrane current (i_m) is the current that when flowing through membrane resistance r_m produces the transmembrane potential difference (V_m). Axial current (i_a) is the current flowing within the intracellular compartment, through r_a, the cytoplasmic resistance.

representation of a squid axon, and is often used as an approximation for other tissues as well (Figure 13).

The simple cable model is a cylinder of membrane separating the cytoplasm from the outside solution. In this theoretical cable analysis, the cytoplasm is represented by an ohmic resistance r_a ($\Omega \cdot cm^{-1}$), which is the intracellular resistance to axial current flow per unit length of cable. The membrane is represented by a sequence of elements corresponding to parallel RC circuits (see above) in which the resistive element is membrane resistance r_m. Since multiple elements with resistance r_m are connected in parallel, actual membrane resistance depends on the length of membrane considered; thus, it is conveniently expressed in value per unit length of fiber ($\Omega \cdot cm$).

Let us first consider the flow of charge along the axis of a cable (axial current i_a) in which r_m is infinitely large (i.e., charge is not lost across the membrane). Under this condition i_a is constant along the fiber, and the relation between the intracellular axial current (i_a) and voltage (V_i) can be represented by Ohm's law:

$$\Delta V_i / \Delta x = -r_a / i_a \qquad (39)$$

where r_a is the resistance of the intracellular medium and x is the distance along the fiber. Here $\Delta V_i / \Delta x$ represents the potential difference generated by intracellular current flow, rather than by transmembrane current. Considering an infinitesimal distance ∂x across which the voltage difference ∂V occurs, the differential form of equation 39 then becomes:

$$\partial V / \partial x = -r_a / i_a \tag{40}$$

By taking the second derivative, we can relate axial potential to axial current gradients:

$$\partial^2 V / \partial x^2 = -r_a \cdot \partial i_a / \partial x \tag{41}$$

The negative sign in these equations derives from the convention that flow of positive charges from low to high values of x is regarded as a positive current. In this case, the voltage must decrease as x increases, so that $\partial V / \partial x$ must be negative when positive current flows.

In cells, membrane resistance, albeit considerably higher than axial resistance, has a finite value (membrane conductance is not null). Thus, a proportion of axial current leaks through the membrane per each unit of fiber length, much as water would flow through a leaky hose. When a current pulse is injected at a point along the fiber, the rate of change of axial current i_a with distance along the fiber is equal to and opposite to the current lost through the membrane (transmembrane current, i_m):

$$\partial i_a / \partial x = -i_m \tag{42}$$

This reasoning can help us answer an important question: how big is the transmembrane current available to depolarize the membrane at various distances from the point of actual current injection (e.g., the point where Na^+ channels open)? The answer can be obtained by combining equations 41 and 42:

$$-i_m = (1/r_a) \cdot \partial^2 V / \partial x^2 \tag{43}$$

i.e., transmembrane current flowing at distance from the primary injection point depends on the second derivative of axial voltage drop and is inversely proportional to axial resistance of the fiber.

As shown in Figure 13, biological membranes also include a capacitative component, arranged in parallel with membrane resistance. Indeed, total transmembrane current is the sum of capacitative and resistive currents:

$$i_m = c_m \cdot \partial V / \partial t + V / r_m \tag{44}$$

Combining the various expressions of i_m, we obtain:

$$1/r_a \cdot (\partial^2 V / \partial x^2) = c_m \cdot \partial V / \partial t + V / r_m \tag{45}$$

The constants r_m, c_m and r_a in this equation refer to membrane resistance, capacitance and axial resistance normalized for the relevant geometrical properties of a unit length of the fiber (assumed to be a cylinder). The relation of normalized to raw constants (R_m, C_m, R_i) is as follows:

$$r_a = R_i / \pi a^2 \tag{46}$$

where a is fiber radius. This means that axial resistance decreases as the cross sectional area of the fiber increases;

$$r_m = R_m/2\pi a \tag{47}$$

and

$$c_m = C_m \cdot 2\pi a \tag{48}$$

i.e., transmembrane resistance and capacitance have opposite relationships to fiber circumference, depending on the opposite consequences of parallel summation of resistive and capacitative elements respectively (see section on parallel and series circuits).

In the experimental setting we can measure R_m, C_m and R_i, but we ignore the geometrical properties of the fiber from which the parameters are measured. Thus, to be practically useful, cable equations must be written using non-normalized values of the parameters. This can be done by including the relations just described in the cable equation:

$$(a/2R_i) \cdot \partial^2 V/\partial x^2 = C_m \cdot \partial V/\partial t + V/R_m \tag{49}$$

or:

$$\lambda^2 \cdot \partial^2 V/\partial x^2 = \tau_m \cdot \partial V/\partial t + V \tag{50}$$

This important equation provides the relations between V, x and t, which are required for the understanding of current spread along a cable (fiber). In this equation,

$$\lambda = \sqrt{r_m/r_a} \tag{51}$$

and

$$\tau_m = r_m \cdot c_m \tag{52}$$

τ_m is the membrane **time constant** (in ms), and is equivalent to the time constant of an RC membrane circuit ($\tau = r_m \cdot c_m$). λ is the membrane **space constant** and has dimensions of a distance (mm). The time constant depends on the ratio of membrane resistance to axial resistance, and expresses the tendency for current to spread along the fiber. When the extracellular resistance r_o is not negligible (e.g., due to narrow intercellular clefts), equation 51 becomes:

$$\lambda = \sqrt{\{r_m/(r_a + r_o)\}} \tag{53}$$

where r_o is the external resistance per unit length of cable.

The meaning of the space constant can be better appreciated by considering a relatively simple case, illustrated in Figure 14. A constant current I is applied for a long time (infinite with respect to τ) at point x_0; this current sets up the

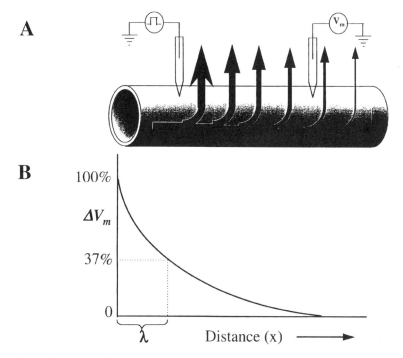

Figure 14 Schematic representation of the attenuation with distance (x) of the membrane potential (V_m) response to current injection. [A] Current injected into the fiber by a microelectrode follows the path of least resistance, causing electrotonic spread of current. [B] The exponential decay of V_m as a function of distance (x). At $x = \lambda$ (the space constant), V_m decays to 37% of its value at $x = 0$.

transmembrane potential $V_0 = IR_m$ at that point. Changes in transmembrane potential (V) at increasing distances x from x_0 are described by the equation:

$$V = \lambda^2 \cdot \mathrm{d}^2V/\mathrm{d}x^2 \tag{54}$$

The relevant solution of this equation is:

$$V_x = V_0\, e^{-x/\lambda} \tag{55}$$

This relationship means that the voltage across the membrane falls exponentially with the distance from the point at which the current was injected (Figure 13 bottom panel). At $x = \lambda$, V_x becomes $V_0\, e^{-1}$, and λ can be defined as the length of fiber over which the voltage across the membrane falls to $1/e$ (or 37%) of its original value (Figure 13). Hence, the higher the membrane resistance (r_m) and/or the lower the axial resistance (r_a) (i.e., less current will "leak" through the membrane), λ will be higher and the decline of voltage along the cable (fiber) will be attenuated. The distributions of V at different values of the space constant are illustrated in Figure 15.

Clearly, as the value of the space constant increases a faster conduction velocity is seen. Due to the dependency of λ on cell diameter, it may be as large as 5 mm in a squid giant axon with a diameter of 500 μm, and as small as 2 mm in a 100 μm frog muscle fiber. Further, in fibers and fine processes of the central nerves system having

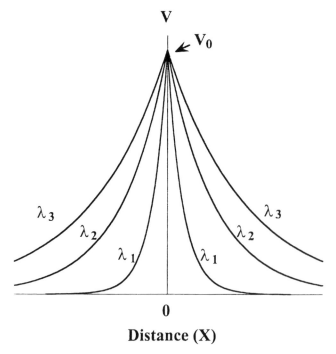

Distance (X)

Figure 15 The effect of different space constants λ ($\lambda_1 < \lambda_2 < \lambda_3$) on the theoretical distribution of membrane potential difference across a one-dimensional cable model. V_0 is the voltage change at $x = 0$. In the presence of a larger space constant, the same amount of transmembrane current depolarizes a greater fiber length (or membrane surface).

a diameter of few microns, λ is only a fraction of a millimeter (Kuffler and Nicholls, 1976).

Finally it must be emphasized that the equations in this section apply only to a linear cable in which r_m, r_a, and c_m are independent of V, x and t. However, except for a small range of membrane potentials (around the resting potential of the cell), the membrane resistance (r_m) is strongly dependent on V and t, and as voltage-dependent channels open (e.g., the fast inward current, I_{Na}), the system becomes highly non-linear. The nature of membrane potential changes under non-linear conditions is described in chapter 3.

The Concept of the Voltage Clamp

The functional properties of ion channels are studied through the analysis of the relationships existing between membrane potential and ionic current flowing through a specific channel. This implies that membrane current needs to be measured at membrane potential values precisely determined by the experimenter.

Biological membranes behave as highly non linear (non-ohmic) conductors for which, due to voltage-dependent channel activation, conductance is a complex function of membrane potential. When a channel is "activated" by an imposed change in membrane potential, the resulting current would instantaneously move membrane potential away from the imposed value. Thus, maintaining membrane potential at a specific value, irrespective of the current flowing through the membrane, becomes a remarkable technical problem. Such a problem has been solved by the technique of **voltage clamp**.

Membrane potential can be held constant ("clamped") if the current flowing through the channels can be compensated by passing through the membrane an equal current of opposite sign. This can be accomplished by a simple feed-back circuit that continuously compares membrane potential (V_m) to a reference value (V_c), set by the experimenter. Every difference between V_m and V_c is amplified and used to inject current in the cell; when V_m becomes equal to V_c, the difference becomes null and current injection ceases. The principle underlying the technique is similar to that of the thermostat, with the difference being that the feed-back signal is represented by transmembrane potential rather than by temperature. Since there are strict limitations to the amount of membrane current that can be accurately compensated, voltage clamp is more easily performed on single cells (having small membrane capacitance) than on multicellular preparations. As described in subsequent chapters, the voltage clamp technique enabled the discovery of individual ion, pump and exchanger currents, all of which contribute to the transmembrane action potential. When applied to a small "patch" of membrane, ideally containing one channel, the voltage clamp technique (thus termed **patch clamp**), has been utilized to investigate specific channel properties such as conductance and probability of open and closed channel states.

CONCLUSIONS

Although a good deal of detail regarding the derivation of mathematical formulas pertaining to electricity and bioelectrical systems has been provided here, this is only a fraction of the work that has been done in relating electricity to electrophysiology. The point to be emphasized to the reader is that cells in general and cardiac myocytes (the subject of this book) in particular truly do function as complex electrical systems containing the machinery (pumps, ion channels, etc.) necessary to generate a signal that ultimately drives the contractile machinery of the cell in an efficient and organized fashion. The reader need not recall the mathematical equations in order to comprehend the electrophysiologic phenomena described in the succeeding chapters, but it is hoped that their presentation here will drive home the important interface that exists between the worlds of physics and of biology in creating the signaling processes that comprise electrophysiology.

2 Molecular Physiology of Cardiac Ion Channels

Paul B. Bennett and J.P. Johnson

FUNCTIONAL MODELS OF CHANNELS

Ion channels are intrinsic membrane proteins that control the flow of specific ions across the cellular membrane. Figure 1 illustrates some of the major properties of voltage gated ion channels deduced from biophysical data. This cartoon shows an ion channel in the cell membrane in three different states: closed, open and inactivated. A kinetic diagram of these states is above each configuration of the channel. Ion channels in the cell membrane open or close depending on the cell membrane potential. When a channel is in an open state, specific ions are allowed to flow down their electrochemical gradient. The process of controlling the flow of ions through the channel is referred to as gating (Hille, 1992). When channels are open, ions can

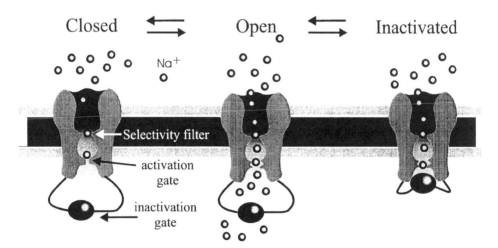

Figure 1 Cartoon of a voltage gated ion channel. The protein is split in half in the membrane to illustrate the ion conducting pore. Three kinetic states of the channel exist: Closed, Open and Inactivated. There are two "gates" that regulate whether the channel is open (ion conducting): an activation gate and an inactivation gate. The selectivity filter discriminates various ions and only allows certain ions through (e.g., sodium for a sodium channel). The activation gate is within the body of the protein and is located intracellular to the selectivity filter. The inactivation gate is depicted as an intracellular peptide loop tethered to between two domains. This idea is based on the "ball and chain" model of inactivation proposed by Armstrong (Armstrong, 1981a; Catterall, 1995b).

flow through a pore and an ionic current can be measured experimentally. From these types of experiments, it has been learned that a channel protein adopts different conformational states depending on membrane potential. From biophysical measurements such as these scientists have deduced that channels can be described in terms of their ionic current, their conductance, their ion selectivity, gating (conformational changes) and pharmacology. Figure 1 assigns these properties to specific regions of the channel. For example, there is a region devoted to ion selectivity; other regions are involved in gating. A great deal of experimental effort has gone into developing and testing models such as this one. More recent data derived from molecular biology and genetic methods have revealed gene and protein sequences, and have provided hope for elucidating protein structure. Definitive measurements of channel structure have not yet been obtained, and thus our knowledge about channel topology is rudimentary. Current efforts are directed at developing a unified description of ion channel structure and function that combines information from different sources.

In this chapter we will briefly review biophysical and molecular data on some of the molecules that control membrane excitability. Because general concepts are emphasized, this is not an exhaustive review of this field, but an attempt is made to present general principles using specific examples. Understanding the properties of ion channels is important not only for understanding the fundamental basis for cellular electrical excitability, but for understanding the molecular basis for certain disorders and diseases as well. Sodium channels are the molecular elements of electrical excitability in nerve and muscle. Opening of voltage gated sodium channels causes the rapid depolarization that occurs during a cellular action potential. Recently, mutations in the cardiac sodium channel gene have been identified as one cause of an inherited cardiac arrhythmia syndrome, the congentital long QT sydrome, which can lead to cardiac arrhythmias and sudden death (Wang *et al.*, 1995a; Wang *et al.*, 1995b; Bennett *et al.*, 1995b). Potassium channels stabilize electrically excitable membranes and counteract the depolarization caused by opening of sodium and calcium channels. They determine resting membrane potentials in some cells, facilitate action potential repolarization and thus regulate the duration of action potentials. In some cells, potassium channels play a major role in refractoriness and automaticity. Important cardiac potassium currents include the transient outward current, and the rapid and slow delayed rectifier currents, I_{TO}, I_{KR} and I_{KS}, respectively. The transient outward current is also referred to as an A-type current and it is likely that the molecular basis of this current involves Kv4 family channel subunits (Dixon *et al.*, 1996). Recent data indicate that subunits known as KvLQT1 and minK underlie I_{KS}, and that a channel subunit known as *HERG* contributes to I_{KR}. Mutations in KvLQT1 and minK have been found in subsets of patients with the congenital long QT syndrome. The *HERG* protein is also clearly important in both normal and pathophysiological states as mutations in *HERG* cause still another variant of the congenital long QT syndrome (Roden *et al.*, 1995). In addition, drugs that inhibit the *HERG* potassium current, such as dofetilide, prolong the human cardiac action potential and in some cases induce a polymorphic ventricular arrhythmia known as Torsades de Pointes that is seen as well in the congenital long QT syndrome (Roden, 1993; Sanguinetti *et al.*, 1995).

Ionic current

As noted above, an ionic current can be measured when ions flow through an open channel. The best method for studying ion channel behavior is the voltage-clamp technique. In this method, the cell membrane potential is controlled by a negative feedback electronic circuit and can be set to any desired level experimentally. Figure 2 illustrates examples of how this is accomplished. The top of Figure 2 shows two principal methods for ionic current measurements. Each involves placement of a saline filled glass pipette onto a cell. The pipette is electrically connected to the voltage clamp amplifier which controls the membrane potential across the pipette tip and allows measurement of ion current. On the left, the pipette isolates a single channel protein in an excised membrane patch. The membrane potential is changed

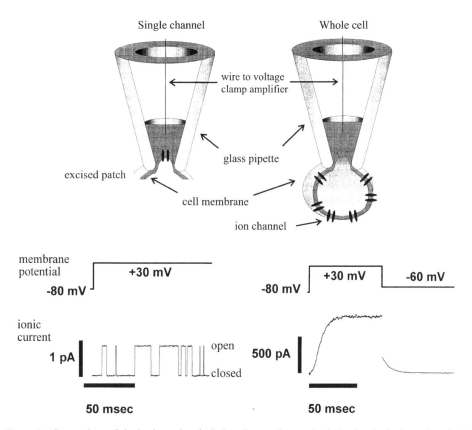

Figure 2 Comparison of single channel and whole cell recording methods. In the single channel method (top left), a glass pipette filled with extracellular solution is pressed against a cell to isolate one channel. The glass forms a giga-ohm (10^{-9} ohm) seal with the membrane. The patch of membrane containing the channel is removed from the cell to give an excised patch. The electrical potential across the patch of membrane is controlled by the voltage clamp amplifier. The current recorded through a single channel is shown on the bottom left. The step change in membrane potential is shown above the current tracing. The right hand panels show the whole-cell recording configuration and the ionic current recorded from a population of ion channels. A giga-ohm seal is formed but instead of removing the patch, the membrane is ruptured by suction to allow the pipette contents to mix with the cell contents. In this case, the pipette is filled with a solution similar to that found in the cytoplasm.

from one value to another as shown below (middle panel) and the opening and closing of an individual ion channel is measured (bottom panel). Note that the ion current appears as random duration rectangular pulses of current that report whether the channel is open or closed. The amplitude of most single channel currents is in the range of 0.1–10 pA (10^{-12} ampere). Single channel recording permits observations of the stochastic opening and closing of an individual ion channel protein and allows direct measurement of the channel elementary conductance. Such analysis permits separation of the channel conductance properties from its gating properties. By analyzing the temporal nature of opening and closing of single channels, direct measurements of transition rate constants can be determined (Sakmann and Neher, 1995).

Alternatively, macroscopic observations of populations of channels are made. This method is illustrated on the right of Figure 2. The most common way in which these measurements are made is referred to as the whole-cell method of voltage-clamp in which the ion channels in the entire cell surface are investigated. In this case the opening and closing of hundreds or thousands of channels is occurring. The current through each channel is summed together with all other channels in the membrane in this measurement. The shape of the whole-cell current waveform as a function of time under voltage-clamp conditions is proportional to the average open probability of the channels. Note how the whole-cell macroscopic current differs from that observed in single channel records. The basis for these differences is discussed below.

Conductance

Ohm's law ($V = I \cdot R$) states that voltage (V, which can be thought of as electrical pressure) is proportional to the current (I, charge flow) times the resistance to that flow (R). Conductance reflects the ease of charge flow and as such it is the reciprocal of resistance. Resistance is measured in ohms and conductance is measured in siemens (1/ohms): one siemen equals $1\,\text{ohm}^{-1}$. Hence Ohm's law can be restated as current equals conductance ($1/R$) times the electrical driving force, voltage ($I = V/R$). As related to ion channels, conductance reflects the ease of ion movement through the open pore of the ion channel. A fundamental property of an ion channel is its unitary conductance. Most ion channels have conductances in the range of 1–200 picosiemens (10^{-12} siemens). The measurements of individual channel currents reveals that a channel randomly flips between non-conducting and ion conducting states. These openings appear as rectangular-shaped current pulses which report the occupancy of the open state of the protein (see Figure 2). Although, the conductance (γ) of an individual ion channel is usually constant, the unitary current (i) changes as a function of membrane potential (E_m) due to differences in the electrochemical driving force for the ions that permeate the pore. This electrochemical driving force ($E_m - E_K$) is the difference between the applied membrane potential and the equilibrium potential (E_K) for the ion of interest (see Chapter 1), in this case potassium. The driving force is both electrical and chemical, due to the voltage gradient (electrical force) and the concentration gradient (chemical driving force) of the ions. The single channel current (i) can be defined in the form of Ohm's law as

$$i = \gamma \left(E_m - E_K \right) \tag{1}$$

Experimentally, the conductance (γ) is determined by measuring the amplitude of the single channel current as shown in Figure 2 and dividing by the driving force.

Selectivity

What is selectivity? Physiologists have long sought to understand the answer to this question and the molecular basis of the ion selectivity is one of the most important questions in ion channel biophysics. Selectivity refers to the remarkable property of an ion channel to identify and allow through its open pore a particular type of ion (e.g., potassium ions), but to exclude all other ions even if they are present at a higher concentration. This process is even more remarkable if one considers the rate of transit of the ions through the channel: $>10^7$ per second.

Ion channel proteins can discriminate among inorganic ions such as sodium, potassium, chloride, and calcium, permitting passage of one type to the exclusion of all others. While the concept of ionic selectivity of a channel seems obvious (some ions traverse the channel better than others) there is no well defined mechanism nor is the molecular basis completely understood. Three major classes of cation selective ion channels have been investigated extensively: potassium, sodium, and calcium selective channels. A calcium selective channel permits passage of a calcium ion and excludes sodium ions even when the sodium concentration is 50–100 times greater than the calcium concentration. Furthermore the ion channel can maintain this exquisite selectivity while permitting millions of ions per second through its pore. Classically this high rate of ion transport through an ion selective pore has distinguished a channel from a carrier or a pump.

Ion size and charge are obvious properties that might provide a physical mechanism for distinction among ions. These alone are not enough, however to explain selectivity and rapid ion flux. The atomic radius of sodium (0.95 Å) is smaller than that of potassium (1.33 Å) and has the same charge. Therefore sodium would flow freely through potassium channels if size and charge were the only criteria for permeation. Clearly more is involved. Note that the charge density of sodium is greater than that of potassium: one positive charge but on a smaller object. Ions in solution are surrounded by a shell of water molecules making them too large to pass through the pore of the channel. Removing these water molecules requires energy. Sodium ions have a relatively greater attraction for water and the energy for dehydration of sodium ions is much greater than that for potassium. It is now believed that an ion channel protein acts as a catalyst for dehydration of the permeant ion (Hille, 1992). The charged or partially charged amino acids of the channel can act as surrogate water molecules in solvating the ion. This makes the dehydration of the ion for passage through the channel energetically possible. An ion that is larger than the preferred ion will not physically fit through the selectivity filter even if it could be fully dehydrated. One that is too small will not be appropriately solvated by the channel walls. The ion will retain its aqueous shell and cannot pass through the selectivity filter. Despite ideas about how selectivity might occur, the actual molecular mechanisms of channel selectivity remained obscure until molecular biological approaches allowed manipulation of ion channel amino acid sequence. The ability to alter the primary amino acid sequence of channels has led to a description of the basic structural motifs that mediate selectivity in sodium, potassium, and calcium channels (Heinemann *et al.*, 1992; Yool and Schwarz, 1991; Yang *et al.*, 1993; Heginbotham and MacKinnon, 1992).

Channel gating (macroscopic and single channel)

The macroscopic ionic current (I) is equal to the product of the total number of channels in the membrane (N), the channel open probability (P_{open}) and the single channel current (i).

$$I = N \cdot P_{\text{open}} \cdot i \tag{2}$$

The power and utility of single channel recordings comes from the ability to simplify this relationship through direct experimental observation. The single channel current (and conductance, see equation 1) are measured directly. If a single channel patch is utilized ($N = 1$), then P_{open} can be readily determined.

The simplest ion channel with voltage dependent gating serves as a switch that is either open or closed. When the ion channel is in the open state, ions are permitted to pass through the pore of the protein from one side of the membrane to the other resulting in an ionic current that can be measured. Measurement of this current under voltage clamp reports the occupancy of the open conformation of the channel. It is informative to first consider how the simplest two state ion channel can gate ion flux as a function of membrane potential and subsequently to use these principles to gain insight into the more complex gating behavior of real ion channels.

Figure 3 illustrates the relationship between single channel (1 channel) and macroscopic (whole-cell, many channels) measurements. In the bottom panel, the occupancy of the open state as a function of time is plotted illustrating the opening and closing of a channel. When only one channel is observed, determination of the open state is unambiguous. The channel was initially in the closed state. Once a channel protein enters a state, it remains there for a period of time which is on average equal to the reciprocal of the rate constant leading away from that state. Because this is a system of molecules, the behavior can be understood using a statistical approach. The period of time the channel spends in any state is random, but the average lifetime can be estimated.

We can carry this molecular example to the macroscopic level by adding more channels (see Figure 3). When additional channels are considered ($N = 3$, 10, 30, 100, 1000) note how the average begins to resemble a whole-cell recording as N increases (compare to Figure 2 right panel). As the number of channels increases, the certainty of the average open probability (P_{open}) increases, however knowledge about the single channel amplitude and the open and closed durations is lost. As N increases the binary opening and closing of an individual channel transforms into the exponential time course of opening observed macroscopically. When N is large the average P_{open} of the channel can be easily estimated.

Channel proteins undergo conformational rearrangements and occupy different kinetic states with a probability that depends upon membrane potential. The theory of reaction rates and transition states used in chemistry provides a definition of the rates and transition probabilities of these macromolecules (Stevens, 1978). This formalism assumes that major conformational states of the channel protein

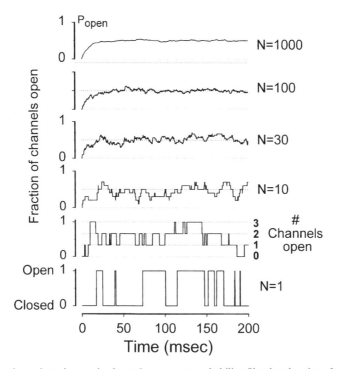

Figure 3 Time dependent changes in channel open state probability. Simulated gating of a two-state ion channel such as shown in Figure 1. Tracings represent changes in the number (N) of channels present from N=1 to N=1,000. The channel is initially in the closed conformation and at time zero, the rate constants were switched to be equal such that the steady state open probability was equal to 0.5. When N=1, there is absolute certainty regarding whether the channel is in the open or in the closed conformation. As the number of channels in a patch increases, the ease of measuring the average steady state open probability increases. However, information about the single channel current levels and open and closed times is lost.

correspond to energetic minima and that transitions among various stable states involves crossing activation energy barriers. Figure 4 depicts such a reaction with two stable states, *C* and *O*. The rate constants that govern transitions among states can be predicted based on the well-to-barrier heights in such a scheme. The channel is in a stable energy minimum when in the *C* state and must cross the barrier to enter the *O* state. The height of this barrier from the well bottom to the barrier top determines the rate of the reaction in the forward direction. A rate constant (α in this case with units of sec^{-1}) characterizes this forward transition. The larger the energy barrier (well-to-barrier height) the slower the reaction. If the height of the barrier or the depth of the well depends on membrane potential, then the rate constant will also depend on membrane potential. The dashed lines in the figure illustrate a change in the energy wells and barriers. Because the energy required to hop over the barrier is changed, the rate constant will change. The effects of this are discussed below.

The partitioning among energetic states of a macromolecule can be defined by the Boltzmann relationship where the likelihood of existing in one state or the other depends on the energy difference (ΔG) between those states.

$$S2/S1 = \exp[-\Delta G/kT] \qquad (3)$$

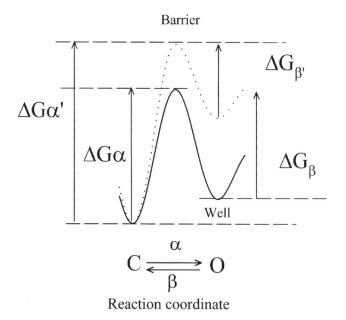

Barrier

Reaction coordinate

Figure 4 Energy barrier transition state diagram of channel gating. C represents the closed conformation, O represents the open conformation. In order for the channel to move between the closed and open
conformation, it must overcome the energy barrier that separates them. The rate constants of a reaction
and hence the rate of the reaction depend on the height of the barrier relative to the well. For voltage
gated ion channels the barrier heights and/or well depths may depend on membrane potential. The barrier
with the dashed lines indicates what might happen to the reaction rate energetics upon changing membrane potential. Other factors such as drugs or assembly with channel subunits may also alter these
barriers and wells. This is discussed in the text.

where $S2/S1$ is the fraction of molecules in state 2 compared to state 1. The thermal
energy of the system is product of the Boltzmann constant (k) and absolute temperature (T); kT has a value of about 0.59 kcal per mole at room temperature.

The difference in free energy between the states (ΔG) determines the equilibrium
distribution. A fundamental expression for a transition rate constant (e.g., α) can be
derived by considering the energy barriers that must be overcome for this transition
to occur. The rate of a given transition is set by the energy barrier and the number of
attempts at crossing the energy barrier (Stevens, 1978). The attempt rate for crossing
the barrier can be calculated from the Boltzmann constant (k), absolute temperature
(T) and Planck's constant (h) as kT/h which has a value of approximately of 6×10^{12}
per second at room temperature. Since only a fraction of the attempts at crossing the
barrier are successful, this number is scaled down by the channel specific energy
barrier. There are at least two types of energetic terms that govern this system. One
represents the free energy changes that occur independently of membrane potential
(ΔG_1) and the other (ΔG_2) depends explicitly on membrane potential (E_m). ΔG can
be divided into $\Delta G_1 + \Delta G_2$ where $\Delta G_2 = z \cdot \delta \cdot e \cdot E_m$. ΔG_2 depends on membrane
potential and contains components influenced by the apparent charge (z) and the
fraction of the electrical field (δ) experienced by the part of the protein that senses
the membrane potential (E_m). e is the elementary electronic charge. The following

equations define the forward (α) and reverse (β) rate constants as a function of membrane potential.

$$\alpha = (kT/h) \exp[\Delta G\alpha + (z \cdot \delta \cdot e \cdot E_m)/kT] \qquad (4)$$
$$\beta = (kT/h) \exp[\Delta G\beta - (z \cdot (1 - \delta) \cdot e \cdot E_m)/kT] \qquad (5)$$

From these equations for each rate constant, the entire set of voltage-dependent kinetic properties of an ion channel can be derived. The only unknowns in these equations are the energy barrier heights in the absence of an electric field ($\Delta G\alpha$, $\Delta G\beta$), and the sensitivity of the voltage sensor to the electrical field ($z \cdot \delta$).

Channel activation (opening from closed states)
Utilizing the voltage dependence for the rate constants derived from the transition state theory, the kinetic behavior of the 2-state ion channel is explored at several different membrane potentials in Figure 5. This figure depicts the behavior of the channel using reasonable estimates for the energetics just described (see Figure

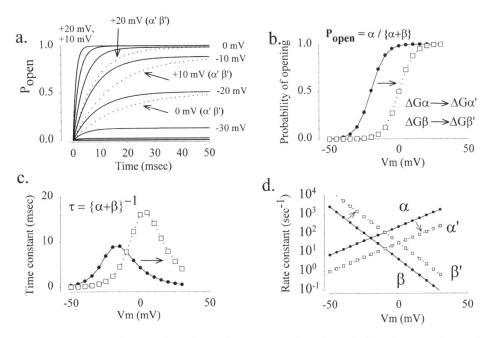

Figure 5 a. Time and voltage-dependence of a two state channel switch. The time-dependence of channel average open probability at different membrane potentials is shown. The records were generated with voltage-dependent rate constants calculated from the equations given in the text. As membrane potential is increased, the rate of the opening increases and the steady state probability of opening changes reaches a maximum at strong depolarizations. Panel b shows the steady state open probability as a function of membrane potential calculated from the ratio of the rate constants as shown c. The system time constant as a function of membrane potential. d. The rate constants α and β as a functional membrane potential plotted on a semi-logarithmic graph. The voltage-dependence of the rate constants were calculated from equations 4 and 5 where $z = 5$, $\delta = 0.35$, $\Delta G\alpha = -24kT$, $\Delta G\beta = -28kT$. These ΔG values correspond to free energy changes of 14.16 kcal/mol and 16.52 kcal/mole, respectively. The dashed lines in each panel indicate the changes in gating that occur when $\Delta G\alpha$ and $\Delta G\beta$ are both changed to $-26kT$ (15.34 kcal/mol).

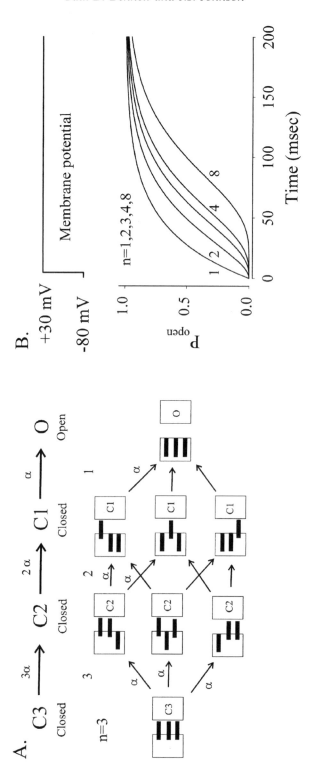

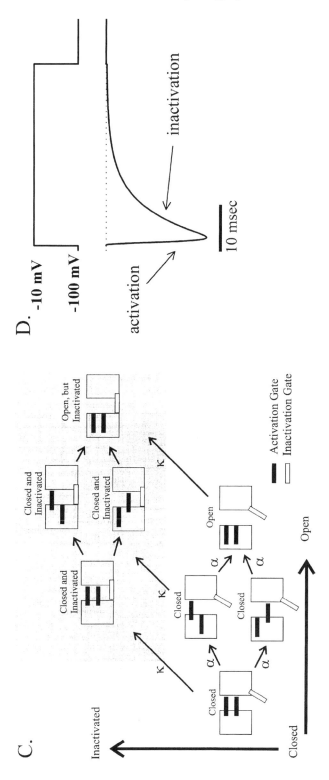

Figure 6 A. Possible gate positions in a channel with three independent gates. The horizontal bars represent the channel gates. The state labeled O has all gates closed and the state labeled O has all gates open. The equivalent kinetic state diagram is shown above. In this representation the forward rate constant α is multiplied by an integer equal to the number of gates that are closed before the transition occurs. B. The effect of the number of gates, n, on the time delay for channel open probability. The average open probability as a function of time was calculated for models with 1, 2, 3, 4 or 8 gates. Adding gates to the reaction increases the delay in the rise of P_{open}. When only one gate is present there is no delay. C. Channel gating scheme with two activation gates and one inactivation gate in series. This independent gate scheme can produce inactivation. In this case the gates attached to the left hand "subunit" are the activation gates and are identical. The gate attached to the right hand "subunit" is a distinct inactivation gate. Each gate functions independently and all gates must be open for the channel to be open. The activation gates are closed and the inactivation gate is open at the resting membrane potential (e.g., $-100\,mV$). The probabilities that an activation gate will open or that the inactivation gate will close both increase with membrane depolarization. The rate constants that govern opening of the activation gates are larger than those of the inactivation gate, hence the activation gates open faster than the inactivation gate can close. Eventually the inactivation gate closes. D. The bottom panel shows the time course of a sodium current generated by this scheme. Upon a step depolarization from $-100\,mV$ to $-10\,mV$ there is a rapid increase of inward sodium current due to opening of the channels. The current decreases again as the channels inactivate.

legend). The figure also demonstrates the effects of small changes in $\Delta G\alpha$ and $\Delta G\beta$ (dashed lines) as might occur when a drug binds to the channel or when an amino acid in the protein is mutated.

Figure 5a plots the average time-course of change in the open probability at different membrane potentials. At membrane potentials more negative than approximately –60 mV, the channels do not open. At less negative membrane potentials, the channels open with a characteristic time-course and reach a steady state level that depends on membrane potential. The rate of change of the current (or P_{open}) at each membrane potential is characterized by a membrane potential dependent time constant (τ). Figure 5b plots the steady state open probability as a function of membrane potential. The shape of this curve as illustrated by the solid line is predicted from the ratio of the rate constants that govern the system ($\alpha/\alpha + \beta$). Likewise, the time constant of this system is calculated from the sum of the two rate constants ($1/\alpha + \beta$) and the voltage dependence of the time constant is illustrated in Figure 5c. Because the system time constant (τ) is derived from the two rate constants, the voltage dependence is bell shaped: the value of τ is dominated by one rate constant at each voltage extreme and τ is greatest (reaction rate is slowest) when α equals β.

The two fundamental rate constants, α and β are plotted as a function of membrane potential in Figure 5d. Note that when plotted on a semi-logarithmic graph, these rate constants are linear functions of membrane potential. Also note the membrane potential where they are equal is the same as the midpoint of the open probability curve as well as the peak of the time constant curve. Thus, in a simple two state system such as this the kinetics are slowest at a membrane potential where half the channels are open and half are closed.

In each panel, the effects of altering the change in free energy for each rate constant are shown by the dashed lines. In this case the well to barrier height was increased for $\alpha(\Delta G\alpha$ from 14.16 to 15.34 kcal/mol) and decreased for $\beta(\Delta G\beta$ from 16.52 to 15.34 kcal/mol). This has the effect of shifting the voltage dependence of channel opening (Figure 5b) and slowing the kinetics (Figure 5a and c). Note the large changes in gating that occur even though the energy changes were rather small (~ 2.4 kcal/mol). The dashed lines in Figure 5a show the changes in the time course of P_{open} at 0, $+10$, $+20$ mV. Note for example that the kinetics at 0 mV are slowed and the steady state level of P_{open} is decreased compared to the control (solid lines).

Experimental observation indicates that the time course of opening of the channels occurs after a delay. A simple 2-state model cannot give rise to a delay in opening. In order to account for this delay seen in the data, Hodgkin and Huxley (Hodgkin and Huxley, 1952b) made a simple assumption that several identical, independent gates exist and each must open before the channel as a whole is in the open state (Hodgkin and Huxley, 1952a). Each gate has a its own probability of being in the open configuration. Figure 6 compares the gate positions of a hypothetical ion channel with three independent gates. The equivalent linear kinetic state diagram is also shown. Note that the rate constants are integral multiples of α(i.e., 1α, 2α, 3α). This can be understood by considering the number of possible new gate configurations from each occupied state. In state C3, there are three possible ways the channel can go to the next state each with a rate constant α. Thus, the aggregate rate for this transition in the whole channel is 3α. When in one of the C2 states however, there are only two possible ways to change to the next state (C1) and when in a C1 state only one gate is left to open before the channel is in the ion conducting open state. This can be easily generalized to a channel with any number of independent gates.

The effect of the number of gates, **n**, on the time course of the average P_{open} is shown in Figure 6B. Note that as **n** is increased there is more of a delay, but the increase in the delay does not increase linearly with **n**. In the original Hodgkin and Huxley model, the potassium channel was assumed to have four such independent gates. The probability of the channel opening is the product of the open probabilities of each of the independent gates. Thus, if any one of the gates remained in a closed state the channel itself would be closed and only when all gates were open was the channel itself open. Kinetically, this configuration gives rise to a delay in the appearance of the open state. In order to envision the delay in channel opening intuitively, it is often simpler to view the channel as transiting a number of closed states prior to entering the open state. In the linear kinetic scheme the channel must go through several closed states prior to entering the open state (see Figure 6). As the number of gates is increased, the number of possible states increases and so does the delay before final opening of the channel. In this case the rate constants have a fixed relationship to one another. This fixed relationship creates a mathematically simple system for analyzing channel kinetics. However, it also provided the first of a number of testable hypothesis which eventually led to the need for more complicated models to describe channel gating.

Inactivation

Another characteristic of some channels that cannot be accounted for by a simple two state switch is the property known as inactivation. During a depolarization under voltage clamp conditions, sodium channels open but then spontaneously close again (see Figure 6C and D). To account for this observation, Hodgkin and Huxley placed another two state switch in series with the switches that govern channel opening (Hodgkin and Huxley, 1952a). They referred to this switch as the inactivation gate. Figure 6C shows the possible gate positions for a channel with 2 activation gates and 1 inactivation gate. Only when all of the activation gates were in the open position and when the inactivation gate was in the open position would the channel conduct ions. If any one of the switches were in a non-open position the channel would be closed. By adjusting the kinetics of these switches, the appropriate time course of the macroscopic sodium current can be obtained. Figure 6D shows Na^+ current computed from the model if Figure 6C. The channels are closed at $-100\,mV$. Upon stepping the membrane potential to $-10\,mV$ the channels open (activate) and then close again (inactivate).

Ion channel inactivation is a mechanism for conservation of energy resources (energy stored as ionic gradients) after a signaling event. Inactivation serves as a molecular form of memory that is useful for numerous important time synchronized events that are required in excitable cells. In addition, the inactivated state of ion channels corresponds to the high affinity state for interactions with some ion channel blocking drugs and as such may represent a target of opportunity for drug development.

At least three kinetically distinct forms of inactivation have been observed. One is the easily visible (rapid) closing of channels that is seen in A-type potassium channels (see Figure 7A), calcium channels and sodium channels (Figure 6D). A second, usually slower type of inactivation exists in many channels. Still another manifestation of inactivation results in an apparent rectification of the current referred to as I_{kr}, which is derived from the potassium channel subunit known as *HERG* (Trudeau *et al.*, 1995; Sanguinetti *et al.*, 1996a; Smith *et al.*, 1996). This type of inactivation is very rapid relative to the activation (opening) of the *HERG* channels and as a consequence the ionic current appears to inwardly rectify during standard current voltage protocols. The simplest kinetic model of a channel with inactivation is shown below.

$$C \rightleftharpoons O \rightleftharpoons I$$

In this model the channel is closed (C) at resting membrane potentials, opens (O) upon membrane depolarization and then inactivates (I). Thus, C states are defined as closed states that are occupied at the resting potential and I states are closed

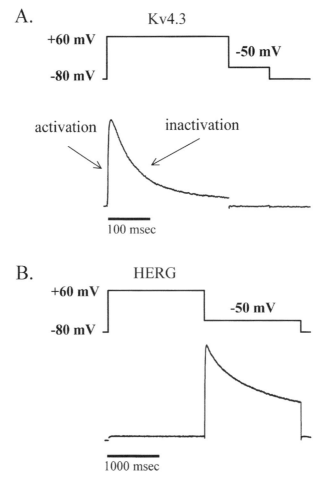

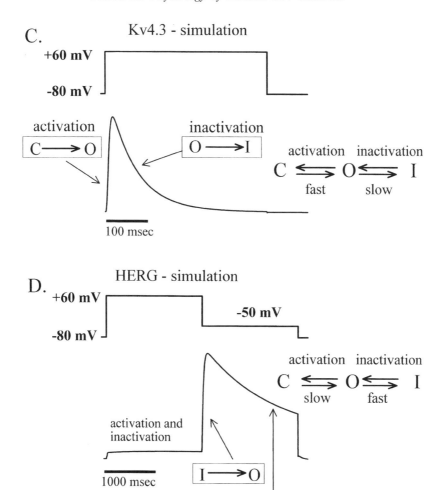

Figure 7 Two types of inactivation gating behavior. A. Expression of recombinant Kv4.3 K^+ channels in CHO cells. The voltage clamp protocol is shown above each record. Upon a step depolarization from –80 mV to +60 mV, Kv4.3 channels open rapidly and then become inactivated. B. Expression of recombinant *HERG* K^+ channels in CHO cells. Upon a step depolarization from –80 mV to +60 mV, *HERG* channels appear to rectify and have little outward current. However, when the membrane potential is stepped to –50 mV a large outward K^+ current is seen that slowly deactivates. K^+ currents in A and B were measured using the whole-cell patch clamp method. The same simple gating scheme can account for channels with classical inactivation behavior such as Kv4.3 (C) as well as the *HERG*-like (D) inactivation. K^+ currents were simulated assuming a K^+ equilibrium potential of –90 mV. The same gating scheme was used in each case only the energy barriers defining the rate constants were changed (see Figure 5 and eqs. 4 and 5).To produce the Kv4.3-type behavior the $C \rightleftharpoons O$ transition rates were greater than the $O \rightleftharpoons I$ transition rates. To produce the *HERG* type behavior the $O \rightleftharpoons I$ transition rates were greater than the $C \rightleftharpoons O$ transition rates.

states that are occupied during depolarization. The observed kinetics depend on the relative rates of transitions from the closed-to-open state and the open-to-inactivated states. Inactivation gating behavior such as that observed in sodium, calcium and

A-type potassium channels can be described when the closed-to-open transition is fast and the open-to-inactivated transition is slower (see Figure 7C). The same gating model can be used to describe *HERG*-like channel behavior when the closed-to-open transition is slow relative to the open-to-inactivated transitions (Figure 7D).

MOLECULAR IDENTITY OF ION CHANNELS

In the 1950s and 60s there was still debate about the chemical and molecular nature of ion transport and the fundamental basis of excitability. During the 1970s calcium and sodium channels had been identified as proteins and their biochemical isolation was underway (Catterall, 1995). Progress was aided by developments in protein chemistry and in pharmacology. However, these methods were not available for potassium channels because there were no high affinity ligands or toxins to aid in their isolation. Developments in molecular biology eventually allowed the cloning of the voltage gated sodium channel (Noda *et al.*, 1984) followed by cloning of the *Shaker* potassium channel (Tempel *et al.*, 1987). These events revolutionized channel biology as they paved the way for detailed structure-function studies that are still underway.

Ion channels are membrane proteins

Proteins, including the ion channels, are made up of the 20 primary amino acids. The physical chemical characteristics of these amino acids determines in part the pattern

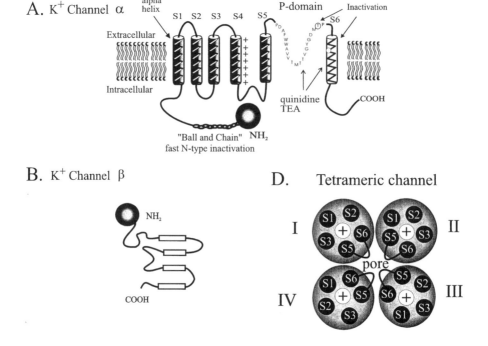

C. Na$^+$ Channel α

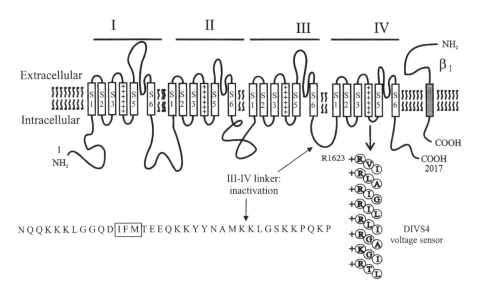

Figure 8   A. Cartoon of K$^+$ channel α subunit. There are six putative trans-membrane segments (S1–S6) that are presumed to be alpha helices connected by intra- or extracellulat loops. The amino acids at the extreme N-terminus have been shown to be involved in fast inactivation. The amino acids connecting S5 and S6 form a part of the ion conducting pore as well as play a role in channel inactivation. Arginines (R) or lysines (K) in the S4 segment (shown as positive charges) play a role in voltage sensing and channel activation. B. Cartoon of K$^+$ channel β subunit. β subunits modify α subunit function and expression. Some Kvβ subunits are believed to have an N-terminus that can act as a fast inactivation gate. C. Cartoon of Na$^+$ channel trans-membrane segments and domains. Four largely homologous domains (DI - DIV) each with six membrane spanning segments (S1-S6) make up the α subunit peptide. Similar motifs as in the K$^+$ channel α subunit are believed to exist. The regions connecting S5 and S6 in each domain make up a part of the ion conducting pore. The intracellular loop linking DIII and DIV is involve in fast inactivation. The amino acids IFM in this region are critical for fast inactivation. Arginines (R) or lysines (K) in the S4 segment (shown as positive charges) also play a role in voltage sensing and Na$^+$ channel activation. The β_1 subunit is a much smaller protein with a single putative trans-membrane segment and an extracellular amino terminus. D. Tetrameric nature of K$^+$ or Na$^+$ channels. Four K$^+$ channel α subunits are assumed to come together as a tetramer with the ion conducting pore in the middle. A similar assembly is envisioned for Na$^+$ channels except all 4 domains are part of the same protein.

of folding of the resultant protein. Each amino acid has a distinct side chain that confers unique characteristics. Protein folding depends on numerous forces. Interactions among the amino acids in the primary sequence of a protein (one dimensional amino acid sequence) including electrostatic interactions, disulfide bonds, hydrophobic interactions and the presence of water all influence folding patterns. Nevertheless, the precise mechanisms that determine folding are not fully understood. One characteristic that biophysical chemists have used to characterize amino acids in proteins is hydrophobicity. Indices of hydrophobicity have been used to predict whether a segment of protein prefers the hydrophobic membrane or a hydrophilic environment. According to this analysis, many ion channels are predicted to have domains with six membrane spanning segments (S1–S6). Proteins generally form characteristic secondary structures, typified by alpha helices and beta sheets. An alpha helix has 3.6 residues per turn which spans approximately 5.4 Å. Thus, a 22 amino acid alpha helix will span 33 angstroms, a distance comparable to the thickness of the lipid membrane.

As noted above, the first voltage gated potassium channel subunit clone was from the *Shaker* locus of *Drosophila melanogaster*. The amino acid sequence deduced from the *Shaker* gene indicated a protein of approximately 70 kDa. Each subunit contains six transmembrane segments (S1–S6) that are presumed to be alpha helical (See Figure 8A). The pore is made of amino acids from the segment (P-domain) connecting S5 and S6 (see Table 1). The amino and carboxy termini are presumed to be intracellular and some potassium channels interact with β subunits (Figure 8B) which are discussed below. A functional potassium channel is believed to be a tetramer consisting of four homologous subunits (See Figure 8D).

Voltage gated sodium and calcium channel α subunits are also believed to consist of four homologous domains, each having approximately the same topology as a single "Shaker-like" potassium channel domain (See Figure 8C). In this case, the four domains reside in the same protein (See Figure 8D). Sodium channels consist of approximately 2000 amino acids (depending on the isoform) with a molecular mass of around 260 kDa.

Table 1 Comparison of potassium channel P-domain amino acid residues

Channel	Amino acid sequence	Ion current phenotype and species
	430 (*Shaker*) 450	
Shaker	PDAFWWAVVTMTTVGYGDMTP	A-type channel drosophila
rKv1.1	PDAFWWAVVSMTTVGYGDMYP	delayed rectifier rat
rKv1.2	PDAFWWAVVSMTTVGYGDMVP	delayed rectifier rat
hKv1.3	PDAFWWAVVTMTTVGYGDMHP	
hKv1.4	PDAFWWAVVTMTTVGYGDMKP	A-type channel human (I_{TO} ?)
hKv1.5	PDAFWWAVVTMTTVGYGDMRP	delayed rectifier human(I_{KUR})
hKv1.6	PDAFWWAVVTMTTVGYGDMYP	
KvLQT1	ADALWWGVVTVTTIGYGDKVP	delayed rectifier human (I_{KS})
Kv2.1	PASFWWATITMTTVGYGDIYP	
Kv3.1	PIGFWWAVVTMTTLGYGDMYP	
Shal	PAAFWYTIVTMTTLGYGDMVP	A-type channel drosophila
mKv4.1	PAAFWYTIVTMTTLGYGDMVP	A-type channel mouse
rKv4.2	PAAFWYTIVTMTTLGYGDMVP	A-type channel rat (I_{TO})
rKv4.3	PASFWYTIVTMTTLGYGDMVP	A-type channel rat (I_{TO})
HIRK	TAAFLFSIETQTTIGYGFRCV	inward rectifier human
AKT1	VTSMYWSITTLTTVGYGDLHP	Arabidopsis thaliana (plant)
SKT1	ITSIYWSITTLTTVGYGDLHP	Solanum tuberosum (potato)
eag	VTALYFTMTCMTSVGFGNVAA	
HERG	VTALYFTFSSLTSVGFGNVSP	delayed rectifier human (I_{KR})

```
                     | ^^^^^^  |
             Internal TEA   |   External TEA site
                     K selectivity
```

The amino acids of the P-domain are aligned from different K^+ channels. The P-domain is the stretch of amino acids linking the S5 and S5 transmembrane segments (see Figure 8). The numbering at the top refers to the *Drosophila Shaker* channel sequence. Amino acids are shown as single letter codes. The sites of external and internal TEA block and K^+ selectivity as determined in the *Shaker* channel are indicated by vertical lines and ^ below the sequence. The glycine-tyrosine-glycine (GYG) motif is in bold as is the Shaker equivalent 449 amino acid that affects external TEA sensitivity and C-type inactivation. A hydrophobic aromatic amino acid (Y, F) in the 449 position confers high sensitivity to TEA and little C-type inactivation. A charged amino acid (R) confers low sensitivity to TEA and much more C-type inactivation.

Molecular basis of function

The three dimensional structure of voltage gated ion channels is unknown at the present time and it has not yet been possible to crystallize channel proteins due to their size and hydrophobic character. Similar problems plague efforts to deduce structure by other methods such as nuclear magnetic resonance spectroscopy. Therefore, the presumed structure has been deduced from knowledge of its amino acid sequence and by mutagenesis experiments which permit a trial-and-error deduction of the role particular amino acid groups play in channel function.

Conductance, selectivity and block

Most models for the structure of voltage gated ion channels place the ion conducting pore at the center of the four homologous domains of an α subunit (see Figures 8 and 9). Thus, each domain contributes one fourth of the pore. Experimental studies have begun identifying the amino acids that make up the pore lining. Understanding the structure, function and placement of these amino acids is important as it holds the key to the ion selectivity mechanism described above and it is known that a number of therapeutically relevant drugs as (well as experimental agents) interact with the pore of the ion channel and inhibit flow of ions. Thus, elucidating structure in this region may help us understand the receptor site for a number of ion channel blocking drugs.

The outer mouth of the potassium channel has been mapped in a series of experiments using site directed mutagenesis as well as drugs and toxins that are known to interact with the outer part of the channel. Tetraethylammonium (TEA) blocks some potassium channels from the external side in a way that appears to depend on a tyrosine residue in the outer part of the pore (Kavanaugh *et al.*, 1992; Heginbotham and MacKinnon, 1992; Po *et al.*, 1993). This residue, located at position 449 in the *Shaker* potassium channel confers high or low affinity interactions with tetraethylammonium, depending on the amino acid located there (see Figure 8 and Table 1). Researchers have also utilized high affinity peptide toxins as a "molecular ruler" to probe and measure the outer mouth of the channel (Park and Miller, 1992; Shimony *et al.*, 1994; Smith *et al.*, 1986; Stampe *et al.*, 1994; Stocker and Miller, 1994; Gross *et al.*, 1994; Hidalgo and MacKinnon, 1995; Krezel *et al.*, 1995). Because the three dimensional structures of some of these toxins are known, it was reasoned that understanding points of contact with the channel would provide molecular information about distances between residues in the channel that interact with the toxin. This approach has proven very successful. For example, the outer pore of the channel must be a vestibule that can accommodate a $25 \times 35\,\text{Å}$ toxin molecule. It seems to be at least 10–15 Å deep and probably has a rather flat "floor". This gives a profile of a large flat bottom funnel that transforms into the narrow ion conduction path ($< 5\,\text{Å}$).

The amino acid residues that confer ion selectivity have likewise been identified. Chimeric potassium channels were created which swap regions of the pore domain among channel types (see Table 1 and Figure 8). It was shown that the single channel conductance, a fundamental characteristic of a particular ion channel, can be transferred with this region. Changes in individual amino acids in this region also have effects on ion selectivity. The threonine at position 441 in *Shaker* appears

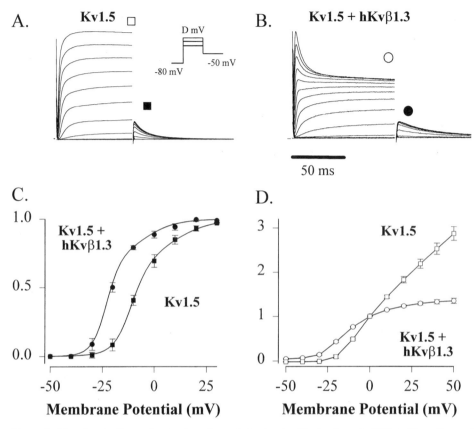

Figure 9 Functional effects of potassium channel β subunits (England *et al.*, 1995a). The effects of the potassium channel Kvβ1.3 subunit on the Kv1.5 α subunit. A. Whole-cell recordings of Kv1.5 K+ currents during voltage clamp steps to different membrane potentials. The voltage clamp pulse protocol is shown as an inset. B. Co-expression of Kvβ1.3 and the Kv1.5 α subunits. The β subunit causes the current to decline during sustained depolarization. This effect resembles inactivation. C. The β subunit causes a negative shift in the voltage dependence of channel opening and gives the appearance of current rectification (D).

critically important (Yool and Schwarz, 1991). Heginbotham *et al.* (Heginbotham and MacKinnon, 1992) first pointed out the high degree of identity in the stretch of amino acids between the S5 and S6 transmembrane segments (see Figure 8, Table 1). That this region in *Shaker* containing the amino acid motif TMTTVGYG is a "signature" for potassium selective channels can be appreciated from Table 1. Comparison of the P-domain of channels from plants to humans reveals the evolutionary conservation of the critically important TTxGYG. In some channels the second threonine (T) is conservatively replaced by a serine (S) or the tyrosine (Y) is replaced by a phenylalanine (F), but overall the conservation is remarkable. The ability to experimentally manipulate the ion conductance and selectivity by changing amino acids in this region and further, to be able to transfer these properties among ion channels strongly support the idea that these residues form a crucial part of the ion channel pore and selectivity filter (see Figure 8, Table 1).

The intracellular mouth of the pore also appears to be an important site of interaction for certain drugs. Local anesthetics may interact in the pore region of the sodium channel (Ragsdale *et al.*, 1996; Ragsdale *et al.*, 1994). The phenylalkylamine class of calcium channel antagonists interact in this region of calcium channels and tetraethylammonium and antiarrhythmic agents such as quinidine interact in the intracellular mouth of the potassium channel pore. Analyses of mutations in potassium channels indicate that tetraethylammonium and related compounds can act from the intracellular side of the membrane and block the channel by interacting with residues in the P-domain as well as the intracellular end of the transmembrane S6 segment. The threonine in position 441 in the Shaker potassium channel also appears to be a critical amino acid for drug block. Biophysical studies have shown that charged compounds such as tetraethylammonium and quinidine traverse approximately 15–20% of the electric field to reach this binding site from the intracellular side (Choi *et al.*, 1993; Yeola *et al.*, 1996).

The local anesthetic agent etidocaine interacts with amino acids in the S6 segment associated with the pore of the sodium channel (Ragsdale *et al.*, 1996; Ragsdale *et al.*, 1994). In particular, two key amino acids have been identified in the rat brain (RBII) sodium channels at positions 1764 and 1771, which appear to be required for interactions with etidocaine. If S6 is assumed to be an α-helix, these two residues are located on the same face, approximately 11 ångstroms apart. Thus, they are sufficiently close in proximity to interact with the drug molecule of this size. However, it is known that the highest affinity interactions with sodium channels involve the inactivated state of the channel in a way that stabilizes it. For therapeutically relevant concentrations of antiarrhythmic agents such as lidocaine, the mechanism of block cannot be described by an open channel block mechanism. However, residues in S6 have also been shown to be important for inactivation, specifically phenylalanine 1764 and valine 1774 play a role in channel inactivation (McPhee *et al.*, 1995; McPhee *et al.*, 1994). It is possible that lidocaine also binds in this region to help promote, facilitate, or otherwise stabilize the inactivated state of the channel and inhibit conduction.

Calcium and sodium channels have also been studied to determine the molecular basis of selectivity. The selective properties of a sodium channel can be converted to those of a calcium channel by point mutations in the pore domain, as can the reverse conversion of selectivity (Heinemann *et al.*, 1992; Yang *et al.*, 1993). Sodium and calcium channels are large proteins that share some important structural features. Both channel types have four homologous regions, each believed to form one fourth of a symmetrical channel protein (see Figure 8C , 8D and Table 2). The location of important amino acids of the outer pore vestibule in sodium channels was first determined by identifying the specific residues that mediate binding of toxins (tetrodotoxin and saxitoxin) and divalent cation block (e.g., Cd^{++}) (Noda *et al.*, 1989; Terlau *et al.*, 1991; Backx *et al.*, 1992). The binding site consists of two negatively charged amino acids, aspartic acid (D) and glutamic acid (E), that are located at homologous positions in the first two of the channel's four internal repeats (see Table 2). Alignment of these regions of the sodium channel amino acid sequence with that of the calcium channel reveals a pattern. The calcium channel has glutamic acids in these positions and in the third and fourth internal repeats as well (Terlau *et al.*, 1991). Thus, the calcium channel uses each of the four negatively charged

Table 2 Amino acids in the pore (SS1–SS2) region of sodium and calcium channels

Sodium channel	*Tetrodotoxin / Cd⁺⁺ site*

Sodium channel												
DI												
Brain II	R	L	M	T	Q	**D**	F	W	E	N	L	Y Q
Heart	R	L	M	T	Q	**D**	C	W	E	R	L	Y Q
Skeletal	R	L	M	T	Q	**D**	Y	W	E	N	L	F Q
E. electricus	R	L	M	L	Q	**D**	Y	W	E	N	L	Y Q
DII												
Brain II	R	V	L	C	G	**E**	W	I	E	T	M	W D
Heart	R	I	L	C	G	**E**	W	I	E	T	M	W D
Skeletal	R	I	L	C	G	**E**	W	I	E	T	M	W D
E. electricus	R	A	L	C	G	**E**	W	I	E	T	M	W D
DIII												
Brain II	Q	V	A	T	F	**K**	G	W	M	D	I	M Y
Heart	Q	V	A	T	F	**K**	G	W	M	D	I	M Y
Skeletal	Q	V	A	T	F	**K**	G	W	M	D	I	M Y
E. electricus	Q	V	S	T	F	**K**	G	W	M	D	I	M Y
DIV												
Brain II	Q	I	T	T	S	**A**	G	W	D	G	L	L A
Heart	Q	I	T	T	S	**A**	G	W	D	G	L	L S
Skeletal	E	I	T	T	S	**A**	G	W	D	G	L	L N
E. electricus	E	I	T	T	S	**A**	G	W	D	G	L	L L

Calcium channel												
DI												
Brain B1	Q	C	I	T	M	**E**	G	W	T	D	L	L Y
Heart	Q	C	I	T	M	**E**	G	W	T	D	V	L Y
Skeletal	Q	C	I	T	M	**E**	G	W	T	D	V	L Y
DII												
Brain B1	Q	I	L	T	G	**E**	D	W	N	E	V	M Y
Heart	Q	I	L	T	G	**E**	D	W	N	S	V	M Y
Skeletal	Q	V	L	T	G	**E**	D	W	N	S	V	M Y
DIII												
Brain B1	T	V	S	T	G	**E**	G	W	P	Q	V	L K
Heart	T	V	S	T	F	**E**	G	W	P	E	L	L Y
Skeletal	T	V	S	T	F	**E**	G	W	P	Q	L	L Y
DIV												
Brain B1	R	S	A	T	G	**E**	A	W	H	N	I	M L
Heart	R	C	A	T	G	**E**	A	W	Q	D	I	M L
Skeletal	R	C	A	T	G	**E**	A	W	Q	E	I	L L

-SS1 ---SS2---

DI, DII, DIII, and DIV refer to each of the four homologous domains of sodium or calcium channels (see Figure 8). Amino acids are given by their single letter code.

glutamic acid (E) residues, one in each of the channels 4 homologous repeats, to coordinate a calcium ion. The corresponding amino acid sequence in the sodium channel is DEKA (see Table 2). It was found that mutating the lysine and alanine (KA) residues of the sodium channel to glutamic acids (as in the calcium channel) caused the channel to conduct calcium ions (Heinemann *et al.*, 1992). This indicated two things. Firstly, the DEKA sequence of the sodium channel and the equivalent

EEEE of the calcium channel are in the respective ion conduction pores. Secondly, these amino acids are critical in determining which species of ions can pass through the channels. These four residues are expected to form a four sided ring in the pore lumen that coordinates binding of the permeant ion thereby dehydrating it and allowing passage through the channel.

Channel activation gating (opening)
Voltage-dependent opening of a channel requires a mechanism for sensing changes in transmembrane potential and coupling this to a conformational change in the protein. Mechanisms by which a channel may permit or prevent passage of ions through the pore range from very subtle rearrangements of the pore structure (to prevent or allow ion passage) to major conformational rearrangements in the protein (Hille, 1992; Stuhmer *et al.*, 1989; Schlief *et al.*, 1996; Heinemann *et al.*, 1994; Heinemann *et al.*, 1992). Mutations in the selectivity filter of the pore do not greatly alter channel activation. These mutations change the single channel conductance and selectivity suggesting that the permeation and selectivity pathway are independent of the region of the channel involved in activation.

The equivalent of 10–12 elementary charges moving across the entire membrane electrical field are required to account for the voltage dependent sensitivity of opening. (Armstrong, 1981; Armstrong and Bezanilla, 1974; Vandenberg and Bezanilla, 1991; Schoppa *et al.*, 1992; McCormack *et al.*, 1993; Hoshi *et al.*, 1994; Hirschberg *et al.*, 1995). The S4 segments in each of the four domains of sodium, calcium and potassium channels contain a number of positively charged amino acids (up to eight) and S4 segments have been hypothesized to be the voltage sensors of channels. These segments have positive charges (either arginine or lysine) in every third position and are presumed to form an α-helix. The evidence that the S4 segment is a voltage sensor derives from mutations in this region that alter the voltage dependence of channel activation and shift the voltage range over which the channel opens (Stuhmer *et al.*, 1989; Auld *et al.*, 1990; Fleig *et al.*, 1994; Yang *et al.*, 1996). Yang *et al* (Yang *et al.*, 1996) have shown that the second and third arginine in the S4 segment move from an internally accessible to an externally accessible location during membrane depolarization. They concluded that this highly charged segment is shielded from the hydrophobic environment of the membrane lipids by a surrounding region of the protein that forms a channel-like structure through which the charged peptide segment can move during the conformation changes that occur during activation and deactivation. The data indicate that the physical distance through which the gating charge moves is quite short, about 5 Å. Because of the presumed hour-glass shape of the protein in this region and the very short segment of protein across which the membrane electrical field drops, the field strength is expected to be extremely high (approximately 10^8 volts per meter). Another important finding in this study(Yang *et al.*, 1996) is that most of the charged residues in the S4 segment appear to remain intracellular and do not cross the membrane electric field and therefore do not contribute directly to charge movement as had been believed previously (see Catterall, 1995; Catterall, 1991; Catterall, 1988; Catterall, 1993; Hille, 1992). Nevertheless, because the second and third arginines move through the entire electrical field and the first arginine moves through part of the field, a total of about 2.5 charges per subunit may be moving. This could account for the 10 elementary charges that seem to move during gating if all four subunits behave in this manner.

As a cautionary note, previous data have indicated that regions other than S4 were involved in voltage-sensing as well (Auld *et al.*, 1990). The fact that mutations in the S4 segment and their modification by sulfhydryl reagents have large and dramatic effects on channel inactivation suggests that additional regions of the protein may be involved in the different types of gating.

Molecular determinants of inactivation gating

Early work on neuronal sodium channels established that fast inactivation was eliminated by intracellular exposure to proteases (Armstrong, 1981; Armstrong, 1992; Armstrong and Bezanilla, 1974; Armstrong and Bezanilla, 1977; Armstrong *et al.*, 1974; Rojas and Rudy, 1976). This led to the the "ball-and-chain" hypothesis that inactivation resulted from a part of the protein that was tethered to the intracellular surface of the channel and acted as a blocker of the open pore (see Figure 1).

Inactivation in Shaker K$^+$ channels   More recently Aldrich and colleagues (Hoshi *et al.*, 1990; Hoshi *et al.*, 1994; Hoshi *et al.*, 1991; Zagotta and Aldrich, 1990a; Zagotta *et al.*, 1990b; Zagotta *et al.*, 1994a; Zagotta *et al.*, 1994b) have shown that the N-terminal 20 amino acids are involved in *Shaker* K$^+$ channel fast inactivation. It was proposed that this region acts as a blocker of the open K$^+$ channel pore similar to the "ball-and-chain" model (see Figures 1 and 8) (Demo and Yellen, 1991). A second type of inactivation has been described in *Shaker*-B (ShB) channels in addition to the amino terminal related (N-type) inactivation. (Choi *et al.*, 1991). These channels display a slower inactivation process associated with the carboxy-terminal half of the *Shaker* channel. The alternately spliced *Shaker* channel variant known as *Shaker*-A (ShA) inactivates primarily by this C-type mechanism; deletions of the amino terminus in ShA do not abolish fast inactivation. Hoshi *et al.* (Hoshi *et al.*, 1991) identified an amino acid residue in the S6 segment at position 463 in *Shaker* as determining which type of inactivation dominates. ShA has a valine in this position; ShB has an alanine. If the A463V mutation is made in ShB, the channel recovers slowly from inactivation like ShA (sec to min). If the V463A mutation is made in ShA, the channel recovers rapidly from inactivation like ShB (msec). This suggests that most or all of the slow time course of recovery from inactivation in channels containing the ShA carboxy terminus is due to the C-type inactivation process and does not result from differences in the stability of the N-type inactivated state. The amino acid at position 449 in *Shaker*-B (threonine, T449) is also known to be critical in determining C-type inactivation (see Figure 8A and Table 1). This residue was originally identified as part of the high affinity TEA binding site in some potassium channel isoforms (MacKinnon and Yellen, 1990). *Shaker*-B is sensitive to block by external TEA, but mutation of T449 to tyrosine results in even higher affinity TEA binding. Mutation of T499 to a charged residue results in loss of external TEA sensitivity. The conversion of the native threonine to a tyrosine (T449Y) also reduces slow C-type inactivation of the channel as does conversion to valine (T449V). Furthermore, internal TEA slows N-type inactivation whereas external TEA slows C-type inactivation suggesting that internal TEA competes with the N-terminal inactivation "ball". The interaction between external TEA interferes and C-type inactivation suggests that C-type inactivation is mediated by amino acid residues in the outer P-domain.

HERG K^+ channel gating　The human ether-a-go-go related gene or *HERG* voltage gated potassium channel has homology with *Shaker*-like channels of the type shown in Figure 8A, but unlike *Shaker* channels *HERG* channels show unusual inactivation gating behavior (see Figure 7B). This channel shows a profound inactivation that causes the ionic current to appear to rectify. *HERG* channel inactivation is much more rapid than activation (see Figure 7D) (Smith *et al.*, 1996; Spector *et al.*, 1996; Trudeau *et al.*, 1996; Trudeau *et al.*, 1995; London *et al.*, 1997). At depolarized membrane potentials, as soon as a channel opens it inactivates, which results in very little outward K^+ current (see Figure 7B). This inactivation process occurs at a rate similar to the fast N-type inactivation of *Shaker*-B potassium channels, but resembles C-type inactivation in other ways. For example, *HERG* inactivation is slowed by external application of TEA but unaffected by internal TEA. Deletion of the cytoplasmic amino terminus of the protein does not affect the rate of channel inactivation. C-type inactivation in *Shaker* and related channels is associated with conformational rearrangements of the outer mouth of the channel pore (Choi *et al.*, 1991). The serine at position 631 (S631) in *HERG* is in a position equivalent to threonine 449 (T449) in the outer pore of the *Shaker* potassium channel (see Figure 8 and Table 1). Mutations at residue S631 have effects on the inactivation of HERG channels. Replacing this residue in *HERG* with a cysteine, S631C, results in increase in the rate of the channels inactivation, but concomitant mutation of a nearby glycine to cysteine (G628C:S631C) leads to loss of inactivation (Smith *et al.*, 1996). The *Drosophila melanogaster* ether-a-go-go (EAG) potassium channel is homologous to *HERG*, but this channel shows essentially no inactivation. The amino acid position equivalent to *HERG* S631 in EAG is an alanine, which may point to the importance of this residue for *HERG* inactivation. Nevertheless, this residue cannot be the sole determinant of inactivation in this channel as three recently identified ERG isoforms all contain a serine at position 631 but show distinct differences in inactivation (Shi *et al.*, 1997). The inactivation process in *HERG* channels also has a distinct voltage dependence, unlike that of N- or C-type inactivation in *Shaker* channels. (Wang *et al.*, 1996; Wang *et al.*, 1997).

Sodium channel inactivation　Recent evidence using molecular biological strategies has implicated the cytoplasmic region that links transmembrane domains III and IV of the sodium channel protein in this fast inactivation process. If this domain is altered by proteolysis or by mutagenesis, channels show altered inactivation ranging from modest defects to very severe loss of fast inactivation (Stuhmer *et al.*, 1989; Moorman *et al.*, 1990; Vassilev *et al.*, 1989; Patton *et al.*, 1992a; Patton *et al.*, 1992b; West *et al.*, 1992; Bennett *et al.*, 1995a; Hartmann *et al.*, 1994; Valenzuela and Bennett, 1994).

Convincing arguments can be developed for the role of the III–IV inter-domain loop as a hinged lid inactivation blocking particle, Although it should be kept in mind that there are experimental clues that this is not the full story. Moorman and colleagues examined the role of charged amino acids in this region of the rat brain (type III) sodium channel (Moorman *et al.*, 1990). Amino acid substitutions that neutralize positive charges, produced either channels that did not function or channels that had faster rather than the expected slower rate of macroscopic inactivation. Another mutation in this region, R1515E, actually slowed activation (channel opening). Patton *et al.* (Patton *et al.*, 1992a) systematically removed ten amino acid segments from this region of the channel or neutralized sets of positive charges. The mutants in which positive charges were neutralized had large shifts in the voltage-dependence of both channel activation and inactivation with little change in the inactivation phase of the current when corrected for differences in voltage. The systematic deletion of segments of this region of the channel revealed amino acids that were important in conveying rapid inactivation on the channel. West *et al.* (West *et al.*, 1992) identified three hydrophobic amino acids, isoleucine, phenylalanine and methionine (IFM) at position 1488-1490 in this III–IV interdomain as being critical in the inactivation process. Substitution of these three amino acids with glutamines (Q) abolished fast inactivation. These experiments provided compelling evidence for the role of this region as a putative inactivation gate (Kellenberger *et al.*, 1996; Kellenberger *et al.*, 1997a; Kellenberger *et al.*, 1997b). If this peptide loop plays such a role, then synthetic peptides corresponding to this region of the channel are predicted to be effective in reconstituting inactivation in a channel where it had been removed (Tang *et al.*, 1996; Eaholtz *et al.*, 1994; Kellenberger *et al.*, 1996). The results of these experiments are somewhat controversial because the full native sequence (see Figure 8C) could not be employed due to solubility problems, but an artificial sequence containing the IFM motif flanked by positively charged lysines (KIFMK) appeared to reconstitute fast inactivation. These experiments can be interpreted differently if the short penta-peptide is assumed to be a novel open channel blocker that is unrelated to the endogenous inactivation process. Evidence in support of the latter hypothesis is the strong voltage-dependent block of the channel caused by this peptide whereas the apparent voltage-dependence of endogenous inactivation is thought to derive largely from coupling to channel activation and not from an intrinsic voltage-dependence of the inactivation step. The importance of hydrophobic residues in this region of the channel suggests that if this region is acting as a gate then interactions with its docking site are likely to be hydrophobic. This is easy to envision since channels do not inactivate readily from the rested state (occupied at negative membrane potentials). Presumably the hydrophobic receptor site would be shielded from the intracellular hydrophilic environment while the channel is closed. The hydrophobic binding pocket would only become accessible after the channel enters the open conformation. This would allow the inactivation process to occur. The return of the channel from the inactivated to the closed resting states would destabilize the interaction between hydrophobic regions of the III–IV interdomain and its binding site and result in recovery from inactivation. This conceptualization provides a basis for the observed coupling between channel activation and inactivation.

Auxilliary subunits of voltage gated ion channels

The pore forming α subunits of ion channels often co-assemble with other "auxiliary" proteins to generate functional channel entities. These auxiliary subunits are named as β, γ, or ζ to signify their relationship to the primary α subunits which contain the ion conducting and gating machinery. These subunits often modify α subunit function or expression levels. Auxiliary subunits are derived from distinct genes and control of their expression is not well understood. Tissue or cell specific expression of these subunits can serve to further expand the diversity of channel function (Adelman, 1995; Isom *et al.*, 1994; Isom *et al.*, 1992).

Sodium channels isolated from brain co-purify with two smaller proteins. These proteins have been designated β1 and β2. Neuronal sodium channels are a heterotrimeric complex of α, β1 and β2 subunits (Hartshorne and Catterall, 1984). The skeletal muscle sodium channel (SkM1) appears to have a β1 subunit but not a β2 subunit (Barchi, 1995). The role of β subunits in heart, if any, is not clear. The β2 subunit is not expressed in heart or skeletal muscle (reviewed by Catterall 1995b).

Nerve and muscle sodium channels inactivate too slowly when the α subunit is expressed alone in *Xenopus laevis* oocytes. Co-expression with the β1 subunit corrects this abnormal gating (Isom *et al.*, 1992; Bennett, Jr. *et al.*, 1993). The β1 subunit seems to do this by promoting conversion of gating from a slow to a fast gating mode (Bennett, *et al.*, 1993; Zhou *et al.*, 1991). This results in an increase in the rate of inactivation of the channel.

In the case of potassium channels, an auxiliary subunit was identified as a protein which co-purified with the dendrotoxin receptor (a potassium channel α subunit). It was dubbed a β subunit to designate its position on electrophoretic gels and to distinguish it from the larger α subunit which actually binds the toxin (Dolly *et al.*, 1994; Parcej and Dolly, 1989; Parcej *et al.*, 1992). Cloning of this β subunit lead to the homology cloning of a family of related auxiliary proteins (Heinemann *et al.*, 1995; Rettig *et al.*, 1994; England *et al.*, 1995a; England *et al.*, 1995b; Morales *et al.*, 1995). Three subfamilies are known thus far and are designated Kvβ1, Kvβ2 and Kvβ3 (see Table 3). Members of the Kvβ1 subfamily are derived from a common gene on human chromosome 3 with the differences among members generated by alternative splicing of the messenger RNA (England *et al.*, 1995a). This group of subunits have amino acid homology with the NAD(P)H dependent oxidoreductase family of

Table 3 Summary of known β subunits for voltage gated potassium channels*

Subfamily	Name	original name	Species and tissue	Human chromosome/ gene name
Kvβ1	Kvβ1.1	Kvβ1	rat brain human brain	3q26.1 KCNA1B
	Kvβ1.2	Kvβ3	human heart ferrert heart	
	Kvβ1.3		human heart	
Kvβ2	Kvβ2.1	Kvβ2	Rat brain bovine brain human brain	1p36.3 KCNA2B
Kvβ3 ?	Kvβ3.1 ?	Kvβ3 Mink, ISK	Rat brain human heart human ear human kidney	? 21q22.1–q22.2 KCNE1

*modified from England *et al.*[104]

enzymes, though no physiological significance has been attributed to this similarity (Chouinard *et al.*, 1995). The β subunits of voltage gated K^+ channels appear to be cytosolic proteins. When co-expressed with α subunits they modify both the function and expression. The effect on channel function depends on the particular combination of Kvα and Kvβ subunits that are co-expressed, but the most common effect is to enhance the inactivation of the channel (England *et al.*, 1995a; England *et al.*, 1995b; Sewing *et al.*, 1996). Some of these subunits have a long amino terminal region which is believed to serve as an inactivation "ball and chain" much like the amino terminus of the fast inactivating *Shaker* potassium channel α subunits (Rettig *et al.*, 1994). C-type inactivation is also enhanced, even in Kvβ subunits which lack the ball and chain amino terminus (Morales *et al.*, 1995).

Kvβ subunits not only alter function but are also involved channel biosynthesis. In transfected mammalian cells, the predominant beta subunit isoform in brain associates with the Kv1.2 alpha subunit early in channel biosynthesis. The Kvβ subunit exerts chaperone-like effects on Kv1.2 including promotion of cotranslational N-linked glycosylation of the nascent Kv1.2 polypeptide, increased stability of Kvβ/Kv1.2 complexes, and increased efficiency of cell surface expression of Kv1.2. The results indicate a fundamental role of Kvβ subunits to mediate the biosynthetic maturation and surface expression of voltage-gated K+ channel complexes (Shi *et al.*, 1996).

The minK or ISK protein is another auxiliary subunit which, until recently, was believed to be an independent pore forming subunit. This small protein has a single transmembrane domain with an extracellular amino-terminus and a cytosolic carboxyl-terminus. Upon expression in *Xenopus laevis* oocytes this subunit induces slowly activating potassium currents which resemble the slowly activating delayed current (I_{KS}) of native myocytes (Takumi *et al.*, 1988; Folander *et al.*, 1990). For this reason the subunit was named minK (minimal K channel) or ISK (after I_{KS}). Attempts to express the current in mammalian cells failed until the cloning of KvLQT1 (the KCNQ1 gene), which encodes a six transmembrane α subunit (Wang *et al.*, 1996; Barhanin *et al.*, 1996; Sanguinetti *et al.*, 1996b). It turns out that minK assembles with KvLQT1 and that *Xenopus* oocytes express an endogenous KvLQT subunit, whereas many mammalian cells used for heterologous expression do not. KvLQT1 is one of the genes that is mutated in the congenital long QT syndrome (Wang *et al.*, 1996). Expression of KvLQT1 alone results in a relatively rapidly activating delayed rectifier potassium channel. Coexpression of KvLQT1 with minK in mammalian cells leads to a slow, I_{KS}-like current much like that observed in native cells. (Balser *et al.*, 1990; Sanguinetti *et al.*, 1996c; Barhanin *et al.*, 1996; Sanguinetti and Jurkiewicz, 1990a).

SUMMARY

Major strides have been made in recent years toward understanding the molecular basis of electrical excitability. The theoretical and biophysical underpinnings of ion channel behavior are largely developed. Many of the molecules that are responsible for electrical excitability have been identified and more are being discovered every day. The next challenges lie in combining these two areas of inquiry. In order to truly understand the electrical precesses that are so intimately involved with everything we do from breathing to thinking, we must understand the cellular environment in which channels exist; we must discover the partner molecules with which α subunits interact and under what circumstances; we must learn how cells regulate the expression of these molecules; and perhaps most challenging, we must learn the true 3 dimensional structure of these molecules so that we can begin to apply the principles of biophysical chemistry and molecular biophysics to understand their dynamic behavior.

ACKNOWLEDGEMENTS

This work was supported by a grants (HL51197, HL46681) from the National Institutes of Health and the American Heart Association.

3 The Cardiac Action Potential

Antonio Zaza

The action potential of a single cardiac myocyte and the electrophysiologic and mechanical function of the heart are interdependent. Hence, just as many aspects of cardiac function are modulated through changes in the voltage-time course of the action potential, alterations in the function of the cardiovascular system strongly influence the contour of the action potential. For the purpose of this discussion I shall first describe the Na-dependent action potential that typifies normal atrial and ventricular muscle and atrial and ventricular specialized conducting fibers. Later I shall describe the characteristics of sinoatrial and atrioventricular nodal action potentials.

The cardiac transmembrane action potential is readily recorded using intracellular glass microelectrodes, containing a low-resistance electrolyte solution (usually ~3 M KCl) and having a tip diameter sufficiently small ($< 1 \mu$) to minimize injury to the cell. The action potential is divided into 5 distinct phases corresponding to clearly recognizable landmarks in its contour (Figure 1):

Phase 0: fast depolarization or upstroke
Phase 1: fast initial repolarization
Phase 2: plateau
Phase 3: fast terminal repolarization
Phase 4: electrical diastole

The term "action potential" most precisely describes phases 0 through 3, while the term "repolarization" includes phases 1 to 3. The magnitude and time course of each phase vary in different types of myocytes; for example, phase 1 is large in action

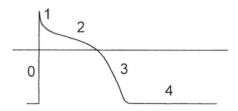

Figure 1 The action potential of a Purkinje myocyte. The numbers refer to the action potential phases (see text).

potentials of ventricular epicardial myocytes and small in ventricular endocardial myocytes.

MEMBRANE CURRENTS AND MEMBRANE POTENTIAL

Specific ionic currents contribute to each phase of the action potential. For phase 0, an inward current carried by Na^+ is the dominant charge carrier. For phases 1–3 several channels are simultaneously active at any instant such that a "net membrane current" is produced. An outward current carried by K^+ is the major determinant of the negative membrane potential during phase 4. In the following discussion I shall first consider the general relation that links net membrane current to membrane potential and then, the ionic mechanisms underlying specific phases of the action potential.

Membrane Potential as a Function of Membrane Current

Any current carried by positive ions (cationic current) that enters the cell (inward current) moves membrane potential in the positive direction (depolarization). The opposite change (i.e., repolarization or hyperpolarization) is caused by any cationic current leaving the cell (outward current). Changes in membrane potential resulting from anionic currents (carried by negative ions) are obviously opposite to those just described.

Ohm's law predicts that the change in membrane potential produced by net membrane current will be proportional to membrane resistance (also referred to as input resistance). The opening of ion channels is influenced by voltage and by time. As a result of these openings, input resistance changes continuously during the action potential; a larger number of active channels, independently of the nature and direction of the currents they carry, will correspond to a lower input resistance. Thus, a magnitude of membrane current that would minimally affect membrane potential when input resistance is low can result in large membrane potential changes when input resistance increases.

Membrane Current as a Function of Membrane Potential

The relation between the current "$I(i)$", carried by a specific ion channel "i", and membrane potential (E_m) can be described by the general equation:

$$I(i) = G(i) \cdot G_{max}(i) \cdot [E_m - E_{rev}(i)]$$

- $[E_m - E_{rev}]$ is the difference between membrane potential and the potential at which the net current through the channel is null (current reversal potential). This term defines the (electrochemical) force driving the ions through the membrane.
- G_{max} is the conductance of the fully opened channel; thus $G_{max} \cdot [E_m - E_{rev}]$ (Ohm's law) describes the maximal current amplitude. G_{max} is determined by the product of the conductance of a single channel protein times the number of proteins expressed on the membrane.

- G is a fractional number (ranging from 0 to 1), that defines which proportion of G_{max} is actually activated; since it can be envisioned as a gate that limits channel conductance, G is often referred to as a "gating variable."

In "voltage-gated" channels (most cardiac channels) the value G is controlled by membrane potential; in "receptor-gated" channels G is modulated by binding of a signaling molecule to the channel protein. In some channels changes of G are instantaneous; these channels carry "instantaneous" or "background" currents (see below). In other channels, G changes with a time course, specific to the channel, that is affected by membrane potential; these channels carry time-dependent currents (see below).

Figure 2 illustrates in a generic sense the function of some voltage-gated channels (e.g., I_{Na}, I_{CaL}) in which G is equal to the product of two independent gating variables, having opposite dependence on membrane potential. Such "activation" and "inactivation" variables define the proportion of channels that are *activated* and *not-inactivated* respectively. The channel can carry current only when activation and inactivation variables are simultaneously different from 0. This may occur transiently after a change in membrane potential, due to different rates of change of the two variables.

Alternatively membrane potential may be within a "window" at which both variables are different from 0 even at steady-state. Within this range of potentials, even quickly inactivating channels such as I_{Na} and I_{CaL} can conduct a sustained current. Such a current, generally representing a small fraction of maximal current, is referred to as "window current."

In summary, current amplitude may depend on membrane potential in two ways:

- deviation of E_m from E_{rev} causes an increase in the driving force; when $E_m = E_{rev}$ the current is null, irrespective of G. This applies to both voltage- and receptor-gated channels.

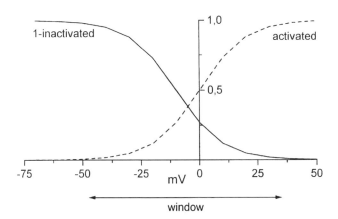

Figure 2 Voltage-dependency of channel conductance. The fractions of total current that are activated and not inactivated (1-inactivated) at steady state are plotted against membrane potential. In the interval of potentials marked by the arrow (window), the product activated × (1-inactivated) is different from 0. Within this window the current may exist at steady state.

- in voltage-gated channels, the value of G and the rate of its changes are determined by E_m. If E_m is such to make $G = 0$, the current is null, irrespective of the driving force.

IONIC MECHANISMS UNDERLYING THE PHASES OF THE ACTION POTENTIAL

In the remainder of this section, the ionic mechanisms underlying each phase of a "prototypical" cardiac action potential (e.g., Figure 1) will be described. The differences between nodal (e.g., sinoatrial) and ventricular action potentials and the underlying ionic currents are shown in Figure 3.

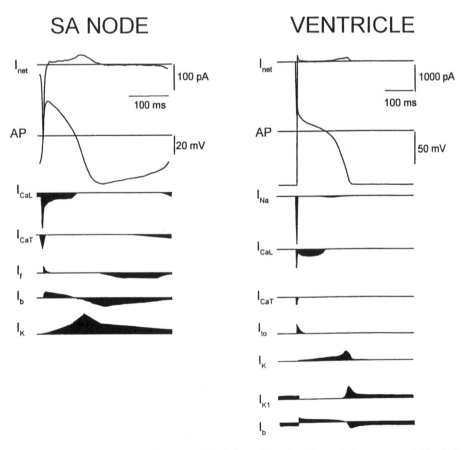

Figure 3 Comparison between action potentials of sinoatrial node and ventricular myocytes. Major ionic currents flowing during each phase are shown below each action potential. Changes in the trace thickness are meant to illustrate approximately the phases of the cycle in which the current prevails; however, the absolute trace thickness does not accurately reflect current magnitude. The background current (I_b) includes Na^+/K^+ and Na^+/Ca^{2+} exchanger currents as well as time-independent Na^+ and Ca^{2+} conductances. Current traces have been drawn by hand to summarize the information provided by experimental results and model simulations. (Modified after Task Force of the Working Group on Arrhythmias of the European Society of Cardiology, 1991).

Ionic Currents During Diastole (Phase 4)

Cardiac myocytes may have pacemaker properties (e.g., SA node) such that during phase 4 there is depolarization of the membrane potential until a threshold voltage is reached and an action potential is initiated. In non-pacemaker cells (e.g., ventricular myocardium) there is no spontaneous depolarization. Here, net membrane current is determined mainly by the balance between a prevailing outward current (I_{K1}) carried by K^+ and smaller, time-independent inward (or "background") currents carried by Na^+ and Ca^{2+} (Figure 3). Currents generated by operation of the Na^+/K^+ pump (I_{NaK}, outward), and the Na^+/Ca^{2+} exchanger (I_{NaCa}, inward) also may contribute, depending on the degree of activation of the respective exchange mechanisms. As a result of such a balance, the resting membrane potential (E_{rest}) is usually several millivolts positive to the K^+ equilibrium potential ($\approx -95\,mV$) and very negative to the equilibrium potentials for Na^+ and $Ca^{2+}(> +70\,mV)$ at physiological ion concentrations.

The most relevant properties of resting membrane current are determined by I_{K1}, a K^+ selective current expressed in many types of excitable and non-excitable cells. As illustrated in Figure 4A, I_{K1} conductance (seen as the slope of the $I-V$ curve) is constant at potentials negative to that at which the current reverses (i.e., crosses the voltage axis $\sim -95\,mV$), but markedly decreases at potentials at which I_{K1} is outward. This voltage-dependency of I_{K1} conductance, commonly referred to as "inward rectification," is generated by blockade of the channel by intracellular cations, such as Mg^{2+}, Ca^{2+} and polyamines (Matsuda *et al.*, 1987; Mazzanti and DiFrancesco, 1989; Lopatin *et al.*, 1994). The consequences of I_{K1} rectification on the time-course of this current during the action potential are shown in Figure 4B. Depolarization is associated with a sharp decrease of I_{K1}. During repolarization, when the potential approaches its resting value, I_{K1} conductance recovers and the current, driven by a large electrochemical gradient, reaches a peak. Completion of repolarization brings potential closer to the I_{K1} reversal potential, causing the current to return to its diastolic value.

The pivotal contribution of I_{K1} rectification to electrical stability and excitability of the cell membrane can be appreciated from Figure 4A, by considering the consequences of stimuli causing deviations of membrane potential from E_{rest}. The increase in I_{K1} that accompanies a small depolarizing stimulus would effectively oppose further depolarization, thus tending to stabilize membrane potential. A larger depolarizing stimulus would move membrane potential to a region of the curve where I_{K1} is reduced, rather than increased, by further depolarization. Thus, if the stimulus is large enough, the stabilizing effect of I_{K1} is removed and the membrane can be efficiently depolarized by relatively small inward currents (i.e., it becomes excitable). In other words, the voltage-dependency of I_{K1} conductance may effectively contribute to determining the voltage "threshold" for activation.

During the cycles of periodic excitation that characterize the beating heart, the level of membrane potential maintained during phase 4 tends to be significantly more negative than E_{rest}, particularly at rapid heart rates. This is largely accounted for by stimulation of the Na^+/K^+ pump (Vassalle, 1970) as follows: with every action potential upstroke, Na^+ enters the cell via the open Na^+ channels. The more rapidly the heart beats, the more Na^+ that enters per unit time. The Na/K pump is

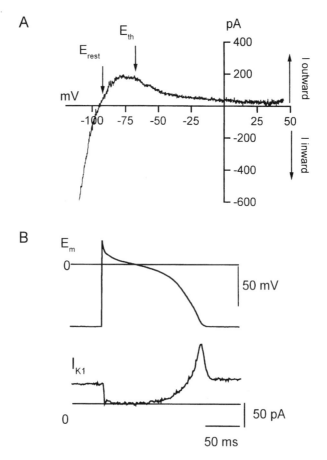

Figure 4 I_{K1} (inward rectifier) in a ventricular myocyte, properties and role. A: I–V relation of I_{K1} measured in a single ventricular myocyte. E_{rest} and E_{th} represent commonly recorded values of resting and threshold membrane potential respectively; the decrease in I_{K1} occurring for depolarization beyond E_{th} and the small current amplitude at plateau potentials can be easily appreciated. B: An action potential recorded from a single myocyte (E_m) and I_{K1} flowing during that action potential. The sharp decrease in I_{K1} during depolarization (inward rectification) and the overshoot occurring during phase 3 can be easily appreciated (modified from Zaza *et al.*, 1998)

exquisitively sensitive to Na^+ elevations and the action of the pump is electrogenic, driving Na^+ out and K^+ in, with a ratio of ~3/2. The pump generates an excess of negative charge inside the cell and a hyperpolarized membrane potential.

Common Causes of Abnormally Depolarized Diastolic Potential
In settings of cardiac disease (see chapter 7) a number of changes occur in the action potential, among them a decrease in the diastolic membrane potential. Because the diastolic potential is largely determined by K^+-selective currents, it is sensitive to changes in the K^+ electrochemical gradient and/or K^+ channel conductance. For example, the conductance of I_{K1}, as that of other K^+ channels, depends on extracellular K^+ concentration $[K^+]_0$ (Figure 5) (Sakmann and Trube, 1984). At $[K^+]_0$ values less than 8–10 mM, channel conductance becomes low enough to cause the

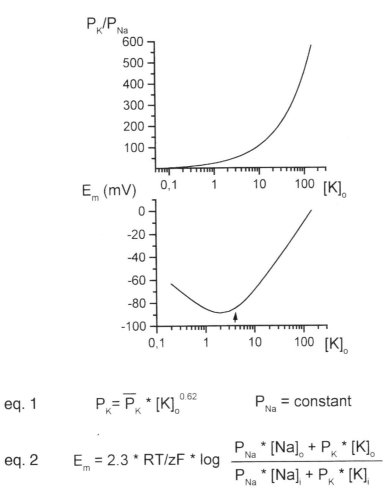

eq. 1 $\qquad P_K = \overline{P}_K * [K]_o^{0.62} \qquad\qquad P_{Na} = \text{constant}$

eq. 2 $\qquad E_m = 2.3 * RT/zF * \log \dfrac{P_{Na} * [Na]_o + P_K * [K]_o}{P_{Na} * [Na]_i + P_K * [K]_i}$

Figure 5 Effect of changes in extracellular K^+ concentration ($[K^+]_o$) on the K^+/Na^+ permeability ratio (P_K/P_{Na}) and on membrane potential (E_m). Changes in P_K/P_{Na} ratio were determined by dependency of I_{K1} conductance on $[K^+]_o$ according to equation 1 shown below (P_{Na} is held constant). E_m was computed from equation 2 (Goldman, Hodgkin-Katz equation, see chapter 1), based on K^+ and Na^+ permeabilities only. Dependency of E_m on $[K^+]_o$ deviates from linearity at low $[K^+]_o$ values; the most negative E_m values are achieved at $[K^+]_o \approx 2\,\text{mM}$. The arrow shows physiological $[K^+]_o$ value. (Computations based on parameters from Sakmann and Trube, 1984).

relation between resting potential and log $[K^+]_o$ to depart from linearity. The interplay between K^+ and Na^+ electrochemical gradients and permeability ratios (Figure 5 upper panel) results in the most negative value of E_m occurring between 2 and 3 mM $[K^+]_o$ (Figure 5 middle panel). Although $[K^+]_o$ levels either above or below normal may cause membrane depolarization, the two settings are functionally different. In both cases I_{Na} availability is reduced by depolarization (see below), but at low $[K^+]_o$ membrane excitability may actually be enhanced by the decrease in I_{K1} conductance. Indeed, oscillations in membrane potential and abnormal automatic firing are commonly observed in the presence of low $[K^+]_o$, possibly accounting for the high incidence of cardiac arrhythmias associated with hypokalemia (Gilmour and Zipes, 1986).

Significant depolarization of diastolic membrane potential may also be induced by blockade of the Na^+/K^+ pump (e.g., by digitalis), with consequent inhibition of the outward current generated by this membrane transport system.

The Action Potential Foot and Threshold

In non-pacemaking cells, membrane excitation requires an external current source, provided by a neighboring, activated cell, that depolarizes the membrane to its threshold potential, after which Na^+ channels are activated to an extent sufficient to initiate phase 0 of the action potential. The change in membrane potential that precedes threshold is electrotonic and is commonly called the "foot" of the action potential. During the foot, the membrane behaves as a passive, parallel RC circuit (see chapter 1), depolarizing along an exponential time course, whose rate of depolarization is proportional to the supplied current and to membrane resistance. Under normal conditions, the supplied current is largely redundant with respect to that actually needed to achieve threshold; thus, the foot depolarizes sufficiently rapidly to bring the membrane to threshold almost instantaneously. However, if the supplied current is only moderately larger than the liminal one (e.g., in some pathological conditions), the foot may require a time on the order of milliseconds (Daut, 1982), or longer. In the presence of slow foot depolarization, a significant number of Na^+ channels may be inactivated before I_{Na} becomes large enough to initiate the action potential upstroke. This may substantially decrease the inward current available during phase 0, thus reducing the velocity of phase 0 depolarization. Thus, even if the action potential upstroke may be considered an "all or none phenomenon," under specific conditions its rate of rise may be a function of the activating stimulus.

Since I_{Na} is the dominant current during the action potential upstroke, the threshold potential is actually similar to the threshold for activation of Na^+ channels; however, the two terms should not be confused. A suitable definition for threshold potential would be that potential at which net inward membrane current becomes large enough to initiate autoregenerative depolarization. Many factors besides I_{Na} threshold determine such a value. These include membrane input resistance, the extent of I_{K1} rectification, the rate-dependent persistence of outward currents activated during the preceding action potential, and the availability of non-inactivated Na^+ channels. Thus, rather than a constant value, action potential threshold is a variable, under the dynamic influence of facts such as heart rate, diastolic potential, ionic environment and intercellular coupling resistance. Since activating currents are largely suprathreshold, fluctuations in the threshold value usually are not perceivable during normal propagation; however, they may acquire relevance when the conditions for propagation become marginal.

IONIC CURRENTS DURING THE ACTION POTENTIAL

The Action Potential Upstroke (Phase 0)

Sodium-Dependent Action Potentials
As stated earlier, the action potentials of atrial and ventricular myocardium and specialized conducting fibers are dependent largely on fast inward Na^+ current. This

current is carried via rapidly inactivating voltage-dependent channels. Both channel opening (activation) and subsequent inactivation are induced by depolarization. The current flows only during the brief interval between channel opening and inactivation (i.e., I_{Na} in Figure 3). Once the channel has been inactivated, it can open again only after having recovered from inactivation, which occurs at negative membrane potentials. The rates of both activation and inactivation are faster at depolarized potentials; recovery from inactivation is enhanced by negative membrane potentials. Although I_{Na} is the major determinant of the action potential upstroke, other currents are involved as well, most notably inward current carried by Ca^{2+} and outward current carried by K^+. For I_{Na} and the low threshold component of the Ca^{2+} current (I_{CaT}) both channel activation and inactivation are purely voltage-dependent processes with thresholds between -70 and -60 mV. Although I_{Na} is much larger than I_{CaT}, both these channels activate very rapidly and, at plateau potentials, both are inactivated within 10–15 ms, thus resulting in sharp spike of inward current (Berman *et al.*, 1989; Vassort and Alvarez, 1994; Hirano *et al.*, 1989). The larger, "high threshold" component of the Ca^{2+} current (I_{CaL}) activates at potentials positive to about -30 mV and inactivates partly through a voltage-dependent mechanism and partly through a process dependent on the increase in subsarcolemmal Ca^{2+} concentration (Ca^{2+}-dependent inactivation) (Lee *et al.*, 1985). The rates of I_{CaL} activation and inactivation are remarkably slower than those of I_{Na} and I_{CaT}; thus, the I_{CaL} transient is more sustained.

Finally, a K^+ current (I_{to}) quickly activates and inactivates upon depolarization positive to about -20 mV (Hiraoka and Kawano, 1989; Josephson *et al.*, 1984). Although this current is predominantly involved in phase 1 repolarization (see below), its activation is fast enough to provide outward current during the terminal portion of phase 0, thus limiting the action potential amplitude (Litovsky and Antzelevitch, 1988).

The rate of phase 0 depolarization (dV/dt) is determined by the net balance between inward and outward currents. Thus, the maximum dV/dt (dV/dt_{max}) is often used as an estimate of the peak net inward current flowing during phase 0. As the dominant current during phase 0, I_{Na} is the main determinant of dV/dt_{max} and is the main source of charge for propagation of the cardiac impulse in normal specialized conducting fibers and working myocardium. Ca^{2+} currents were thought to contribute to normal propagation only in sinoatrial and atrioventricular nodes (in which I_{Na} is minimally expressed) and to abnormal propagation in markedly depolarized specialized conducting tissues and myocardium, where I_{Na} is largely inactivated. However, it has recently been appreciated that, when a large activation delay occurs between two cells (e.g., in the presence of high intercellular coupling resistance), propagation may become crucially dependent on I_{CaL}, even if I_{Na} is normal (Sugiura and Joyner, 1992; Rohr and Kucera, 1997). Under such conditions, the duration of the action potential "foot" in a cell downstream may last longer than the entire duration of the I_{Na} transient in an upstream cell. In this setting, the long duration of I_{CaL} may contribute charge during the time required for the achievement of threshold potential in the cell to be activated (Sugiura and Joyner, 1992; Rohr and Kucera, 1997).

As a result of I_{Na} inactivation after phase 0 of an action potential, a second action potential cannot be initiated until the membrane has repolarized from the previous activation to values negative to -60 to -70 mV. The time during which the membrane remains refractory to activation by currents of any magnitude is referred to as the absolute refractory period. Absolute refractoriness is followed by a period of "relative" refractoriness, in which, due to partial I_{Na} availability, action potentials with slow upstrokes and conduction velocities may be elicited. Under normal conditions, I_{Na} recovery is fast and the end of the relative refractory period precedes the termination of the action potential. However, if diastolic potential is partially depolarized, the recovery from inactivation of I_{Na} may outlast repolarization and a variable portion of diastole may be characterized by decreased excitability (post-repolarization refractoriness). Under such conditions, conduction may become crucially dependent on the duration of diastolic interval (rate-dependency of conduction).

Ca^{2+}-Dependent Action Potentials

The normal SA and AV nodes manifest depolarized diastolic potentials (e.g., -60 to $-40\,mV$) (Figure 3). Such low diastolic potentials may also be seen under certain pathologic circumstances in cardiac myocytes that routinely would show high membrane potentials and Na-dependent upstrokes. In the strongly depolarized setting I_{Na} may be completely inactivated, but propagation can still occur, entirely supported by I_{CaL}.

In SA and AV nodal cells, in which the primary cause of membrane depolarization is a reduced I_{K1} expression (Noma *et al.*, 1984), the unavailability of I_{Na} during phase 0 is compensated by a marked increase in membrane input resistance (about 16 times higher than that of ventricular cells), thus resulting in preservation of membrane excitability. Also, lack of the stabilizing effect of I_{K1}, makes such cells prone to spontaneous activity. Due to the smaller magnitude and slower kinetics of I_{CaL}, as compared to I_{Na}, Ca^{2+}-dependent action potentials have dV/dt_{max} and conduction velocities on the order of $5–50\,V/s$ and $1–10\,cm/s$ respectively; these values are substantially lower than those measured in highly polarized cells (up to $1000\,V/s$ and $2\,m/s$ respectively in Purkinje fibers). Accordingly, Ca^{2+}-dependent action potentials are also referred to as "slow responses." Since recovery from inactivation of I_{CaL} is slow, the refractory periods of these action potentials may exceed action potential duration, and the velocity of propagation may decrease at short diastolic intervals (rate-dependent propagation).

Phase 1 Repolarization

Phase 1 (Figure 1) is determined by activation of a transient outward current (I_{to}) (Figure 3). I_{to} has two components, I_{to1}, carried by K^+, and I_{to2}, which has K^+ and/or Cl^- components, is Ca^{2+} activated, and is opened by the large rise in sub-sarcolemmal Ca^{2+} that is initiated by activation of I_{CaL} (Hiraoka and Kawano, 1989; Tseng and Hoffman, 1989; Zygmunt and Gibbons, 1991; Zygmunt and Gibbons, 1992; Escande *et al.*, 1987). The "transient" nature of this current is due to the coexistence of depolarization-induced fast activation and inactivation, similar to that just described for I_{Na}. I_{to1} activates late in phase 0, at potentials positive to about $-20\,mV$ (Hiraoka and Kawano, 1989); (Josephson *et al.*, 1984). Complete recovery of I_{to1} from inactivation may require up to hundreds of milliseconds at diastolic potentials, thus extending through the early portion of diastole (Cohen *et al.*, 1986;

Tseng and Hoffman, 1989). As a result, for action potentials with short coupling intervals (high heart rate or premature responses) I_{to} is only partially available for activation (Litovsky and Antzelevitch, 1988).

The magnitude of phase 1 repolarization varies widely among action potentials recorded across the ventricular myocardial wall and is of variable magnitude in atrium, as well. Whereas phase 1 is minimally present in subendocardial myocytes, a large phase 1 "notch" attaining voltages of 10–20 mV can be easily appreciated in subepicardial myocytes (Litovsky and Antzelevitch, 1988). In these cells, the prominent phase 1 is followed by a further depolarization, giving rise to a typical "spike and dome" morphology (Figure 6). Transmural differences in phase 1 repolarization

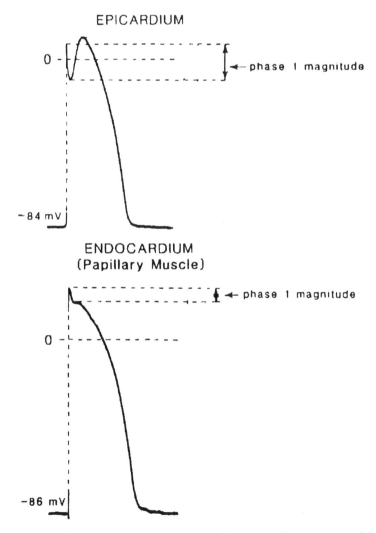

Figure 6 Comparison between action potentials recorded from epicardial and endocardial ventricular muscle. A large phase 1, leading to a spike and dome morphology, differentiates epicardial from endocardial action potential. (Modified from Litovsky and Antzelevitch, 1988).

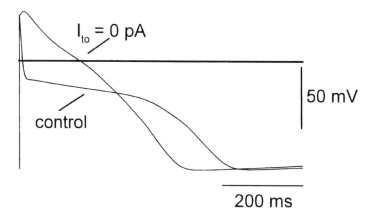

Figure 7 Paradoxical effect of I_{to} blockade on action potential duration. Model simulation of Purkinje fiber action potentials before (control) and after removal of $I_{to}(I_{to} = 0)$. Blockade of I_{to} causes loss of phase 1 repolarization and "pradoxical" shortening of action potential duration (see text for explanation).

correlate well with differences in the expression of I_{to1}, which is negligible in sub-endocardial myocytes and maximal in subepicardial myocytes (Liu *et al.*, 1990).

The contribution of phase 1, and of the underlying currents to total repolarization is very complex. One would expect that blockade of a repolarizing current, such as I_{to1}, should be uniformly followed by a prolongation of action potential duration. Contrary to such expectation, I_{to1} blockade by 4-aminopyridine may shorten repolarization (Kenyon and Gibbons, 1979; Litovsky and Antzelevitch, 1988). This can be accurately reproduced by the model simulation shown in Figure 7. Nonetheless, a reduced expression of I_{to1} is often the only membrane abnormality described in dis-eased human myocytes, in which repolarization is consistently prolonged (Tomaselli *et al.*, 1994; Boyden and Jeck, 1995) (see chapter 7). Such apparent inconsistencies, may arise from the influence of I_{to1} on the membrane potential level at which the subsequent phase of repolarization begins. A positive displacement of such a potential, as the one resulting from I_{to1} blockade, may produce secondary changes in the kinetics and magnitudes of inward and outward currents contributing to the plateau phase (see below). The net effect of such secondary changes on action potential duration might vary according to the type and properties of currents contributing to repolarization.

Phase 2 Repolarization

A major feature distinguishing cardiac action potentials from those of nerve and skeletal muscle is the presence of a sustained plateau during which repolarization occurs at a slow rate, the membrane potential remaining at rather positive values (between $+10$ and $-20\,\mathrm{mV}$) for up to hundreds of milliseconds (Figure 1). This plateau is a determinant of the long refractory period that characterizes cardiac myocytes (see above). The proportion of the cardiac cycle spent at a depolarized potential strongly affects transmembrane Ca^{2+} influx and efflux (Bers, 1993); thus the duration and amplitude of the plateau are relevant to modulation of contrac-tion. The plateau is determined by a fine balance among several small inward and outward currents (Figure 3). Due to the absence of the stabilizing effect of I_{K1} during the plateau, such relatively small currents can significantly affect the time and trajectory of phase 2.

Inward Plateau Currents

Inward plateau currents are carried by Na^+ and Ca^{2+} ions. However, at variance with the transient nature of currents underlying phase 0, the persistent plateau duration requires sustained inward current flow (Figure 3). The slowly inactivating Na^+ currents are small and are carried via channels with intrinsically very slow or incomplete inactivation (Kiyosue and Arita, 1989; Gintant *et al.*, 1984). Moreover, the Na^+ and Ca^{2+} currents have the property of partially activating, yet incompletely inactivating even at steady-state over a restricted range of membrane potentials (Figure 2) (Hirano *et al.*, 1992; Attwell *et al.*, 1979). Within this "window" of potentials, these channels pass a sustained, albeit small current, often referred to as "window current." The plateau phase spans through values that are within the "windows" of both I_{Na} and I_{CaL}; thus, Na^+ and Ca^{2+} window currents may contribute to the plateau.

Outward Plateau Currents

Cardiac myocytes express voltage-dependent K^+ channels that are activated by depolarization (Figure 3). Early voltage-clamp studies identified a single K^+ conductance that, due to its slow kinetics of activation and rectifying properties (less pronounced than those of I_{K1}), was named "delayed-rectifier" current (I_K). Only recently, has it been appreciated that I_K is the sum of at least three components, carried by channels with different kinetics, pharmacology and structure (Sanguinetti and Jurkiewicz, 1990a; Li *et al.*, 1996; Yue *et al.*, 1996). These three major currents are rapidly activating (I_{Kr}), slowly activating (I_{Ks}) and "ultrarapidly" activating (I_{Kur}, also referred to as I_{sus}). Whereas I_{Kr} and I_{Ks} are expressed in atria and ventricles, I_{Kur} is largely limited to atrial myocardium.

I_{Kr} and I_{Kur} activate during the action potential upstroke, upon depolarization positive to approximately $-40\,mV$ (Sanguinetti and Jurkiewicz, 1990; Yue *et al.*, 1996). A large proportion of the steady-state amplitude for these currents is generally achieved within the duration of the action potential plateau. A significant extent of almost instantaneous inactivation (the proportion of channels that inactivate does not even contribute a macroscopic current) limits the amount of I_{Kr} available at positive potentials, thus mimicking an inward-rectifier type of behavior (Spector *et al.*, 1996). I_{Ks} is activated at slightly more depolarized potentials (positive to $-20\,mV$) (Sanguinetti and Jurkiewicz, 1990a) and with much slower kinetics, but, due to little rectification, its amplitude at positive potentials is substantially larger than that of I_{Kr}.

The contribution of I_{Kr} and I_{Ks} to an action potential elicited in a Purkinje myocyte after a period of quiescence is illustrated in Figure 8. The left panels refer to an action potential elicited after quiescence (CL = infinity), the right panels to steady state stimulation at a rate of 60 bpm (CL = 1000 ms). The I/I_{max} ratios (Figure 8) show that a large proportion of total I_{Kr} channels is activated early during the action potential; repolarization is followed by quick and complete deactivation of I_{Kr}. After quiescence, the plateau duration is adequate to activate only approximately

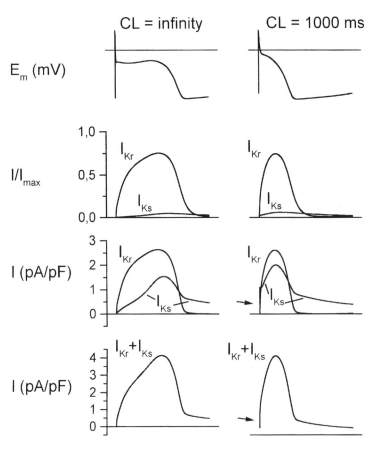

Figure 8 Delayed rectifier currents (I_K) during the action potential and their rate-dependency. Top row: model simulations of a Purkinje action potential stimulated after a long quiescent period (left panel) and during steady-state stimulation at a cycle length (CL) of 1000 ms (right panel). Second row: proportion of maximal I_{Kr} and I_{Ks} currents (I/I_{max}) activated at each instant during the action potential. Third row: density (current per unit membrane area) of I_{Kr} and I_{Ks} at each instant during the action potential. Fourth row: global density of the delayed rectifier current ($I_K = I_{Kr} + I_{Ks}$) at each instant during the action potential. During simulation at CL = 1000, deactivation of I_{Ks} during diastole is not completed. The channels that persist in the activated state at the end of the diastole carry an additional "instantaneous" I_K component (arrow). Thus, at shorter CL, the density of I_K necessary for repolarization is achieved in a shorter time and the proportion of total I_K generated by I_{Ks} is increased. Also notice that, due to incomplete recovery of I_{to} from inactivation, the amplitude and rate of phase 1 repolarization are reduced at CL = 1000.

10% of I_{Ks} channels (small I/I_{max} ratio) (Sanguinetti and Jurkiewicz, 1990a); however, since its fully activated conductance is relatively large, I_{Ks} may still achieve a substantial amplitude during the action potential. At variance with I_{Kr}, deactivation of I_{Ks} is slow and outlasts full repolarization. As shown in the right panels of Figure 8 (CL = 1000 ms), a significant proportion of I_{Ks} channels may persist in the open state at the end of diastole and may thus provide a sort of "instantaneous" current (arrow) during the following action potential. The shorter the diastolic interval, the larger the amplitude of this instantaneous component. Thus, I_{Ks} may actually accumulate through subsequent cycles leading to an increase in the proportion of total I_K carried by this channel at faster heart rates (Jurkiewicz and Sanguinetti, 1993). This phenomenon might account for the "reverse" rate-dependency of the effect on action potential duration of selective I_{Kr} blockers (see chapter 6). Finally, I_{Ks} is enhanced by high intracellular Ca^{2+} levels and by β-adrenergic stimulation (Nitta *et al.*, 1994) (Sanguinetti *et al.*, 1991). This may account for shortening of action potential duration induced by digitalis, by hypercalcemia and by catecholamines.

The outward movement of charge through the Na^+/K^+ pump should be favored by depolarization. Thus, I_{NaK} may contribute outward current during the plateau in excess of that generated at diastolic potentials (Luo and Rudy, 1994). Due to the systolic rise in intracellular Ca^{2+} activity, plateau potentials should be very close to the equilibrium value for the Na^+/Ca^{2+} exchanger (Bers, 1993; Luo and Rudy, 1994). Thus, $I_{Na/Ca}$ is expected to provide very little current during the plateau. Moreover, Ca^{2+} extrusion from the cell is minimal, or even reversed, during the plateau (Bers, 1993), allowing efficient reuptake of Ca^{2+} by intracellular stores.

Phase 3 Repolarization

The plateau is terminated, more or less sharply in different cell types, by the onset of a more rapid repolarization, that returns membrane potential to its diastolic values (Figure 1). The transition to fast repolarization reflects a sudden change of the net current balance toward outward currents, determined by both time- and voltage-dependent processes (Figure 3). These include more complete activation of I_{Ks} and, possibly, full inactivation of I_{CaL}. The slow repolarization taking place during phase 2 may move membrane potential out of the I_{CaL} and I_{Na} window ranges, thus removing the window inward current components.

Once fast repolarization has been initiated, membrane potential returns to a range in which I_{K1} conductance becomes significant and increases steeply with further hyperpolarization; thus, although I_{K1} is almost negligible during phase 2 repolarization, it significantly contributes to phase 3 repolarization (Figures 3 and 4).

Depending on the fine balance among relatively small currents, the transition between phases 2 and 3 is a very delicate one. Prolongation of phase 2, resulting from either decreases in K^+ currents (Sanguinetti *et al.*, 1996a; Antzelevitch *et al.*, 1996), or increases in inward plateau currents (Wang *et al.*, 1995a; Bennett *et al.*, 1995b), may induce fluctuations of membrane potential, known as "early afterdepolarizations" (EADs). It has been suggested that EAD may result from undue persistence of membrane potential within the window of I_{CaL} (January and Riddle, 1989). Under such conditions, a small proportion of Ca^{2+} channels might recover from inactivation and immediately reactivate, providing enough inward current to interrupt repolarization. If K^+ currents, including I_{K1}, are markedly inhibited, the transition between phases 2 and 3 may even fail to occur; this can result in a permanently depolarized state, characterized by instability of membrane potential leading to abnormal impulse initiation.

Rate-Dependency of Action Potential Duration

Due to the long action potential plateau, action potential duration may occupy a significant proportion of the cardiac cycle. Were action potential duration unvarying it would have the potential to limit heart rate by diminishing the diastolic interval to a point where succeeding action potentials would arise during phase 3. However, changes of cycle length over a wide range are accompanied by corresponding variations in action potential duration; this tends to preserve the diastolic interval, thus allowing action potential activation to occur from fully repolarized membrane potentials, even at rapid heart rates. The mechanisms of the rate-dependency (or adaptation) of action potential duration have been thoroughly investigated (for review see Boyett and Jewell, 1980; Surawicz, 1992).

Under steady-state conditions, the relationship between action potential duration and cycle length is well described by a saturating (e.g., hyperbolic) function, reaching a plateau at cycle lengths exceeding those occurring under physiological conditions (Figure 9, top panel). As illustrated in the bottom panel of Figure 9, adaptation of action potential duration is not instantaneous. Upon a step change in cycle length, duration varies with a time course that includes a fast, dominant component and a smaller slow one. The biexponential course of adaptation is better appreciated from the semilog plot shown in the Figure 9 inset. The faster component is completed in

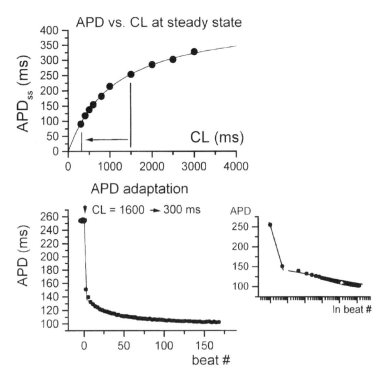

Figure 9   Rate-dependency of action potential duration (APD) in a Purkinje fiber. Upper panel: APD as a function of cycle length (CL) during steady state stimulation; data points are fitted (solid line) by the hyperbolic function $APD_{CL} = APD_{max} \cdot CL/(CL_{50} + CL)$ in which APD_{max} is APD at an infinite CL and CL_{50} is the cycle length at which 50% of APD_{max} is achieved. Lower panel: time course of APD adaptation upon a step change in CL from 1600 to 300 ms; APD shortened with a biexponential time course, better appreciated from the semilog plot shown in the inset, whose fast component was completed within the first 2–3 beats (time constant = 0.45 beats). The overall change in APD observed at steady state corresponds to the one marked by the two lines in the upper panel. (Data from Zaza, unpublished observations).

less than 1 second, i.e., one or a few cycles, according to cycle length. The ionic mechanism underlying this phase is probably represented by incomplete deactivation of delayed rectifier currents, activated during the preceding action potential (see Figure 8). Incomplete recovery from inactivation of I_{CaL} and of I_{to} may also contribute. The same ionic mechanisms underlying the fast component of adaptation are probably responsible for "electrical restitution," i.e., the progressive recovery of duration of premature action potentials elicited at increasing coupling intervals.

The slower component of adaptation, accounting for approximately 20% of the process, occurs over several seconds. It is attributed to progressive changes in the Na^+/K^+ pump current, secondary to cycle-length dependent variations in the rate of Na^+ influx.

The rate of adaptation of action potential duration is increased by adrenergic influences (Zaza *et al.*, 1991). This might cause a more rapid shortening of refractoriness upon a sudden change in activation rate (e.g., an ectopic tachycardia), a phenomenon potentially relevant to the genesis of reentry.

IONIC CURRENTS CONTRIBUTING TO SPONTANEOUS IMPULSE INITIATION

Normal Automaticity

Under physiological conditions, the property of generating spontaneous electrical activity is restricted to cells in the sinoatrial (SA) and atrioventricular (AV) nodes and to myocytes within the conducting system (e.g., Purkinje myocytes). The activity of such "pacemaker" cells is said to result from "normal automaticity," to distinguish it from the "abnormal automaticity" that can occur in all types of cardiac myocytes depolarized by pathological conditions (Figure 10).

Automaticity is spontaneous impulse initiation that results from progressive depolarization of diastolic membrane potential (diastolic depolarization) from the negative value achieved at the end of an action potential (maximum diastolic potential $= E_{max}$) to the activation threshold (E_{th}) for the following one (Figure 10). In SA nodal myocytes, the difference between maximum diastolic potential and threshold potential is usually less than 30 mV and, within the range of physiologic automatic rates, the duration of the diastolic interval may vary between about 100 and 800 ms. Thus, the average rate of membrane potential change (dV/dt) during diastolic depolarization may vary between 0.04 and 0.3 V/sec. The amount of current required to support a change in membrane potential of 0.3 V/sec can be estimated by using the following equation:

$$I/C_m = -dV/dt \approx -0.04 \text{ to} -0.3 \, pA/pF$$

This would amount to $-9 \, pA$ in a single SA myocyte (membrane capacity $= C_m \approx 30 \, pF$) and to -30 pA in a Purkinje myocyte ($C_m \approx 100 \, pF$). At least in the early two thirds of diastole, the rate of depolarization is rather constant (Figure 11A). Therefore, a small, roughly constant net inward current (I_{net} in Figure 11B) is required to support diastolic depolarization in pacemaker cells. Since the driving force for inward current decays slowly due to depolarization, a matching increase in

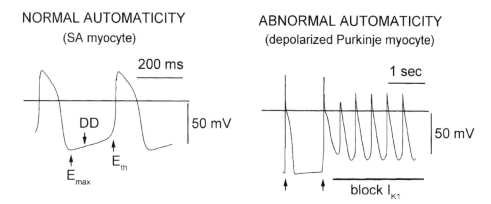

Figure 10 Comparison between normal and abnormal automaticity. Left panel: Automatic impulse initiation in a SA myocyte; almost linear diastolic depolarization (DD) extends from maximum diastolic potential ($E_{max} = -65\,\text{mV}$) to threshold potential ($E_{th} = -40\,\text{mV}$). Action potentials have a slow upstroke (20 V/s) indicating Ca^{2+}-dependent activity. Right panel: a Purkinje myocyte is stimulated under normal conditions (first 2 action potentials) and during blockade of I_{K1} (marked by the horizontal bar). During I_{K1} blockade the membrane fails to repolarize completely and spontaneous activity is initiated. This activity has an oscillatory character and, as in SA node, is supported by Ca^{2+}-dependent action potentials (note the difference in upstroke velocity and shape comparing the two types of action potentials).

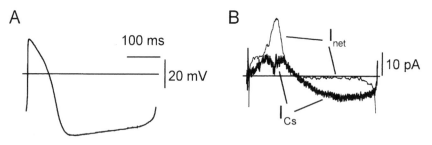

Figure 11 I_f recorded during pacemaking in a sinoatrial myocyte. The current sensitive to 1 mM Cs^+ (I_{Cs}, panel b) was recorded during repetitive activity reproduced under action-potential clamp conditions (a). Inward I_{Cs} recorded during diastolic interval, reflecting I_f, was much larger than the net inward current required to support depolarization (I_{net}) in the same cell. Inward I_f appears at the very onset of diastolic depolarization. (Modified from Zaza *et al.*, 1997).

inward conductance is required to keep diastolic current constant (as an alternative, a constant inward conductance may superimpose on decaying outward conductance).

During diastole, as in other phases of the action potential, net transmembrane current reflects a balance between outward and inward components. Various time-dependent and independent (background) currents are activated in the range of diastolic potentials. In Figure 3, the background currents, including exchanger currents and time-independent Na^+ and Ca^{2+} currents (Hagiwara *et al.*, 1992; Guo *et al.*, 1995), have been summed and are represented by the I_b trace. As shown, during diastole I_b is inward and may provide an additional current superimposed on outward (I_K, I_{KDD}), and inward (I_{CaT}, I_f) time-dependent currents.

Currents Contributing to Pacemaker Activity

All the conductances activated during diastolic depolarization can contribute to pacemaking; therefore assigning the role of "pacemaker current" to any one of them uniquely may be misleading. Nevertheless, a detailed description of all currents flowing during diastole is tedious and unnecessary to the present purpose. Thus, the following discussion will focus on diastolic currents that are either selectively expressed in pacemaker tissues, and/or appear to be involved in functionally important properties of normal automaticity.

I_f is a cationic current that is carried mainly by Na^+ ions in the range of pacemaking potentials (DiFrancesco, 1981a). It becomes available at the end of phase 3 repolarization, thus potentially contributing to the initiation of diastolic depolarization (Zaza *et al.*, 1997). Expression of I_f is detected in all cardiac cells at early stages of development, but is preserved only in normal pacemaker elements when growth and development are complete (Maltsev *et al.*, 1994).

Unlike all other depolarizing cardiac currents, I_f is turned on by hyperpolarization, i.e., the extent and rate of its activation are larger at more negative potentials. At pacemaking potentials, I_f activation is very slow; thus, during diastolic depolarization only a small proportion ($< 10\%$) of total I_f channels may be open. Nonetheless, recent evidence, illustrated in Figure 11B, suggests that an amount of I_f exceeding net pacemaker current (I_{net} in the Figure) may actually be available during pacemaker activity in isolated SA myocytes (Zaza *et al.*, 1997). I_f is exquisitely sensitive to autonomic agonists and adenosine (Zaza *et al.*, 1996a and b), making it a suitable effector for autonomic modulation of heart rate.

A time dependent outward K^+ current, distinct from I_K, but with features similar to it, has been described recently in Purkinje myocytes and SA node, and named I_{KDD} (Vassalle *et al.*, 1995). Slow deactivation of I_K and I_{KDD} during diastole contributes an outward decaying current, potentially relevant to determining the time dependency of membrane conductance during phase 4. Receptor modulation of I_{KDD} remains to be investigated.

The low threshold component of Ca^{2+} current (I_{CaT}) is densely expressed in nodal myocytes (Hagiwara *et al.*, 1988). According to its voltage dependency, this current should be largely inactivated at diastolic potentials. Thus, only a very small proportion of I_{CaT} channels should be open during slow diastolic depolarization. However, in nodal cells inhibition of I_{CaT} significantly slows pacemaker rate, by depressing the later portion of diastolic depolarization. Thus, possibly due to its high channel density, I_{CaT} may carry a significant amount of inward current during the late phase of diastolic depolarization, thus contributing to the achievement of activation threshold.

The abovementioned currents are expressed to a great extent (but not uniquely) in pacemaker tissues. In contrast, the acetylcholine- and adenosine-activated K^+ currents (I_{KACh} and I_{KAdo} respectively), which are expressed in both atrial and nodal myocytes, play a specific role in neurohumoral modulation of the function of SA- and AV-nodes. I_{KACh} and I_{KAdo} have very similar properties and both belong to the family of channels directly activated by a receptor linked G-protein (GIRKs). The gating mechanism of these channels is operated by a receptor-dependent biochemical reaction (G-protein binding), rather than by membrane potential. This mechanism is different from that governing other cardiac currents that, although

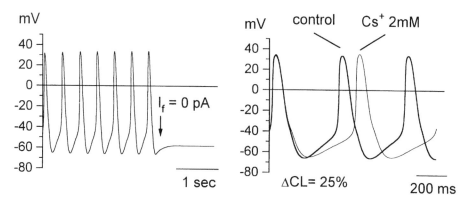

Figure 12 Expected effect of I_f inhibition on I_f-dependent SA pacemaking. SA pacemaker activity was simulated by a numerical model (OXSOFT HEART 4.2, Oxsoft Ltd, Oxford UK). A: Model parameters were set to make pacemaking crucially dependent on I_f, indeed activity stopped when I_f was completely removed ($I_f = 0\,\text{pA}$). B: Voltage dependent blockade of I_f by $2\,\text{mM}$ Cs^+, determined experimentally, was incorporated in the model. I_f inhibition at diastolic potentials exceeding 80% was associated with only a 25% increase in pacemaker cycle length. (Zaza *et al.* unpublished observations).

modulated by intracellular messengers, are voltage activated. Only a very small proportion of I_{KACh} is activated in the absence of acetylcholine; thus, this current has been omitted from Figure 3.

Activation of I_{KACh}/I_{KAdo} supplies an instantaneous outward current, with relatively little rectification, flowing during the entire pacemaker cycle. This current shortens action potential duration, hyperpolarizes E_{max} and depresses diastolic depolarization; activation threshold may also be increased. All these actions contribute to reduction of pacemaker rate. A recent report indicates that knockout of the I_{KACh} gene in mice is associated with a dramatic reduction of heart rate variability (Wickman *et al.*, 1998). This finding suggests that I_{KACh} is pivotal to modulation of heart rate in vivo.

A fascinating and functionally relevant property of SA pacemaking, resulting from its complex ionic mechanisms, is its stability. This is well illustrated by the relatively small reduction of rate induced in SA myocytes by extensive blockade of I_f (Denyer and Brown, 1990). Numerical simulations of SA pacemaking activity, made to be critically dependent on I_f (Figure 12) , show that the increase in pacemaker cycle length expected from an 80–90% reduction in the amplitude of this current does not exceed 25% (Zaza *et al.* unpublished observations). This is accounted for by a sort of negative feedback, supported by changes in other diastolic currents, occurring as a consequence of cycle length prolongation. For instance, prolongation of the diastolic interval, the initial consequence of I_f inhibition, allows for more complete deactivation of time dependent K^+ currents (e.g., I_K). This, in turn, reduces the amount of outward current opposing diastolic depolarization and lowers activation threshold.

Differences Between Normal Automaticity in Nodal Cells and Purkinje Myocytes
Late stages of differentiation of cardiac myocytes are associated with development of a high level of I_{K1} expression in extra-nodal myocytes only (Maltsev *et al.*, 1994). This accounts for the difference in maximum diastolic potential between Purkinje

($E_{max} \approx -90\,\text{mV}$) and SA myocytes ($E_{max} \approx -60\,\text{mV}$). The peculiar contours of nodal action potentials are in large part accounted for by this difference in I_{K1}. Nonetheless, the consequences of the different diastolic potentials on pacemaking are partly compensated by phenomena that might be viewed as "adaptive." For instance, the threshold for I_f activation is more negative in Purkinje myocytes (about $-80\,\text{mV}$) (Yu *et al.*, 1995) than in SA myocytes (-40 to $-60\,\text{mV}$) (DiFrancesco, 1993), apparently conforming to the different potentials at which pacemaking occurs. Thus, the contribution of I_f to normal automaticity in SA node and in Purkinje myocytes may be similar.

The action potential upstroke is supported mostly by I_{Na} in Purkinje myocytes and I_{CaL} in nodal myocytes. When Purkinje myocytes are driven at rates faster than their intrinsic rates, discontinuation of stimulation is followed by a prolonged pause. The mechanism of this phenomenon, termed "overdrive suppression", has been interpreted as follows (Vassalle, 1970). At high rates (i.e., more activations per unit time) Na^+ influx is increased, thus leading to faster Na^+ extrusion through the Na^+/K^+ pump. The extra outward current, generated by the pump, tends to hyperpolarize E_{max} and to increase the activation threshold; this tends to suppress pacemaker activity until the excess Na^+ has been extruded. The same mechanism underlying overdrive suppression may exert a negative feed-back control that limits the maximum rate of impulse initiation in auxiliary pacemakers in which I_{Na} is highly expressed.

Abnormal Automaticity

The term abnormal automaticity refers to the spontaneous activity acquired, under abnormal conditions, by all types of cardiac cells (Figure 10, right panel). Abnormal automaticity is generally induced by membrane depolarization, especially when the loss of polarization is associated with an increased membrane input resistance (Gilmour and Zipes, 1986). This can be obtained either by directly blocking K^+ currents, as in the example of Figure 10, or by displacing membrane potential (through the injection of external current) to voltages positive to $-50\,\text{mV}$ at which I_{K1} is negligible due to rectification.

The coexistence of multiple conductances, with different voltage and time dependencies, makes the genesis of "voltage oscillators" very likely in cardiac myocytes. Thus, the absence of spontaneous activity might be viewed as a specialized function of non-pacemaking cells in which diastolic potential is stabilized by a high level of I_{K1} expression. An example of a voltage oscillator, active at depolarized potentials, may be based on the interplay between I_K, I_{CaL} and/or any other conductance providing the small amount of inward background current that is required to support diastolic depolarization in the absence of I_{K1} (e.g., Ca^{2+} or Na^+ background currents, window currents etc.) (Imanishi & Surawicz, 1976). Membrane depolarization beyond I_{CaL} threshold triggers a Ca^{2+}-dependent upstroke that, in turn, leads to activation of I_K. The resulting increase in outward current and inactivation of I_{CaL} cause membrane potential to repolarize and initiate I_K deactivation. When I_K is decreased enough to make inward current prevail, diastolic depolarization ensues, thus starting a new cycle. The Ca^{2+} dependency of activity arising from depolarized diastolic potentials may account for many features of abnormal automaticity, including sensitivity to modulators of I_{CaL}, insensitivity to Na^+-channel blockers, and lack of overdrive suppression (Wit and Rosen, 1992).

REGIONAL DIFFERENCES IN ACTION POTENTIALS AND AUTOMATICITY

There is impressive heterogeneity of action potential characteristics and impulse initiation in various regions of the atria and ventricles. Detailing the full extent of these is well beyond the scope of this volume. However, two examples will be presented here: the first is the variations in automaticity that occur in regions of the sinus node; the second is the variations in action potential duration that occur transmurally in the ventricles.

Variations in Automaticity in Regions of the SA Node

Sinoatrial pacemaker cells in different regions of the node are characterized by different firing rates and different sensitivities to autonomic agonists (MacKaay *et al.*, 1980). Mapping and microelectrode studies have revealed that exposure to autonomic agonists is associated with shifts, within the SA nodal area, of the earliest activation site (Figure 13). Thus, cells with a lower intrinsic rate, but having lower acetylcholine sensitivity, may assume primary pacemaker function during strong vagal activation. This may represent a useful escape mechanism under conditions of excessive vagal activity and may account for migration of the dominant sinoatrial pacemaker observed during vagal activation.

Transmural Variations in Repolarization of the Ventricle

Differences in action potential characteristics of epicardial and endocardial myocytes in ventricle have long been recognized (Figure 6). The epicardial myocyte has a deep phase 1 notch and – over a wide range of cycle lengths – a longer action potential duration than that in endocardium. The prominent epicardial notch is the result of a large I_{to} in epicardium and a minimal I_{to} in endocardium (Litovsky and Antzelevitch, 1988). The shorter endocardial action potential duration may reflect in part the earlier activation of I_{CaL} and subsequent repolarizing currents.

In the last 10 years, investigators have called attention to a population of cells in midmyocardium (M cells) that have like epicardium, a prominent phase 1 notch and large I_{to} (Sicouri and Antzelevitch, 1991). In contrast to epi- and endocardium, M cells have a very steep rate-dependency of action potential duration, leading to long action potential duration at slow rates. This property is possibly accounted for by a lesser I_{Ks} expression than occurs in the other cell types (Liu and Antzelevitch, 1995). Whereas there is a prominent difference in action potential duration between M cells and epi- and endocardium in isolated tissues and disaggregated cells, the transmural gradient of refractory periods (representative of APD) is far less in the intact heart, no doubt reflecting electrotonic interactions among these diverse cell types (Anyukhovsky *et al.*, 1996). Despite the fact that the transmural gradient in

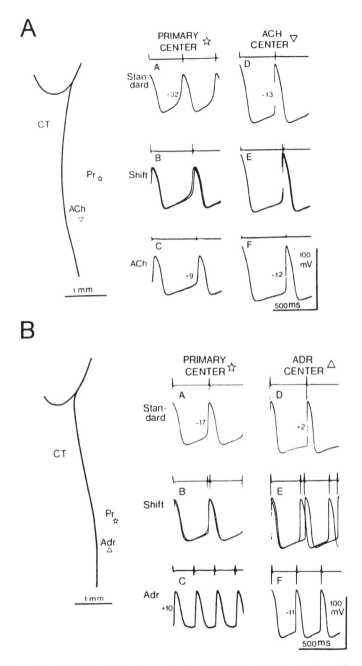

Figure 13 Pacemaker shifts induced by autonomic agonist effects on the sinus node. A diagram outlining the position of the earliest activation site with respect to the christa terminalis (CT) is shown in each panel. "PRIMARY CENTER" is the site of earliest activation under control conditions; ACH /ADR center is the earliest activation site during exposure to agonists. The atrial extracellular electrogram (upper trace) and a transmembrane recording of the local action potential (lower traces) are shown in each record. Shifts in the earliest activation site can be appreciated by taking the atrial electrogram as a time reference. A: exposure to 11 μM acetylcholine (ACH); B: exposure to 1.5 μM adrenaline (ADR). (From MacKaay *et al.*, 1982).

refractory period among cell layers in the normal heart is small ($\sim < 30$ msec at a cycle length of 1500 msec in vivo) it is likely that in settings where tissues become uncoupled (e.g., ischemia, infarction) marked disparities in action potential duration will be expressed and may contribute to arrhythmias.

CONCLUSIONS

The emphasis in this presentation has been the contributions of various ion channels to the cardiac action potential of myocardial and pacemaker tissues. The multiplicity and intricate interdependency of such ionic conductances makes the relation between action potential contour and any individual current very complex. Indeed, the "primary" change in the time trajectory of membrane potential induced by inhibition of a specific current, is likely to produce a number of "secondary" changes in other currents. This will lead to a new action potential shape, possibly very different from the one reflecting the primary change.

This and other aspects of the information presented in this section can be fully appreciated only by working with the action potential, either in actual experiments or via use of a computer model. The reader is encouraged to work with the computer model in chapter 8 – understanding that the model is of the Purkinje fiber action potential, which is only one of the action potentials described in this chapter. Nonetheless, by relating the various perturbations of ion channels to their effects on the action potential the reader will be best able to appreciate the contributions of the channels both as individual populations and as an ensemble to the electrical signal of the myocyte.

4 Propagation Through Cardiac Muscle

José Jalife and Mario Delmar

INTRODUCTION

The propagation of the cardiac impulse is a multifactorial process that depends on the electrical properties associated with cell excitability, the degree of cell-to-cell communication, the geometrical arrangements of intercellular connections and the gross three-dimensional anatomical structure of the atria and ventricles, as well as the heart rate. This chapter is concerned with the way in which electrical activity is transmitted throughout the heart. The discussion starts with a general description of how the ionic currents that move across a given patch of membrane lead to propagation along the membrane, so that the electrical signal originated at one site can spread within a cell and from cell to cell to induce the electrical activation of the entire heart. Subsequently, the contributions of each of the above factors to the phenomenon of propagation are discussed, particularly in regards to their individual roles in normal and abnormal propagation in one-, two- and three-dimensional cardiac muscle. However, it is necessary to emphasize that in this chapter the reader will not find a comprehensive quantitative analysis of the biophysical, biochemical or electrophysiologic process involved in cardiac impulse propagation. The goal, in fact, is to introduce the uninitiated to basic concepts on the electrophysiology of continuous and discontinuous cardiac impulse propagation, as well as to the mechanisms of rate-dependency of propagation, and to the lesser known ideas of nonlinear dynamics and chaos, as applied to the understanding of cardiac conduction abnormalities.

ELECTROTONIC PROPAGATION

The activity generated by cardiac tissues propagates through electrotonic (i.e., local circuit) currents carried by charge bearing ions moving from cell to cell (Hodgkin, 1937a, b; Weidmann, 1952; Jack et al., 1975; Jalife and Moe, 1981). To understand how this happens, consider the cartoon presented in Figure 1, where we have depicted a linear and homogeneous bundle of myocardial cells, arranged end-to-end and connected by low resistance pathways (Delmar and Jalife, 1990). In this *discretized* cable of cells, impulse propagation will occur in such a way that, when cell 1 in the bundle reaches threshold and fires (panel A), it supplies depolarizing current

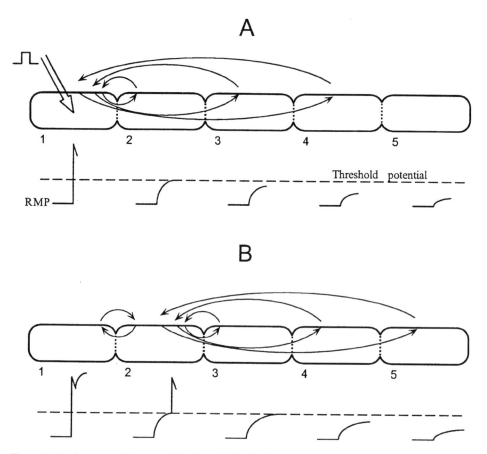

Figure 1 Action potential propagation through local circuit currents in an idealized excitable cable composed of five discrete unit cells. The bottom trace in both panels shows transmembrane potential at each cell. A. Suprathreshold depolarizing current is injected into cell 1 and an action potential upstroke ensues. This establishes an intercellular potential gradient between cell 1 and the rest of the cable. Intracellular depolarizing currents (arrows) move through gap junctions (broken lines) to depolarize cells downstream; extracellular currents move to repolarize cell 1. B. Sometime later, the action potential has propagated to cell 2. RMP, resting membrane potential.

for cell 2, which fires after a small but discrete interval. Cell 2 in turn provides depolarizing current to bring cell 3 to threshold for its action potential (panel B), and so on. As such, this cartoon illustrates the fact that, when viewed microscopically, propagation in this homogeneous bundle of identical cells is stepwise (Spach *et al.*, 1981; Antzelevitch *et al.*, 1980; Jalife and Moe, 1981; Jalife, 1983), with the electrotonic currents propagating from cell to cell, to initiate a local "all-or-none" action potential in each cell as the impulse moves downstream in the bundle. This form of propagation is the result of the connection of each cardiac myocyte to neighboring cells through gap junction channels (Barr *et al.*, 1965; Beyer *et al.*, 1995).

Cell-to-cell propagation can also be explained in terms of basic principles of electricity. Indeed, traditionally the *passive* electrical properties of a patch of membrane of any cell are represented by an equivalent circuit consisting of a resistor in parallel with a capacitor (Figure 2A). The resistor (R) represents an ion channel and the capacitor (C) represents the lipid bilayer of the cell membrane. When a change in voltage is applied across this *RC circuit*, current will flow through the resistor. Consequently the number of charges accumulated across the membrane capacitor will change, and the transmembrane potential will also change. On the basis of these simple principles, an *excitable* cell can be modelled by a set of variable resistors, each one representing an ionic current and connected to a specific voltage source (a battery), and in parallel with a capacitor (Figure 2B). Current moving through any of the resistors either charges or discharges a single capacitor, thus modifying membrane potential. In this model, however, electric charge entering the cell has only one possible return path to complete the circuit; that is, through the membrane capacitor. In other words, according to the model depicted in Figure 2B, all ionic currents move across the cell membrane (Jack *et al.*, 1975; Noble, 1975).

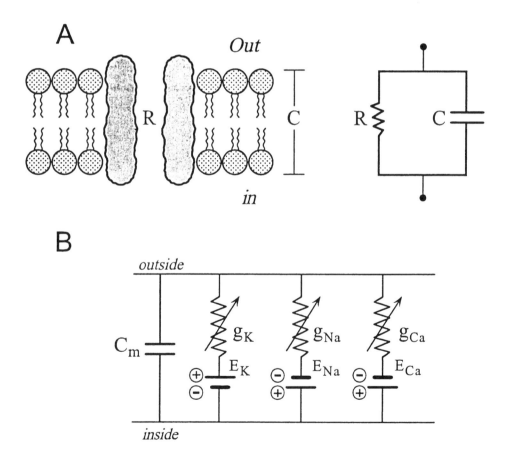

Figure 2 Equivalent circuit of a membrane patch. Panel A, left: diagram represents a patch of membrane lipid bilayer with an ion channel. Right: equivalent electrical circuit of the same patch; R = resistance; C = capacitance. B. equivalent circuit of a patch of active membrane. Three major ion channels are represented, each with its respective driving force (equilibrium potential, E) and variable conductance $g = 1/r$; C_m = membrane capacitance.

The above condition is valid only for the case of single cells in isolation. Since cardiac tissue is a conglomerate of millions of cells, all of which are interconnected through low-resistance intercellular channels, the gap junctions (Barr *et al.*, 1965; Beyer *et al.*, 1995), current entering the cytoplasm of a given cell not only charges the capacitor of that individual myocyte, but also must move in all directions to depolarize neighboring myocytes (Figure 3). The end result will be a gradual decay of voltage change amplitude (ΔV) with distance from the original site of current entry (I_0). The time course of the change in membrane potential produced by that current also will change with distance, as shown in Figure 3 by the tracings at $V_1 - V_3$.

Let us now consider the spread of current in terms of the equivalent *passive* linear array (cable) of parallel RC circuits depicted in Figure 4, where all resistors are ohmic; i.e., there are no "active currents". As shown in Figure 4A, there are four different types of resistors represented in this model (Jack *et al.*, 1975; Sperelakis, 1994): r_m is the membrane resistance; r_i is the "intracellular resistance", equivalent to the lump sum of the axial resistance of the cytoplasm (r_c) and the resistance of the

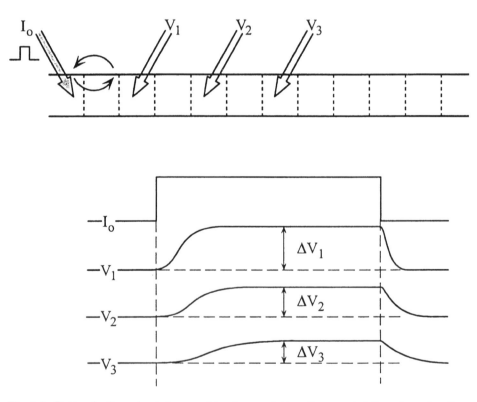

Figure 3 Decay of voltage signal along a cable of nonexcitable cells connected through gap junctions (broken lines). A rectangular pulse of depolarizing current (I_0) is injected at one end of the cable. The voltage change (ΔV) is recorded at three different distances (V_1, V_2, V_3) from the injection site. As shown by the voltage traces, the amplitude of ΔV rapidly falls off with distance because the space constant (λ) is relatively short (~ 2 mm in Purkinje fibers) with respect to the length of the cable. Note that voltage does not change instantaneously at the make or break of the pulse. This is because of the RC properties of the membrane.

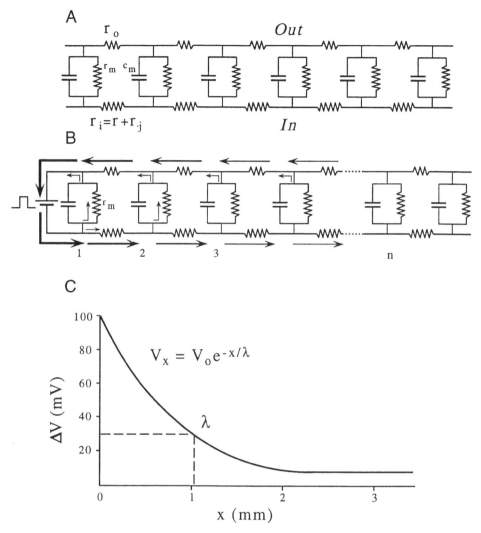

Figure 4 Decay of voltage along a passive cable of infinite length. Panel A, equivalent circuit of cable; r_0, extracellular resistance; r_m, membrane resistance; r_i, intracellular resistance; r_c, cytoplasmic resistance; r_j, gap junction resistance; c_m, membrane capacitance. Panel B, when a transient potential difference (square pulse) is established at one end of the cable; local circuit currents move along the cable but decay very rapidly with distance. Panel C, plot of voltage change (ΔV) as a function of distance (x). V_0, voltage at $x = 0$; λ, space constant.

gap junctions (r_j); r_c is considered to be much lower than the gap junction resistance, and thus r_j predominates. The term r_0 represents the resistance of the extracellular space; i.e., the extracellular solution bathing the cable. As shown in Figure 4B, the current generated by a brief *depolarizing* pulse applied across the membrane of cell 1 will divide to propagate simultaneously a) across the capacitor of cell 1 to depolarize the membrane of that cell; and b) across the intercellular resistances to depolarize neighboring cells. In cell 2, the charges will once again divide; some of these charges will move across the RC circuit of that cell to induce (see Figure 4) membrane depolarization, while some others will continue across r_i and into cell 3; and so on. The same process repeats at each site; yet as the current moves farther along the fiber, less current is available to depolarize cells downstream, in such a way that no current reaches site n. As shown by the graph in panel C, the amplitude of the depolarization decays exponentially with a relatively short space constant (λ), which is determined by the following relation:

$$\lambda = \sqrt{\frac{r_m}{r_i + r_0}} \tag{1}$$

for a cable bathed in a large volume conductor, r_0 is negligibly small and equation 1 reduces to

$$\lambda = \sqrt{\frac{r_m}{r_i}} \tag{2}$$

The intracellular resistance decreases as the cross sectional area πa^2 of the cable increases (Jack *et al.*, 1975; Sperelakis, 1994). Hence r_i is related to the specific resistivity, R_i, of the lumped intracellular compartment by

$$r_i = R_i/\pi a^2 \tag{3}$$

and equation 2 reduces to

$$\lambda = \sqrt{\frac{R_m a}{2R_i}} \tag{4}$$

where R_m is the membrane resistance normalized for cell length. According to equation 4, the greater the membrane resistance and the smaller the intracellular resistance (including gap junction resistance), the greater the space constant. In any case, for a cable of infinite length, the equation describing the voltage at any distance (x) from the applied voltage (V_0) is

$$V_x = V_0\,e^{-x/\lambda} \tag{5}$$

Notice in Figure 4 that all of the current that moves across the membrane returns, through r_0, to the site of injection, so that the circuit can be completed. This is called "the local circuit" or "electrotonic" current and describes the way in which currents travel along linear arrays of cells (Hodgkin, 1937a, b; Weidmann, 1952; Jack *et al.*, 1975; Jalife, 1983).

As the current spreads laterally from its site of application, it discharges the capacitors of neighboring cells, with a consequent slowing of the membrane potential change (see Figure 3). In fact, because of the relatively large capacitance of the cell membrane, the membrane potential does not change instantaneously at any distance from the site of pulse application. Membrane potential changes slowly at the make and the break of the pulse. Thus upon charging (discharging) the membrane capacitance (C_m), the time at which the voltage reaches 63% (37%) of the maximal (initial) value gives the membrane time constant τ, where

$$\tau = R_m C_m \tag{6}$$

The circuit illustrated in Figure 4 would be more or less equivalent to the case of a thin, unbranched Purkinje fiber to which a subthreshold current pulse is applied. A different situation arises when the current pulse elicits an action potential, as illustrated in Figure 1 above. Figure 5 depicts the changes in membrane potential that are observed in a similar passive cable when a square *hyperpolarizing* current pulse is applied to one end of the fiber. Clearly, the largest voltage deflection is observed at the site of current application. As current density decreases with distance, so does the change in membrane potential; at a very large distance, membrane potential is unchanged by the current pulse (Hodgkin, 1937a, b; Weidmann, 1966).

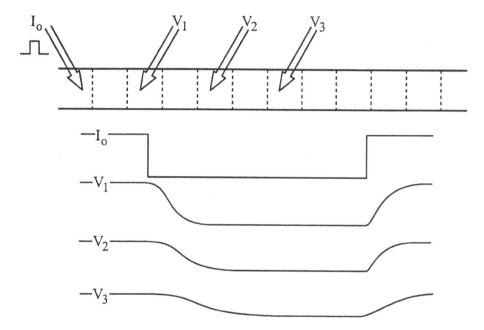

Figure 5 Decay of voltage along a cable of infinite length during application of hyperpolarizing current (I_0) at the left end of the cable. The tracings show the rapid decay of ΔV with distance from injection site.

PROPAGATION OF THE ACTION POTENTIAL: "SINK" AND "SOURCE"

Consider again the simple case of a thin, unbranched, uniform array of cardiac cells (e.g., a free-running false tendon containing a single Purkinje fiber bundle). In panel A of Figure 6, a depolarizing input is applied to the left end of the cell array, thus eliciting an action potential at that site. When cell one depolarizes, an electrochemical gradient is established between that cell and its immediate neighbors. Thus the current generated by the action potential in cell 1 acts as the excitatory current for the cells downstream. The action potential becomes the *source* of current, and the resting potential of cells downstream is the *sink*. The depolarizing current generated by the action potential propagates electrotonically, in the form of a local

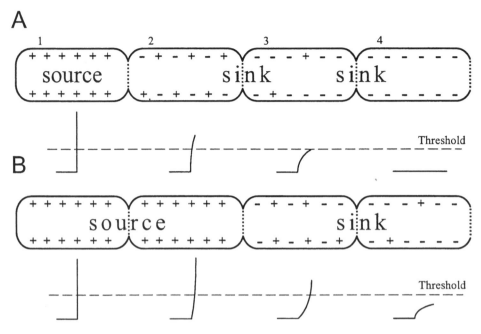

Figure 6 Distribution of intracellular charges during propagation of an action potential from depolarized (source) to resting cells (sink). A. The source is located in cell 1. B. The source has extended to cell 2.

circuit current. For cells that are far away from the source, the electrotonic potential is *subthreshold*, and its amplitude decays exponentially with distance (Jack *et al.*, 1995; Sperelakis, 1994). However, for cell 2, the current source causes sufficient depolarization to bring that cell to its threshold potential. In panel B, the initiation of an action potential in cell 2 generates a new influx of inward current downstream in the array. Cell 2 now becomes a source of current for those cells that are further downstream, and the process repeats itself as the action potential "travels" along the fiber. Note that, as opposed to the case of a single myocyte where all inward current that enters the circuit discharges that cell's capacitor, in the case of the multicellular cable only a fraction of the current depolarizes each cell. A good proportion of the current is used to depolarize the cells downstream. In other words, there is a "loading effect" imposed by the cells downstream on the cell that is being activated (Jack *et al.*, 1975; Spach *et al.*, 1982a). The loading effect draws charges away from the local capacitor (i.e., the capacitor at the site of excitation) and, consequently, prevents depolarization.

CURRENT LOAD AND THE CONCEPT OF LIMINAL LENGTH

From Figure 6, it is clear that when the membrane potential of a cell is brought above threshold, an inward ("all or none") depolarizing current will ensue. However, when the initial depolarization does not attain threshold, then an outward repolarizing current will result, which will force the membrane potential toward rest.

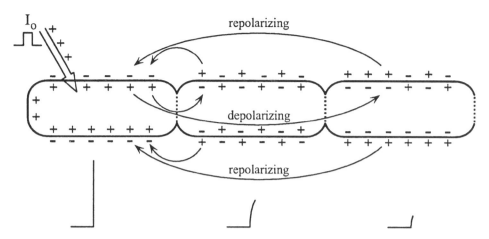

Figure 7 Local circuit currents established upon depolarization of cell 1 in a section of infinitely long cable.

This occurs because the resting potential is determined primarily by a background potassium conductance (I_{K1}; see Delmar *et al.*, 1991), such that depolarization of a given cell in an array moves its membrane potential away from the equilibrium potential for potassium (E_K). However its potassium channels remain conductive, and thus outward flow of potassium ensues and repolarizes the cell. As illustrated in Figure 7, this repolarizing current opposes the depolarizing influence of the current source. Thus, in the case of the propagated action potential, there are both inward and outward currents moving at the same time in opposite directions at different points of the multicellular cable. While at the site of excitation there is an influx of charge, at distal sites charges are leaving the fiber as the repolarizing currents oppose the depolarizing influence of the current source. In this regard, the current sink is not a purely passive element in the propagation circuit; it plays an important active role in dynamically opposing the depolarization of the fiber (Rushton, 1937; Jack *et al.*, 1975; Spach *et al.*, 1982a).

In 1937, Rushton developed the concept of *liminal length* to describe analytically the interplay between depolarizing and repolarizing forces in the propagated action potential. Simply stated, in the case of a unidimensional cable-like structure, this concept defines *the length of fiber that needs to be raised above threshold so that the depolarizing influence of the currents generated within that length exceed the repolarizing influence of the fiber downstream.* A propagated action potential occurs when the density of the depolarizing current overcomes the repolarizing influence exerted by the outward current that is elicited away from the site of excitation. This is illustrated graphically in Figure 8. In the upper panel, the ordinate represents the amplitude and polarity of the current flowing through the membrane. In the bottom panel the ordinate shows the value of membrane potential at a particular site in a cable. In both panels, the distance (x) from the site of current injection is plotted on the abscissa. A pulse of depolarizing current is delivered inside the cell at $x = 0$. The amplitude of the depolarization decays with distance as predicted by the cable equations (see equation 5). Between points A and B, the depolarization is large

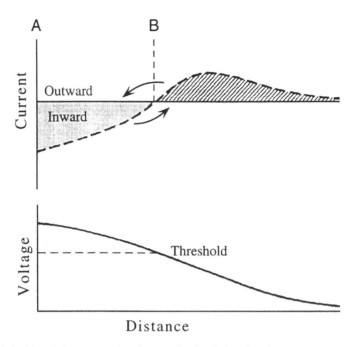

Figure 8 Liminal length for propagation. See text for detailed explanation.

enough to bring the membrane potential above the threshold for sodium current activation. However, for cells to the right of point B, depolarization is subthreshold. In the top graph, the distribution of current is such that, while for the cells between points A and B an inward current is elicited (shadowed area), the cells downstream only respond with repolarizing current (hatched area). According to the liminal length concept (Rushton, 1937), success or failure of propagation would be determined by whether the density of depolarizing current can overcome the repolarizing influence of cells downstream.

FACTORS REGULATING ACTION POTENTIAL PROPAGATION IN CARDIAC TISSUES

The concept of liminal length (Rushton, 1937) is very useful as a didactic tool to explain the interaction between sink and source forces during propagation of the action potential. One can summarize the process of propagation of the cardiac action potential as being dependent on a) the balance between the magnitude of the current source and the magnitude of current needed to depolarize cells downstream, and b) the ability of the current to move along the fiber through gap junction channels. Conduction velocity, and in general, the success or failure of propagation, can be affected by changes in either or both of these two factors.

The magnitude of the current source (the amplitude and velocity of the action potential upstroke) is determined, for the most part, by the amplitude of the active inward currents. In working atrial and ventricular muscle cells, as well as in the ventricular specialized conduction system, sodium currents provide the largest fraction of the excitatory current (Weidmann, 1955; Dominguez and Fozzard, 1970; Catterall, 1988a). In the sinoatrial (Noma and Irisawa, 1976; Nakayama *et al.*, 1984) and AV nodes (Shrier *et al.*, 1995), on the other hand, inward current during the action potential upstroke is largely provided by the calcium channels. As reviewed in Chapter 6 pharmacological manipulations that decrease the amplitude of these currents can drastically impair propagation.

Propagation can also fail because the tissue acting as a sink is not excitable. Administration of sodium channel blockers (or calcium channel blockers in the case of nodal tissue) significantly impairs cell excitability (Zipes and Mendez, 1973; Catterall, 1988b). Thus, even if an excitatory input invades the cell acting as a current sink, that cell cannot become a source of current unless inward channels are available locally to produce all-or-none depolarization. In other words, administration of sodium (or calcium) channel blocking agents has the double effect of decreasing the amplitude of the current source, and impairing the responsiveness of the cells acting as the current sink.

There are other conditions that affect cell excitability without impairing inward currents. A good example is the increase in background outward conductance that follows activation of ATP-sensitive potassium channels in cardiac cells during hypoxia (Noma, 1983; Daut *et al.*, 1990). The outward conductance of the K_{ATP} channel opposes the depolarizing influence of the excitatory current (see above). Thus, a cell whose ATP-sensitive potassium current has been activated requires a larger excitatory input to generate an action potential. In addition, the decrease in membrane resistance effected by the K_{ATP}-channel opening results in a decrease in the space constant (see equation 4) and an increase in the liminal length, thus further impairing excitability.

Propagation can also fail because of a loss of intercellular communication (Delmar *et al.*, 1987; Jalife *et al.*, 1989). Indeed, the heart is a functional syncytium (Weidman, 1952; Barr *et al.*, 1965), and excitatory current has to move from cell to cell across gap junction channels. Conditions such as an increase in proton concentration in the intracellular space (which is likely to occur during myocardial ischemia) can cause the closure of gap junction channels (Liu *et al.*, 1993; Ek-Vitorin *et al.*, 1996) and, consequently, prevent electrical charges from moving from the source to depolarize cells downstream.

In summary, propagation is a highly dynamic process in which individual cells can act, alternatively, as sources of current or as sinks; charges move in the direction of the more negatively polarized tissue to bring about cell depolarization and, if of enough intensity, an action potential. To successfully maintain propagation, current also must move from the source to the sink across permeable low resistance pathways; as the charges return to the source through the extracellular space, propagation of local circuit current is attained.

THE CONCEPT OF "SAFETY FACTOR" FOR PROPAGATION

From the foregoing it is clear that, in a linear cable composed of electrically interconnected excitable cells, impulse propagation is determined primarily by the ratio of the current available to excite cells downstream (the source) and the current required by those cells to be excited (the sink). Among the factors that influence the source, we can include the maximum rate of rise of the action potential upstroke, the action potential amplitude, and, under certain conditions, the action potential duration. Passive membrane properties such as gap junction resistance may also modulate the amount of excitatory current delivered by the source. On the other hand, the factors that influence the sink include the membrane resistance, the voltage threshold, and the difference between voltage threshold and membrane potential. Thus, the *safety factor* for propagation in a one dimensional cable is proportional to the excess of source current in relation to the magnitude of the sink (Jack *et al.*, 1975). Slow conduction, and even block may result from a decrease in the safety factor. Geometrical factors may lead to an *impedance mismatch* between sink and source which will result in propagation disturbances (Spach *et al.*, 1988; Stockbridge, 1988; Rohr *et al.*, 1997). For instance, an action potential may effectively propagate through a cable but block at a branching site as a result of a sudden increase of the repolarizing load at that site (see below). Similar rules apply here for the initiation of a propagated response as those discussed above. In this case also, a liminal length of cable (Rushton, 1937) has to be excited simultaneously to overcome the repolarizing ("loading") effect of neighboring resting cells distal to the branching site.

PROPAGATION IN TWO DIMENSIONS AND THE CONCEPT OF CURVATURE

The discussion thus far has centered on the characteristics of propagation in continuous and discontinuous unidimensional cables of cardiac cells coupled electrically through gap junctions. However, except for the Purkinje fibers, action potential propagation in the heart can hardly be considered a unidimensional process. When propagation of the impulse occurs in two dimensions, additional factors come into play. For example, the shape (i.e., curvature) of the wave front is thought to be a major determinant of the success or failure of propagation (Zykov, 1980; Cabo *et al.*, 1994; Fast and Kleber, 1997). The more convexly curved a wave front is, the lower its velocity of propagation. Beyond a certain critical curvature, propagation of the wave front cannot proceed. This concept of critical curvature is very much related to the existence in two-dimensional cardiac muscle of a *liminal area* for propagation, equivalent to the liminal length in a one-dimensional cable (see above). This is easily appreciated when one considers that the relative area of tissue to be excited (the sink) ahead of a convexly curved wave front (the source) is larger than the area forming the sink in front of an equivalent plane wave.

The relationship between curvature and propagation was predicted theoretically in the 1980's and confirmed experimentally in other excitable media (Winfree, 1987; Zykov, 1987). Its study has just began in cardiac muscle. Indeed, recently published computer simulation and experimental studies have demonstrated that conduction velocity in two-dimensional cardiac muscle is steeply dependent on the curvature of the wave front (Cabo *et al.*, 1994; Fast and Kléber, 1997), and that there is a critical wave front curvature beyond which propagation stops (see below). A convenient way of illustrating this concept is to follow the propagation of a wave front across a narrow isthmus of cardiac tissue as done by de la Fuente *et al.* (1971) in canine atrium. Although their study did not address wave front curvature, they demonstrated a range of isthmus widths of 0.5 to 1 mm at which conduction block occurred. More recently, Fast and Kléber (1995a) studied propagation through narrowing groups of cells in patterned rat myocyte cultures. They found that an action potential emerging from a strand 5–8 cells wide always propagated to a large growth area, albeit at a reduced velocity. The latter would suggest that, in this monolayer cell culture model, the critical isthmus was less than 65–130 μm. Cabo *et al.* (1994) recently investigated the characteristics of propagation through an isthmus, as well as the influence of anisotropy in both computer simulations and experiments in isolated cardiac tissue. In the numerical experiment reproduced in Figure 9, they simulated an isthmus in a two-dimensional array of excitable cardiac cells by placing an impermeable screen with a hole at the center of the array. Propagation was initiated by planar stimulation in the proximal side (left) with the resulting wave front being parallel to the screen. The velocity of propagation of the planar wave was 41 cm/sec. The size of the isthmus was reduced gradually until a critical isthmus was found through which the wave failed to propagate from the proximal to the distal side. Figure 9A illustrates the relation between curvature and conduction velocity during longitudinal propagation across a relatively narrow (e.g., 250 μm) isthmus. Panel A1 shows an isochronal map with isochrone lines representing the position of the wave front every 5 msec as it moved from left to right. Panel A2 depicts the local conduction velocity along a line in the direction of propagation through the center of the isthmus. Proximal to the isthmus, the velocity of the wave front increases as it approached the isthmus. The velocity decreases to a minimum (25 cm/sec) after the isthmus and then, progressively increases again, towards the value of the velocity of a planar wave. Panel A3 shows the changes in wave front curvature as a function of space. Cabo *et al.* (1994) demonstrated that the changes in the curvature correlated very well with changes in the conduction velocity: because of the high resistivity at the barrier, the increase in the conduction velocity just before the isthmus corresponded to that of a wave front of negative curvature (concave). On the other hand, the decrease in the conduction velocity beyond the isthmus (right) corresponded to wave fronts of positive curvature (convex). The minimum velocity occurred at a distance of 0.5 mm distal to the isthmus and coincided with the site of maximum curvature.

Propagation through a wider isthmus (950 μm) is presented Panel B of Figure 9. Qualitatively, the results are similar to those shown in panel A: velocity and curvature were again related to each other. However, there were some quantitative differences: minimum velocity and maximum curvature occurred further away from the isthmus and over a wider range of distances.

The critical size of the isthmus for propagation was strongly dependent on the excitability of the medium. In fact, if the maximum value of the sodium conductance of all cells in the array was decreased there was a decrease in the velocity of a planar wave (longitudinal conduction velocity = 31 cm/sec) and an increase in the size of the critical isthmus.

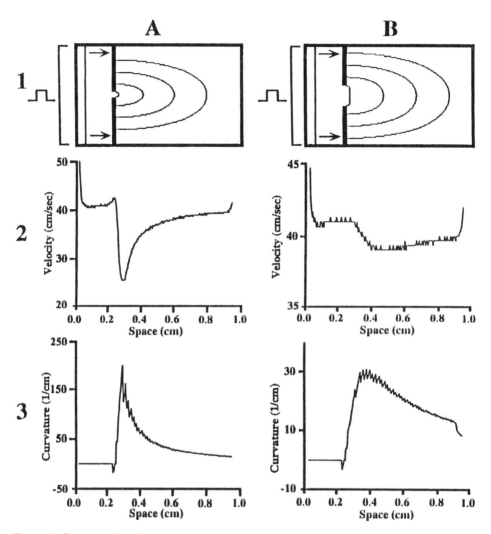

Figure 9 Computer simulation showing longitudinal propagation through narrow (width, 250 μm; A1 through A3) and wide (width, 950 μm; B1 through B3) isthmuses. The isthmus was located 0.25 cm from the left border (A1 and B1); electrical activity was initiated by planar stimulation of the left border of the matrix. A1 and B1 show isochronal maps for each condition; the spacing between isochrones was 5 milliseconds. A2 and B2 are graphs showing the changes in the velocity of propagation along a line in the direction of propagation (left to right) through the middle of the isthmus. A3 and B3 are graphs showing the changes in the curvature of the wave front along the same line. The simulations correspond to a case with normal excitability. Modified from Cabo, C. *et al.* (1994) Wave-front curvature as a cause of slow conduction and block in isolated cardiac muscle. Circ. Res. 75:1014–1028, by permission of the American Heart Association.

It is important to stress that, in this model, conduction block occurs at an appreciable distance away from the isthmus. Right at the isthmus propagation velocity was normal because the wave front was flat; the minimum velocity of propagation occurred at some distance beyond the isthmus where the convex curvature of the wave front was maximal. At a further distance away from the isthmus, the velocity was still slower than that of a planar wave because the wave front was curved. Thus, according to the results of Cabo *et al.* (1994), the most important effect of the isthmus was to diffract the planar wave front into an elliptic curvature. As confirmed by Cabo's experimental results, the local changes in curvature themselves were responsible for the corresponding changes in velocity. It follows from these results that, since a large curvature of the wave front causes a reduction in velocity, propagation may be possible only for wave fronts whose curvature is less than critical.

ANISOTROPIC PROPAGATION

One of the fundamental characteristics of cardiac muscle is its structural anisotropy (Sano *et al.*, 1959; Clerc, 1976; Spach *et al.*, 1983; Barr and Plonsey, 1984). Such anisotropy results from the rod-like shape of adult cardiac myocytes, the heterogeneous distribution of gap junctions on the surface of the membrane and the orientation of cell bundles along the long axis of the cells (Spach *et al.*, 1979; 1981; 1982a; 1982b; Spach and Kootsey, 1985). Thus, activation maps of two-dimensional cardiac muscle demonstrate that the activation fronts that emanate from suprathreshold stimulation by a point source at the center of the muscle are elliptic (Figure 10). As a consequence, any quantitative measurements involving spatial dimensions are, necessarily, directionally dependent. Parameters that are directionally dependent include, among others, space constant, conduction velocity, width of the wave front and, of course, curvature (see above). In the case of conduction velocity, an action potential generated in the center of a sheet of anisotropic cardiac muscle travels faster in the direction that is parallel to the axis of the fibers than in the transverse direction (Sano *et al.*, 1959; Clerc 1976; Spach *et al.*, 1983). In fact, not only is conduction velocity directionally dependent, but also, propagation may be more likely to fail in one direction than in the other (Spach *et al.*, 1981; 1982a; Spach and Kootsey, 1985). The direction in which propagation fails (i.e., longitudinal or

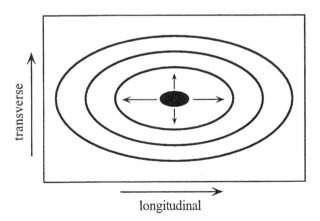

Figure 10 Idealized ellipsoidal wave fronts expected from point stimulation in the center of a rectangular two-dimensional sheet of anisotropic cardiac muscle. The long axis of the cardiac fiber is represented horizontally.

transverse to the fiber axis) varies depending on the conditions used to challenge the propagation properties of the tissue (Spach *et al.*, 1985; Delmar *et al.*, 1987; Delgado *et al.*, 1990). However, it seems clear that lines of propagation block that are associated with the anisotropic properties of the tissue can serve as a substrate for the generation of cardiac rhythm disturbances.

Observations by Spach and Kootsey (1985) in anisotropic ventricular muscle, studied under conditions in which there was uniform depression of active membrane generator properties (i.e., quinidine perfusion or ischemia) suggested that, as a result of a greater upstroke velocity (dV/dt_{max}) of action potentials propagating transversely in cardiac muscle, longitudinal conduction is more vulnerable to block. On the other hand, experimental results by other investigators (Delmar *et al.*, 1987; Delgado *et al.*, 1990) have shown that an increase in intercellular resistance leads to conduction block in a clearly anisotropic manner and can possibly set the stage for longitudinal dissociation. However, in contrast to what was found by Spach and Kootsey (1985), when cell-to-cell uncoupling occurred, propagation in the transverse (T) direction often was blocked at a time when longitudinal (L) propagation was maintained (Delmar *et al.*, 1987); that is, the margin of safety for propagation was greater along the longitudinal axis of the fibers.

In a normally excitable tissue immersed in a homogeneous extracellular fluid with low resistivity, successful propagation should occur if the amount of current offered to a given patch of membrane is large enough to bring that patch to threshold. This condition might not be fulfilled if a) the depolarizing current offered by the source to the recipient patch is too weak and/or b) the longitudinal resistance is too high. Hence, in anisotropic cardiac muscle, action potential propagation should be critically related to dV/dt_{max} if coupling resistance is relatively low and unchanged, in such a way that propagation depends mainly on the amount of inward current generated by each cell or patch of membrane in the conducting pathway. Accordingly, if starting conditions are such that coupling resistance is low and dV/dt_{max} is higher for T than for L, it is conceivable that block can occur more easily for an action potential propagating longitudinally than for one propagating transversely. Such a possibility has been partially supported by experimental results showing L block and T propagation in cardiac muscle exposed to high concentrations of potassium (Tsoubi *et al.*, 1985). On the other hand, if coupling resistance is increased homogeneously throughout the tissue, conduction must depend primarily on the ability of the current to flow from one cell to the next (Jalife *et al.*, 1989), regardless of the change in dV/dt_{max}. In this regard, computer simulations using unidimensional arrays of cardiac muscle cells, have shown that electrical uncoupling can lead to conduction velocity decrease even in the presence of an increased dV/dt_{max} (Fozzard *et al.*, 1982; Spach *et al.*, 1982; Jalife *et al.*, 1989). Further simulations using bidimensional arrays of simple double-conductance model cells (van Capelle, 1983) have predicted that, when coupling resistance is increased homogeneously throughout the array, propagation should be more vulnerable to block transversely than longitudinally. Both theoretical predictions were borne out by experimental results (Delmar *et al.*, 1987; Delgado *et al.*, 1990) which demonstrated in addition that transverse block can be achieved, even in the absence of significant longitudinal propagation changes. Such an anisotropic blockade can be explained readily by the higher initial level of axial resistance in the transverse direction.

Spach *et al.* (1981) have postulated that the higher dV/dt_{max} value observed during transverse propagation is the result of the higher side-to-side resistivity of the cardiac muscle. Under these conditions, the electrotonic propagation of inward current associated with the action potential at each patch of membrane would be reduced, thus reducing the "leak" and leading to increases in the amplitude and velocity of discharges of the membrane capacitors of cells acting as current source. Computer simulations support this hypothesis (Van Capelle, 1983; Spach and Kootsey, 1985). Hence, from a theoretical standpoint, dV/dt_{max} should increase when the gap junction resistance is increased. Yet, the variations in dV/dt_{max} observed experimentally usually do not follow a constant pattern. As shown by Delgado *et al.* (1990), in some experiments, dV/dt_{max} tended to decrease during transverse propagation while increasing longitudinally when gap junction resistance was increased.

PROPAGATION IN THREE-DIMENSIONAL CARDIAC MUSCLE

The myocardium is essentially three-dimensional and thus a full understanding of propagation requires knowledge of what happens in the thickness of the atrial or ventricular wall, as the electrical impulse moves through that wall. Frazier *et al.* (1988), carried out a detailed study of transmural propagation in the right ventricular outflow tract of the dog. These investigators convincingly demonstrated that, in the presence of the deeper layers of myocardium, epicardial surface propagation of an impulse initiated by point stimulation of that surface was different from that which would be manifest if the tissue were two-dimensional. While, as expected from anisotropic cardiac muscle (see Figure 10), the activation fronts near the epicardial site of stimulation were elliptic, most were asymmetrical and had folds and undulations. In addition, the ellipses in each plane rotated clockwise toward the endocardium. The rotation was less than expected from the transmural rotation of the fibers (Streeter, 1979). More recently, Taccardi *et al.* (1994) confirmed that complex anatomical factors significantly affected three-dimensional propagation in the ventricles. Stimulation of the canine left ventricular epicardium resulted in ellipsoidal wavefronts propagating transmurally toward the endocardium and rotating more and more in the different planes. However, upon reaching the endocardium the impulse propagated rapidly across that layer and then moved from endocardium to epicardium in such a way that activation of some regions distant from the stimulus site occurred as epicardial breakthroughs emerging from the deeper layers of myocardium. Such an extremely complex pattern of three-dimensional propagation is explained in part by the intricate anatomical structure of the ventricles. In addition to the elongated shape of and asymmetrical connections among myocardial fibers, which results in anisotropy of propagation, the muscle fiber axes rotates transmurally as much as 120 degrees in some areas (Streeter, 1979; Greenbaum *et al.*, 1981; Hunter and Smail, 1988). Moreover, excitation patterns are also affected by the Purkinje fiber network in the subendocardium and by macroscopic discontinuities and connective tissue septa separating muscle bundles.

Plane wave propagation

Unfortunately, experimental tools available today do not permit a thorough quant-itative understanding of the multiple factors involved in the propagation of the cardiac impulse across the three-dimensional myocardium. Therefore, Keener (1991); Keener and Panfilov (1995) and Colli Franzoni *et al.* (1993a, b) have independently developed simplified but physiologically accurate mathematical models of three-dimensional cardiac impulse propagation based on so-called "eikonal-curvature" equations that track the location of the action potential front, while ignoring the fine ionic mechanisms involved in propagation. This front tracking method is derived from the original work of Christian Huygens who in the 17th century suggested that light travels along rays, which can be tracked perpendicularly to the wave front surface. The method can be used when the propagated signal has an identifiable front. As applied to the heart, the eikonal-curvature equation views the action potential upstroke location as a curve or surface in the myocardial wall, and seeks to determine its location in time, while ignoring the quantitative details of the upstroke or the rest of the action potential. While the derivation of the equations used by these authors is beyond the scope of this chapter, we illustrate some of their results in Figures 11 and 12, and encourage those interested in this modelling approach to consult the original papers (Keener, 1991; Keener and Panfilov, 1995; Colli Fran-zone *et al.*, 1993a, b). In Figure 11, we illustrate results of Keener and Panfilov (1995) who carried out simulations of propagation of a plane wave in a 5 cm × 5 cm slab of ventricular muscle, with thickness of 1 cm and 120 degrees of rotational anisotropy, from endocardium (top) to epicardium (bottom). A plane wave was

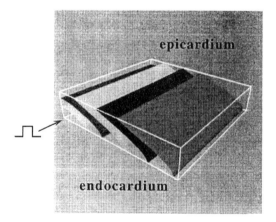

Figure 11 Computer simulation of the propagation of plane wave in a slab of tissue with 120 degrees of rotational anisotropy from epicardium (bottom) to endocardium (top). The slab's dimensions are 5 cm × 5 cm × 1 cm; the speed of propagation along fibers is 0.5 cm/sec; the ratio of plane wave velocities in the longitudinal and transverse directions is 3:1. Plane waves were initiated at 10 msec intervals by stimulation of the left epicardial border. Note that velocity is faster in the epicardium than in the endocardium. In the transmural direction waves are not planar because of rotational anisotropy. For further details see Keener and Panfilov (Keener, J.P. and Panfilov, A.V. (1995) Three-dimensional propagation in the heart: The effects of geometry and fiber orientation on propagation in myocardium. In D.P. Zipes and J. Jalife (eds.), *Cardiac Electrophysiology: From Cell to Bedside*, W.B. Saunders Co., Philadelphia, pp. 335–347.) Reproduced by permission of publisher and authors.

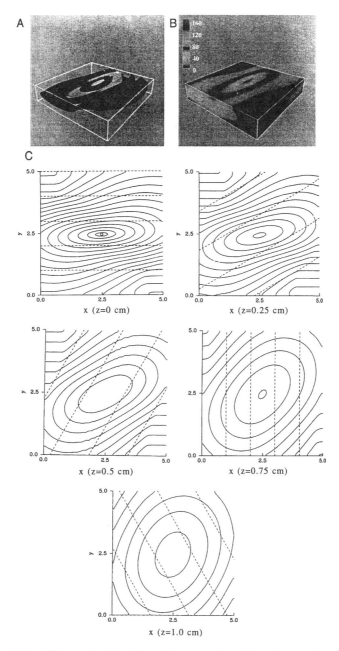

Figure 12 Panels A and B, computer simulation of the propagation of wave front surfaces (A) and arrival time on edges (B) for a three-dimensional tissue slab of 5 cm × 5 cm × 5 cm, after point stimulation at the epicardium (top). Rotational anisotropy from epicardium to endocardium is $2\pi/3$. Wave fronts were initiated at 10 msec intervals. Panel C, cross sectional views of the wave front locations after point stimulation at the epicardium. Broken lines indicate fiber direction at each plane. Modified from Keener, J.P. and Panfilov, A.V. (1995). Three-dimensional propagation in the heart: The effects of geometry and fiber orientation on propagation in myocardium. In D.P. Zipes and J. Jalife (eds.), *Cardiac Electrophysiology: From Cell to Bedside*, W.B. Saunders Co., Philadelphia, pp. 335–347, by permission of publisher and authors.

defined as any wave whose intersection with any constant layer of the myocardial wall between endocardium and epicardium was a straight line. Plane waves were initiated by stimulation of the leftmost endocardial border of the slab. Wave fronts propagated first transmurally toward the epicardium and then toward the right border. As shown in Figure 11, plane wave fronts move as two-dimensional surfaces in three-dimensional space; in the transmural direction, these waves are not planar because of the tissue anisotropy.

Point Stimulation

The data in Figure 12 were taken also from the article by Keener and Panfilov (1995). Here they used the same slab of muscle to simulate three-dimensional propagation of a wave front emanating from a point stimulus applied to the epicardium (top) in the center of the slab. In panel A are shown five wave front profiles at 20 msec intervals; panel B is a grayscale rendering of the time of arrival on the edges of the slab. Panel C shows isochronal maps (10 msec intervals) at five constant levels in the z axis, from epicardium ($z = 0$) through endocardium ($z = 1.0$). As discussed in detail by Keener and Panfilov (1995), there are some interesting features in this Figure. First of all, it is clear from the isochrone maps that the expanding oblong wave fronts do not follow the direction of fiber orientation (dotted lines). For example, on the epicardium ($z = 0$) the long axis of the wave front is about 5 degrees from the fiber direction and on the endocardial surface ($z = 1.0$) it is rotated about 30 degrees from the fiber direction. From epicardium to endocardium there is approximately a sixty degree rotation of the oblong isochrone maps with the 120 degrees of fiber rotation (with respect to $z = 0$), which corresponds well to previous experimental estimates in the dog heart (Frazier *et al.*, 1988).

Scroll waves

In all types of excitable media which have been studied thus far, it has been demonstrated that a particular perturbation of the excitation wave may result in vortex-like activity (Gerisch, 1965; Gorelova and Bures, 1983; Lechleiter *et al.*, 1991). During such activity the excitation wave acquires the shape of an archimedean spiral (Winfree, 1972; Krinsky, 1978) and is called a spiral wave or vortex, organized by its **core**. Recently, the application of nonlinear dynamics theory to the study of wave propagation in the heart (Winfree, 1994; 1995), together with high resolution mapping techniques (Salama, 1976; Dillon, 1991; Davidenko *et al.*, 1991) has enabled investigators to demonstrate spiral wave activity on the surface of ventricular muscle. This has led to the application of new experimental and numerical approaches to the study of the two- and three-dimensional spatio-temporal patterns of excitation that result in cardiac rhythm disturbances (Davidenko *et al.*, 1991; Davidenko, 1993; Pertsov *et al.*, 1993; Gray *et al.*, 1995a; 1995b). However, since the myocardium is spatially three-dimensional, the activity observed on the surface of the ventricles can only be used as a rough approximation to the real-life situation. Thus an appropriate three-dimensional representation of the activity is needed for a meaningful study of the mechanisms of arrhythmias in the whole heart. The theory of wave propagation in excitable media provides some additional tools which allow

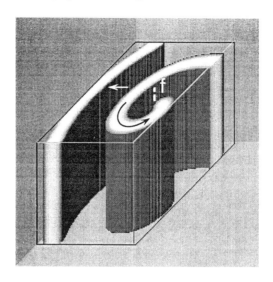

Figure 13 A snapshot of a three-dimensional scroll wave in a computer simulation using the FitzHugh-Nagumo equations (Pertsov and Jalife, 1995). The model consisted of an array of $48 \times 48 \times 48$ elements connected to each other by a diffusion term. The cuboidal array was anisotropic in that element size in the x-axis was twice as large as those in the y and z axes. Nonexcited areas are transparent. The rotation axis f (filament) is shown by the broken line. White arrow indicates direction of propagation. Modified from Pertsov, A.M. and Jalife, J. (1995) Three-dimensional vortex-like reentry. In D.P. Zipes and J. Jalife (eds.), *Cardiac Electrophysiology: From Cell to Bedside (2nd edition)*, W.B. Saunders Co., Philadelphia, pp. 403–410, by permission of the publisher.

such a representation (Jalife and Gray, 1996). If, in a hypothetical experiment, one were to stack many thin sheets of cardiac muscle, one on top of the other, it might be possible to observe the three-dimensional representation of the spiral wave activity occurring synchronously in all the stacked sheets. The three dimensional electrical "object" formed in such an experiment would be a scroll wave. Connecting the cores of all stacked spirals to one another results in a "filament" (f) around which the scroll wave rotates (Figure 13).

There is some information in the electrophysiological literature about whether the myocardium is able to sustain three-dimensional scroll waves. For example, the experiments of Frazier *et al.* (1989) obtained transmural recordings of the activation patterns of right ventricular outflow tract of the in situ canine heart, during and immediately after the application of cross field stimulation (Pertsov *et al.*, 1993) through long orthogonally located electrodes sutured to the epicardial surface over the recording electrodes. The isochrone maps obtained from epicardium, mid-myocardium and endocardium demonstrated vortex-like activity (period 110 msec) throughout the thickness of the outflow tract wall (Frazier *et al.*, 1989), suggesting that the stimulation protocol resulted in the formation of a scroll wave whose filament was nearly perpendicular to the surface (see also Pertsov and Jalife, 1995).

Recently, video imaging technology that permits recording from two orders of magnitude more sites than traditional methods, has been used to study spiral waves on the surface of the whole heart (Gray *et al.*, 1995b; Jalife and Gray, 1996). Similar to Chen *et al.* (1988) and Frazier *et al.* (1989) we used stimulation protocols derived from spiral wave theory developed by Winfree (1973) to initiate scroll waves whose filaments remained perpendicular to the heart surface. Spiral waves were observed on the heart surface of the rabbit heart and these spiral waves tended to drift (Figure 14). The degree of movement of the spiral waves related to the irregularity of the electrocardiograms (ECG's) with the episodes displaying the largest movement resulting in the largest changes in the ECG (Gray *et al.*, 1995a; 1995b;

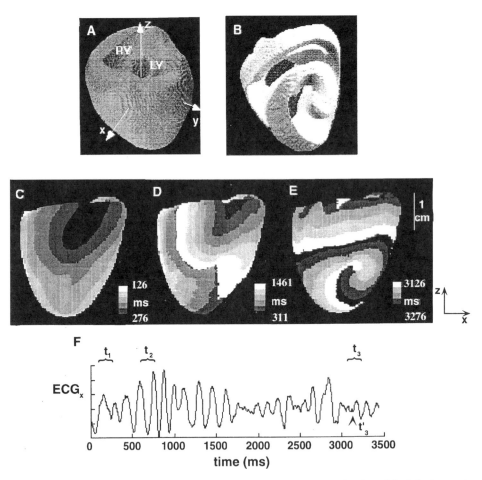

Figure 14 Computer simulation of scroll wave activity in a three-dimensional model of the heart. A, Realistic geometry of right (RV) and left (LV) ventricles. B, Three-dimensional isosurface of activity (variable *e* analogous to normalized membrane potential) at time t_3 reveals a (scroll wave) shown in white (the red heart was made transparent to visualize the three-dimensional structure). C to E, Isochrone maps from the right ventricular epicardial surface at three different time intervals. White denotes earliest activation times and dark gray denotes late activation. C, At time interval t_1 a "V-shaped" collision pattern is evident on the surface. D, at time interval t_2 the scroll wave filament has moved to the lateral surface of the left ventricle and the waves emanating from the scroll wave filament move upwardly in a "V" pattern and also propagate from the bottom. E, at time interval t_3 a spiral wave pattern with a (clockwise) rotation period of 125 msec is manifest on the RV surface. F, a simultaneous horizontal lead (*x*) ECG displaying irregular period and morphology. Modified from Jalife, J. and Gray, R. (1996). Drifting vortices of electrical waves underlie ventricular fibrillation in the rabbit heart. *Acta Physiol. Scand.*, **157**, 123–131, by permission of the publisher.

Jalife and Gray, 1996). These results confirmed the predictions of Winfree (1994), showing that a spiral wave moving over a large portion of the heart gave rise to undulating ECG's characteristic of torsades de pointes, as well as ventricular fibrillation.

To determine whether the spiral waves observed on the epicardial surface of the ventricles corresponded in fact to three-dimensional scroll waves spanning the entire ventricular wall, we carried out computer simulations based on an electrophysiological computer model of the right and left ventricles of the canine heart, which was developed using anatomical geometrical data (Nielsen *et al.*, 1991). The dynamics of the excitable tissue were represented using the FitzHugh-Nagumo equations (Panfilov and Keener, 1995), and the results obtained were scaled such that the average period of activation of an individual site during fibrillation matched the rotation period (133 ms) of spirals recorded from the surface of the rabbit heart (Gray *et al.*, 1995a; 1995b; Jalife and Gray, 1996).

In Figure 15, we have reproduced modelling predictions of vortex-like activity in the whole heart (Jalife and Gray, 1996). Panel A shows a snapshot of the ventricular model with realistic three-dimensional morphology and spatial coordinates. In panel B, the simulated heart was made transparent to present an image of a scroll wave spanning the thickness of the ventricular wall at time t_3 (see below). In C, at time t_1

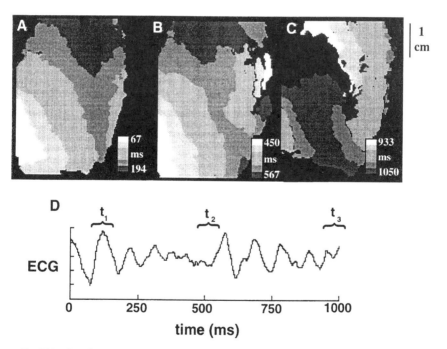

Figure 15 Video imaging experiment showing spiral wave activity on the epicardial surface of the isolated rabbit heart. Isochrone maps from the surface of the free wall of the left ventricle at three different time intervals. White denotes earliest activation times and dark gray denotes late activation. A, time t_1 a "V-shaped" collision pattern is evident on the surface; B, an altered collision pattern; C, a spiral wave pattern with a rotation period of 117 ms. D, simultaneous horizontal ECG. Notice the similarity to the simulation results shown in Figure 14. Modified from Jalife, J. and Gray, R. (1996) Drifting vortices of electrical waves underlie ventricular fibrillation in the rabbit heart. *Acta Physiol. Scand.*, **157**, 123–131, by permission of the publisher.

three-dimensional scroll wave spanning the left ventricular wall was hidden from view. It was manifest on the right ventricular epicardial surface as a collision of two upwardly moving waves in a "V" pattern. This pattern resulted from the waves emanating from the reentrant source on the left ventricle wrapping around the heart. In D, at time t_2, the scroll wave had moved to the posterior surface and the pattern on the right ventricular surface was altered with a central breakthrough band (white) giving rise to V-shaped wave fronts moving upward and to the right, and S-shaped wave fronts moving downward and to the left. Finally, in E, At time t_3, the three-dimensional scroll has moved to the wall of the right ventricle and was manifest on the external ventricular surface as a spiral wave. Panel F illustrates an ECG in the x direction showing complex patterns of activation that cannot be distinguished from ventricular fibrillation.

Although the spatial patterns on the epicardial surface and the myocardial wall exhibited organized scroll wave activity, the signal at individual sites was irregular, as the scroll wave moved throughout the heart. The simulated ECG (Gray *et al.*, 1995a; 1995b; Jalife and Gray, 1996) obtained during this simulation displayed patterns characteristic of fibrillation. Overall, the experimental and numerical results, illustrated respectively in Figures 14 and 15, provide strong support to the idea that complex patterns of excitation during polymorphic ventricular tachycardia and ventricular fibrillation are the result of three-dimensional scroll wave dynamics.

CONTINUOUS VERSUS DISCONTINUOUS PROPAGATION

When viewed microscopically, cell-to-cell propagation in the heart is stepwise with the electrotonic currents propagating to initiate in each cell a local "all-or-none" action potential as the impulse moves downstream in the bundle (see Figure 1 above). This form of propagation is the result of the connection of each cardiac myocyte to neighboring cells through gap junction channels, whose resistance, r_j, is higher than r_i. Yet, at the macroscopic level, the action potential appears to travel at a uniform and continuous velocity. In other words, in the case of a discretized but uniform cable of cells connected by low resistance gap junctions (Figure 16A), the distance traversed by the action potential may be considered to be a linear function of time (Figure 16B), with a slope dx/dt that defines the velocity.

It is important to note, however, that unlike the idealized system depicted in Figure 16, cardiac tissues are not uniform and propagation through them is discontinuous, not only because of the presence of gap junctions but also because of differences in cell geometry, as well as nonuniform three-dimensional distribution of gap junctions connecting neighboring myocytes. In the normal heart, an important source of discontinuity is provided by the large anatomical and electrophysiological variations that exist within and between the various types of cardiac tissue. Severe discontinuities in action potential propagation can indeed occur at branching regions of cell bundles and at the junctions between tissue types as a result of these variations. A case in point is the atrioventricular conducting system. To reach the ventricle, an impulse originated in the atrium must propagate across the AV node and the His-Purkinje network. This impulse has therefore to travel across several areas connecting tissues that may have very different properties from each other in terms

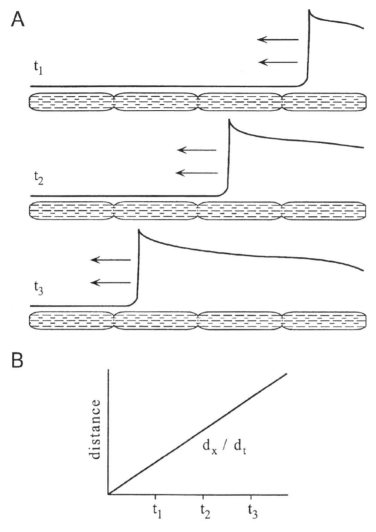

Figure 16 Continuous propagation of action potentials in an idealized homogenous cable of cardiac cells. A. the action potential wave front moves from right to left at constant speed. B, the distance traversed by the action potential is a linear function of time elapsed. The slope dx/dt defines velocity.

of excitability, refractoriness, and cell-to-cell communication, as well as a great variability in the geometrical arrangement of their respective component cells. However, severe discontinuities usually do not become manifest electrophysiologically unless active generator properties (i.e., excitability) are impaired (Jalife *et al.*, 1989; Delgado *et al.*, 1990) or when premature impulses occur in partially recovered tissues (Spach *et al.*, 1981; Spach *et al.*, 1982). The wave front may thus find several obstacles in its path. As such, an electrical impulse generated in the atria or ventricles may reach a junction (atrium-node, node-node, node-His, etc) in which propagation is not possible because the tissue has not yet recovered from a previous depolarization. The ensuing impulse may stop at such a junction and become extinguished or may

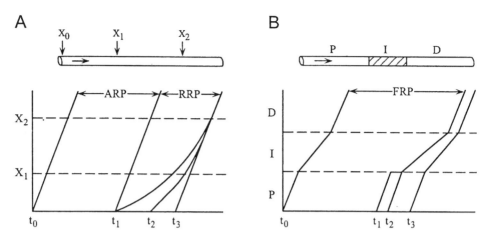

Figure 17 Impulse propagation across homogeneous (A) and nonhomogeneous (B) cables. Panel A, X_0: site of impulse initiation; X_1 and X_2: sites of recording; t_n: times of impulse initiation; y: time of arrival at X_2; ARP: absolute refractory period; RRP: relative refractory period. In B, the impulses are initiated at a site (P) that is proximal to an intermediate area of depression (I), and the functional refractory period (FRP) is measured at the distal (D) element of the cable. Modified from Jalife, J. (1983) The sucrose gap preparation as a model of AV nodal transmission: Are dual pathways necessary for reciprocation and AV nodal echoes? *PACE*, **6**, 1106–1122, by permission of the publisher.

renew its journey, but only after a delay imposed by the time necessary for recovery of excitability of all the tissues involved (see Figure 17).

In the late 1950's, Arturo Rosenblueth (1958a) defined the functional refractory period (FRP) *as the time that must elapse after the propagation of an impulse in an excitable tissue before another impulse can propagate.* The diagrams in Figure 17, adapted from one of Rosenblueth's papers (Rosenblueth, 1958a), illustrate the laws of propagation across continuous (panel A) and discontinuous (panel B) uni-dimensional cables. In Figure 17A, the cable on top is considered to be continuous and homogeneous with respect to all properties of excitable tissues, including excitability, gap junction conductivity and refractoriness. X_0 is the site of impulse initiation; x_1 and x_2 are the location of recording electrodes at two different positions along the cable. In the bottom graph, the distance travelled by the impulse is plotted on the ordinate and time is plotted on the abscissa. In this system, an impulse initiated at X_0 and time t_0 propagates across fully recovered tissue at a uniform velocity (i.e., dx/dt is constant). A second impulse, initiated at the same site at time t_1, will travel at a gradually increasing velocity, until it meets fully recovered tissue (y).

If the monotonic curve $t_1 - y$ defines the conditions for propagation during the relatively refractory period (Figure 17A), then in a continuous cable, an impulse t_2 initiated at any time between t_1 and t_3 will encounter tissue less refractory and will travel faster and faster, but it could never reach any point $X < x_2$ at the same time or earlier than the impulse initiated at t_1. Thus, if two premature impulses are initiated at different moments during the relatively refractory period (RRP) and reach $X < x_2$ simultaneously, their concordance cannot be explained by a slowing of conduction. This is illustrated in Figure 17B, in which the cable at the top is discontinuous in that it contains a central area of depressed excitability (I) separating two fully excitable zones (P, proximal; D, distal). As shown by the bottom graph, in this cable, velocity of propagation is not uniform (i.e., dx/dt is not constant) regardless of the timing of the stimulus. Moreover the impulse initiated at t_1 must have stopped at least for some time at some place (the P–I junction) in the course of its propagation – i.e., its velocity was zero – so that it reached the D segment at the same time as the impulse initiated at t_2. This could not occur in a continuous system, in which the relationship between input and output (see Figure 18A), obtained during programmed P1–P2 stimulation, with P2 stimuli applied at progressively more premature intervals, must terminate on the left in a curve of diminishing slope. If, as in the case of Figure 18b, at any point the slope becomes zero or changes sign – i.e., if the impulse initiated at t_2 reaches $X > x_2$ at the same time or earlier than that initiated at t_1 – the conditions for propagation must be different and the cable cannot be continuous (Rosenblueth, 1958a; Jalife, 1983). As illustrated in Figure 17B above, the region that determines the functional refractory period (FRP) of the entire system is that where the recovery of excitability takes longer (I). In both panels A and B of Figure 18, the FRP corresponds to the minimum attainable D1–D2 interval.

The above concepts indicate that the mechanisms of rate-dependent and intermittent block processes such as during Wenckebach periodicity in atrioventricular transmission (see below) cannot be explained merely on the basis of slow or decremental conduction (Hoffman *et al.*, 1958; Hoffman and Cranefield, 1960), and are not compatible with the behavior expected from a continuous cable. These cyclic processes can be more readily explained by discontinuous propagation across non-homogeneous systems in which an impulse stops at some junctional site (Figure 17B) and resumes propagation after a delay imposed by the FRP of the less excitable element. We tested this concept using an experimental model of nonuniform propagation (Jalife and Moe, 1981) in which a Purkinje fiber was placed in a three chamber tissue bath (Figure 19A). A narrow zone of depressed excitability was

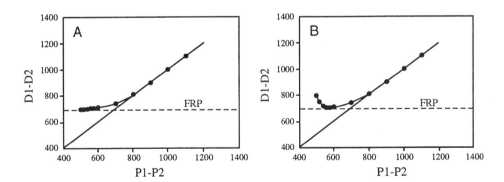

Figure 18 Input-output plots. A. Homogeneous system; e.g., a cable of cardiac cells connected by gap junctions. Experiment is carried out by applying programmed stimulation to the proximal end of the cable at progressively shorter input (P1–P2) intervals. Output (D1–D2) intervals are plotted on the ordinate against the corresponding P1–P2 intervals, both expressed in msec. At long P1–P2 intervals, D1–D2 falls on the identity line. At very short P1–P2 intervals, P2–D2 conduction time increases and thus D1–D2 falls above the identity line following an asymptote toward the function refractory period (FRP). B. An inhomogeneous system; i.e., the AV node or a Purkinje-fiber sucrose gap preparation, the D1–D2 to P1–P2 relation presents a hook at very early intervals because the impulse stops for some time at a junctional site. Under these conditions very short P1–P2 intervals may yield very long D1–D2 intervals.

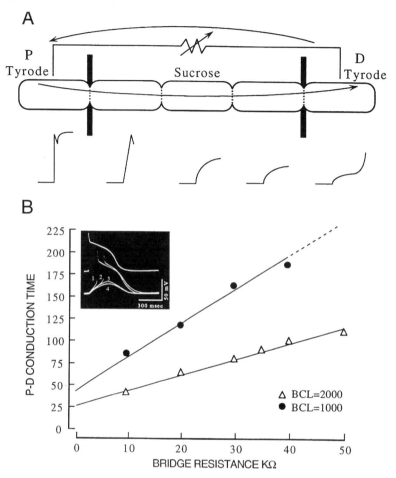

Figure 19 Dependence of conduction on the external impedance between proximal (P) and distal (D) segments of a calf Purkinje-fiber in the sucrose gap. A. Diagram of the preparations. The fiber is placed in a tissue bath divided into three compartments by two rubber membranes (dark vertical bar). The two outer segments are superfused with Tyrode's solution and the central segment is superfused with ion-free sucrose solution. A variable resistor is used to bridge the sucrose chamber. B, Ordinate: P–D conduction time expressed in msec. Abscissa: bridge resistance value expressed in KΩ. Triangles: P–D conduction time at a basic cycle length (BCL) of 2000 msec. Circles: data at BCL = 1000 msec. The black lines were drawn by eye. The dotted line extending the upper curve (BCL = 1000 msec) indicates the development of Wenckebach periods with variable conduction times and followed by complete block. Inset: upper traces are transmembrane potentials from P; lower traces are from D. BCL = 1000 msec. Four superimposed traces are shown at bridge resistance values of 20 KΩ (trace 1); 40 KΩ (trace 2); 50 KΩ (trace 3); and 60 KΩ (trace 4). Calibrations: 300 msec and 50 mV. Modified from Jalife, J. and Moe, G.K. (1981) Excitation, conduction and reflection of impulses in isolated bovine and canine cardiac Purkinje fibers. *Circ. Res.*, **49**, 233–247, by permission of the American Heart Association, Inc.

created by superfusing the central segment of the fiber with an ion-free sucrose solution. Continuous microelectrode recordings were obtained from the two segments in the outer chambers, which were superfused with normal Tyrode's solution. Impulses initiated in the proximal (P) chamber propagated to the distal chamber with delays that depended on the frequency of activation and on the degree of conduction impairment imposed by the unexcitability of the central segment. Note in Figure 19A the discontinuity in the action potential upstroke of the D segment, which exhibits a double component. The first component corresponds to passive electrotonic spread from the unexcitable element, which leads to eventual excitation of the distal end. The latter was modulated by bridging the two outer segments with a copper wire connected to a potentiometer (i.e., a variable resistor), in such a way that a complete "local circuit" was established from the wire through the solution in the proximal bath, the membranes of cells in that bath, the intracellular space, the cell membrane and solution in the distal bath, and then back to the distal end of the wire. As shown in Figure 19B, by changing the resistance of the bridge it was possible to modulate the degree of block and control the P to D delay of electrical impulses initiated in the proximal segment. Moreover, as shown by the different symbols in the plot relating conduction time to bridge resistance, the degree of conduction impairment was dependent on the basic cycle length of stimulation.

Rate-dependent conduction block is a property of the atrioventricular conducting system (Mobitz, 1924; Rosenblueth, 1958b), which is exemplified by the so-called "Wenckebach point". Rate-dependent block also occurs in experimentally depressed cardiac tissues (Jalife and Moe, 1981; Rozanski *et al.*, 1984), as well as diseased human ventricle (El-Sherif *et al.*, 1974). In many cases, periodicities in conduction have been shown to correlate with changes in the amplitude of prepotentials recorded in fibers within or just beyond a region of low excitability (see Jalife, 1983 for review). In Purkinje fibers, these changes may be the result of time-dependent changes in amplitude of electrotonic (subthreshold) depolarizations and active (suprathreshold) responses during diastole (Jalife and Moe, 1981). The change in the magnitude of subthreshold events in nonhomogeneous or depressed atrial or ventricular myocardium reflects a concomitant delay in the recovery of excitability that, in turn, determines the frequency dependence of conduction (Jalife, 1983). This hypothesis was tested in the model of discontinuous propagation depicted in Figure 20. The

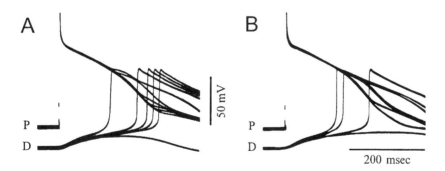

Figure 20 Two examples of second degree block in the sucrose gap model (dog). P = proximal; D = distal transmembrane potential recordings. BCL = 1500 msec and no bridge resistance between P and D. Panel A, six superimposed oscilloscope sweeps show 6:5 block with "typical" Wenckebach structure, i.e., maximum increment of delay occurs after first P–D interval, with progressive decrease in subsequent beats. In panel B, the four superimposed sweeps illustrate "atypical" Wenckebach and 4:3 block. In all cases, the distal activation delay is electrotonically mediated, and is determined by the amplitude and rate of rise of the action potential "foot". Reproduced from Jalife, J. (1983) The sucrose gap preparation as a model of AV nodal transmission: Are dual pathways necessary for reciprocation and AV nodal echoes? *PACE*, **6**, 1106–1122, by permission of the publisher.

superimposed tracings in panel A of Figure 20 illustrate the pattern of P:D propagation achieved at a critical basic cycle length of stimulation of the proximal segment. The 6:5 typical Wenckebach pattern was stable as long as the conditions remained unchanged. In panel B, when the basic cycle length of P stimulation was abbreviated, the pattern changed to a typical 4:3 Wenckebach periodicity. Thus, when the safety factor for conduction was reduced to a relatively low level (as in panel A), conduction aberrations emerged. As the frequency of stimulation increased further (as in panel B), there was further impairment of propagation due to changes in diastolic current requirements (sink) of depressed tissue, as well as in the magnitude of current supplied (source) by the invading activation front.

POSTREPOLARIZATION REFRACTORINESS

Propagation of the action potential across cardiac tissue depends on the excitable properties of the cells and requires appropriately low values of intracellular and extracellular resistances (Weidmann, 1952; Weidmann, 1955a; Barr *et al.*, 1965; DeMello, 1977; Jalife and Moe, 1981). The sucrose gap preparation described above was used as a convenient method to illustrate the effects of changes in some of the above parameters on propagation and its frequency dependence. As shown in the previous section, when the central segment of the fiber was superfused with low resistance sucrose solution, connecting the two outer segments by a bridge provided an alternate low resistance extracellular pathway for the local circuit currents and restored P to D propagation. However, when the resistance of the bridge was set at a constant but relatively high value, P to D propagation became critically dependent on the interval of stimulation. This is illustrated in Figure 21, modified from an experiment in which a calf Purkinje fiber was placed in the sucrose gap chamber (Jalife *et al.*, 1983). At a basic cycle length of 2000 msec, action potentials (P_1) initiated in the proximal segment were transmitted to D at a constant $P_1 - D_1$ interval of 55 msec (panels A–D). Test stimuli (P_2) applied after every 10th basic beat at progressively earlier intervals activated the distal segment with progressively longer $P_2 - D_2$ delay (panels A and B) until, at a $P_1 - P_2$ interval of 530 msec (panel C), complete action potential block occurred. Yet, even though action potentials no longer reached the distal segment, the local circuit (i.e., electrotonic) currents responsible for propagation did not die out abruptly at the site of block (i.e., the sucrose gap), but were manifest in the distal segment as a subthreshold depolarization, an appreciable distance away from that site. Note also that as the distal response was delayed to longer and longer $P_2 - D_2$ intervals (panels A and B), the foot of the action potential in that segment became more apparent. When block occurred (panel C), this foot failed to bring the membrane potential to threshold, and appeared as a depolarization that coincided with the P_2 action potential. Similar foot potentials have been shown to occur in the AV node and other discontinuous systems when block occurs as a result of rapid pacing or premature stimulation (Paes de Carvalho and de Almeida, 1960; Rozanski *et al.*, 1984; Fast *et al.*, 1996). These subthreshold depolarizations are the electrotonic images of action potentials generated by tissues proximal to the site of block.

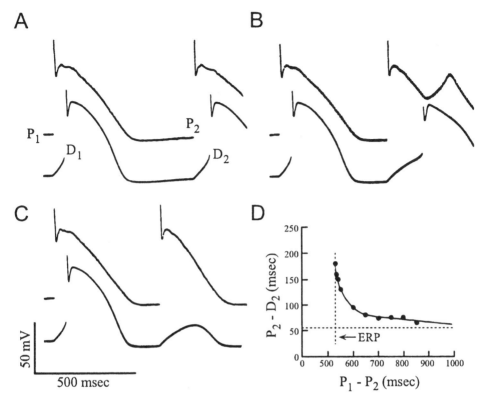

Figure 21 Post-repolarization refractoriness in a calf Purkinje fiber-sucrose gap preparation. Panels A, B, and C show analog recordings. The proximal segment (P; top traces) was driven at a basic cycle length of 2000 msec. Single test stimuli applied after every tenth basic beat at progressively earlier P_1-P_2 intervals yielded increasing delays in distal segment (D; bottom traces) activation. Complete P–D block (panel C) occurred at P_1-P_2 of 525 ms; P–D "refractoriness" outlasted action potential duration. Panel D illustrates complete scan of same experiment. ERP = effective refractory period. Horizontal broken line is control P_1-D_1 interval at P_1-P_2 2000 msec and constant bridge resistance between P and D of 20 KΩ. Spikes have been retouched. Reproduced from Jalife, J., Antzelevitch, C., Lamanna, V., and Moe, G.K. (1983) Rate-dependent changes in excitability of depressed cardiac Purkinje fibers as a mechanism of intermittent bundle branch block. *Circulation* **67**, 912–922, by permission of the American Heart Association, Inc.

The time course of the recovery of excitability after an action potential has propagated through a given heterogeneous pathway may be approximated by measuring the effective refractory period (ERP) of the pathway. ERP may be defined as the longest premature interval at which stimulation at a proximal site fails to generate a distal response (Figure 21D). When the pathway between P and D is highly discontinuous, the ERP can greatly outlast action potential repolarization. This phenomenon, known as *postrepolarization refractoriness*, is an invariable manifestation of discontinuous propagation. It occurs normally in the AV node but is also characteristic of all nonhomogeneous systems in which a local electrophysiological or structural alteration interferes with the normal transmission of the electrical impulse (see Jalife, 1983 for review).

CELLULAR MECHANISMS OF DISCONTINUOUS PROPAGATION

An important question that arises from the foregoing discussion is whether the imbalance between sink and source properties underlying discontinuous propagation and postrepolarization refractoriness represents primarily an alteration in the active generator properties (e.g., inhomogeneous excitability) or in the electrical coupling between cells, or both. In this regard, the development of new optical techniques for measuring membrane potential with high spatial and temporal resolution has enabled investigators to study propagation at the microscopic level, as well as the role of discontinuities in cell-to-cell connections in establishing imbalances between sink and source leading to conduction block. Recently, Fast *et al.* (1996), investigated the role of tissue discontinuities in the activation spread in neonatal rat heart cell monolayers cultured on a growth-directing substrate of collagen (see Figure 22A). The average cell dimensions in such monolayers were smaller than in adult canine myocardium but the degree of cellular anisotropy and connectivity were similar (Figure 22B).

Fast *et al.* (1996) measured the spread of the activation front (i.e., the action potential upstroke) using an array of 100 photodiodes to detect the fluorescence emitted by a voltage-sensitive dye embedded in the membranes of the cultured myocytes. Such a recording system enabled them to determine membrane potential

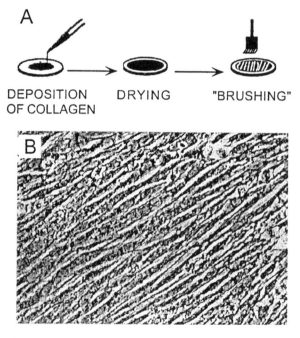

Figure 22   A schematic presentation of the technique used by Fast *et al.* (1996) for anisotropic cell growth. The diagrams show the essential steps in the preparation of glass coverslips covered by a growth-directing matrix. B, phase-contrast image of anisotropic monolayer. Reproduced from Fast, V.G., Darrow, B.J., Saffitz, J.E. and Kléber, A.G. (1996) Anisotropic activation spread in heart cell monolayers assessed by high-resolution optical mapping. Role of tissue discontinuities. *Circ. Res.*, **79**, 115–127, by permission of the authors and the American Heart Association, Inc.

changes with a spatial resolution ranging between 7 and 15 μm, and to directly correlate the constructed activation maps with the cellular architecture, the distribution of gap junctions obtained by immunostaining of the gap junction protein connexin43 and the presence of discontinuities created by the inclusion of non-myocyte cells. Their results showed that the presence of small intercellular clefts (less than one cell in length) did not disturb the general pattern of propagation, except for local changes in upstroke velocity of the action potential as a result of microcollisions of wave fronts propagating in opposite directions around the cleft (Fast *et al.*, 1996). However, as shown in Figure 23, taken from their study (Fast *et al.*, 1996; their Figure 1), large intercellular clefts, of the order of 150 μm or longer, created the substrate for discontinuous conduction and block. Panel A shows a phase-contrast image of the cell culture with a mask of the photodiode array overlaid to indicate the recording sites. The two clefts in the middle interrupted the monolayer structure, leaving a narrow isthmus, about 40 μm wide, interconnecting the upper and lower parts. Panels B and C show the activation maps obtained during longitudinal and transverse propagation. Since the clefts were oriented longitudinally with respect to myocytes, longitudinal propagation (from right to left in panel B) was not markedly affected. However, in panel C, during transverse propagation (top to bottom) the clefts produced major delays in the activation front. Conduction was blocked at the clefts and the activation front passed to the lower part of the mapped region only through the isthmus. Moreover, as shown by the high density of isochronal lines, in this area conduction was exceedingly slow near the tip of the clefts. In panel E, action potential upstrokes recorded at the isthmus (traces 4 through 8) exhibited a double component shape. As shown in panel D, no double component upstrokes were recorded during longitudinal conduction at the same points, which ruled out the possibility that the conduction delay was the result of an inherent heterogeneity in the excitability of cells.

Hence while the results obtained by Fast and his associates (1996) were somewhat different from those presented in the previous section (see Figures 20 and 21), they both point to sink-to-source mismatch as the underlying cause of the slowing of conduction and complex upstroke shapes. In one case, heterogeneities in active generator properties, brought about by the interposition of an unexcitable element between two active sites, results in discontinuous propagation (Figure 20) and frequency dependent block (Figure 21). In the other case, resistive obstacles, forming an isthmus of critical width sets the stage for discontinuous propagation (Figure 23) and block. In the latter case, depression of excitability increases the likelihood of block (Fast *et al.*, 1996).

UNIDIRECTIONAL BLOCK

Unidirectional block is essential for the development of ectopic foci as well as reentrant arrhythmias, but its fundamental mechanisms are not well understood. At the end of the 19th century, Engelmann (1896) concluded that, under appropriate conditions, unidirectional block can occur in single skeletal muscle fibers, and made the generalization that an impulse propagates more easily from rapidly conducting

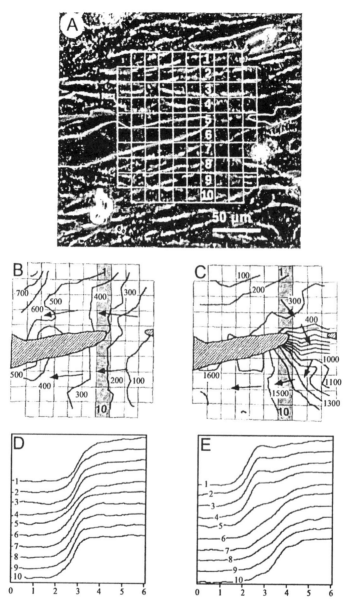

Figure 23 Activation spread in a region with several large intercellular clefts. Panel A shows a phase-contrast image of the cell culture with overlaid photodiode array mask. The numbers 1 to 10 on the diode array correspond to the locations of the signals shown in panels D and E. In panels B and C, the location of these signals is indicated by the gray area. The two clefts in the central area (white outline) from a narrow isthmus of $40\,\mu$m. Activation maps of longitudinal and transverse conduction are shown in panels B and C, respectively. Note slowing and deviation of the wave front at the isthmus. Selected recordings of action potential upstrokes during longitudinal and transverse conduction are shown in panels D and E, respectively. Note discontinuity in the action potential upstroke at the expansion site during transverse propagation only. Reproduced from Fast, V.G., Darrow, B.J., Saffitz, J.E. and Kléber, A.G. (1996) Anisotropic activation spread in heart cell monolayers assessed by high-resolution optical mapping. Role of tissue discontinuities. *Circ. Res.*, **79**, 115–127, by permission of the authors and the American Heart Association, Inc.

tissues to slowly conducting tissues than in the reverse direction (see also Erlanger, 1908; Lewis, 1925). On the other hand, in 1914, Mines suggested that one-way block may result from asymmetric decremental conduction in a depressed region. Later, Schmitt and Erlanger (1928–29) exposed isolated turtle heart muscle strips to localized changes in the ionic environment, but were unable to find any rules predicting the directionality of conduction. They therefore suggested that unidirectional block results from longitudinal dissociation in the area of depression and from the development of multiple pathways with differing conduction characteristics. Microelectrode recordings in apparently normal Purkinje fiber and muscle bundles usually show some degree of asymmetrical propagation, which is not surprising since one would expect absolute symmetry of conduction only in a completely uniform and homogeneous cable (see Figures 16 and 17A above). In the heart, such cable properties are probably the exception rather than the rule because three-dimensional interbundle connections, frequency and distribution of gap junctions and branching are not uniform either along the His-Purkinje network or in the ventricular syncytium, and there are variations in passive and active properties as well. Thus, it should be expected that any isolated segment of heart tissue would conduct more rapidly in one direction than in the other. Such an asymmetry may be exaggerated by agents that depress excitability, including cold, pressure, high KCl, external electrical blocking currents or sucrose superfusion. However, historically, unidirectional block sufficiently stable to allow detailed investigation has been difficult to produce experimentally, and only a handful of examples have been reported. Cranefield *et al*. (1971) showed that it was possible to obtain unidirectional block, slow conduction and reentrant activity in bundles of Purkinje fibers depressed by partial encasing of a false tendon in agar containing 47 mM KCl. The same year, Sasyniuk and Mendez (1971) showed that, at the level of the Purkinje-muscle junction, the margin of safety for orthodromic impulse propagation is lower than in the antidromic direction, thus allowing the conditions for unidirectional block and reentry. As shown 10 years later by Jalife and Moe (1981), unidirectional block can also be obtained when a Purkinje fiber bundle is positioned asymmetrically across a sucrose gap-apparatus. If the proximal segment of the bundle is longer than its counterpart, action potentials will propagate in the proximal-distal direction, but they may be blocked in the opposite direction. Finally, numerical solutions for unidimensional cable equations representing a cardiac strand were carried out by Joyner *et al*. (1980). These authors found major effects of asymmetry in cell diameter and electrical coupling in the development of one-way block.

From the foregoing it is clear that the establishment of the unidirectional block that leads to reentrant and ectopic pacemaker arrhythmias seems to depend on a number of factors whose relative importance has not been completely delineated. One common factor seems certain, however, and that is that there has to be some degree of spatial asymmetry in one or more electrophysiological parameters. In this regard, recently, Rohr *et al*. (1997) demonstrated that spatially uniform reduction of electrical coupling can lead to successful bi-directional conduction in asymmetrical discontinuous cardiac structures exhibiting unidirectional block. This study calls attention to the need of considering the interplay of structural and electrophysiological factors when attempting to establish the cause(s) of unidirectional block under a given set of circumstances.

CELLULAR MECHANISMS OF WENCKEBACH PERIODICITY

Rate-dependent heart block was first demonstrated by His in 1889 and subsequently studied in detail by Wenckebach (1899). The so-called Wenckebach phenomenon in second degree heart block occurs when the atrial rate is abnormally high or when AV conduction is compromised. In its "typical" manifestation, Wenckebach periodicity is characterized by a succession of electrocardiographic complexes in which AV conduction time (the P–R interval) increases progressively in decreasing increments until transmission failure occurs. Following the dropped ventricular discharge, propagation is re-initiated and the cycle is repeated (Figure 24). Several hypotheses have been put forth to account for such an interesting cyclic phenomenon, and perhaps the most plausible is that originally proposed as early as 1924 by Mobitz

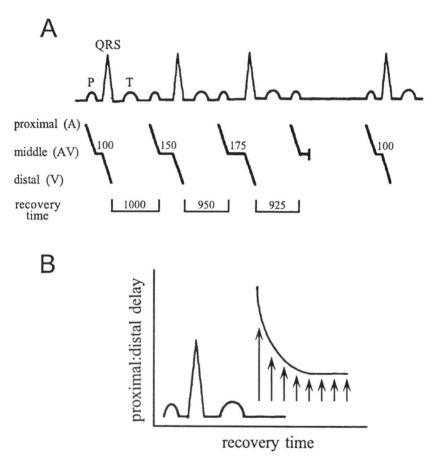

Figure 24 Schematic diagram of electrocardiographic recording illustrating the dynamics of Wenckebach periodicity. A, electrocardiogram and Lewis diagram of a 4:3 Wenckebach cycle. Numbers are in msec. (A), atrium; (AV), atrioventricular node; (V), ventricle. B, recovery curve. The upward arrows indicate timing of atrial discharges. Reproduced from Jalife, J. and Delmar, M. (1991) Ionic basis of the Wenckebach phenomenon. In L. Glass, P. Hunter and A. McCulloch (eds.), *Theory of Heart*, Springer Verlag, New York, NY, pp. 359–376, by permission of the publisher.

(1924) who brought attention to the fact that the progressive lengthening of the P–R interval occurs at the expense of the subsequent R–P interval (recovery time; Figure 24A), which shortens concomitantly after every ventricular discharge. Consequently, the pattern must be associated with a progressive shortening of the time for recovery of ventricular excitability. As the AV conduction time increases progressively on a beat-to-beat basis, the impulse finds the ventricles less and less recovered, until failure occurs (Figure 24B). In the late 1950's, Rosenblueth (1958b) confirmed Mobitz's contention. His experiments in the canine heart further suggested that the progressive delay and eventual failure, leading to recovery and to the start of a new cycle, were in fact the result of discontinuous propagation across the AV conduction system (see above).

Subsequent microelectrode studies in the isolated rabbit AV node by Merideth *et al.*, (1968) provided strong support to Mobitz's and Rosenblueth's hypotheses. In addition, Merideth and his collaborators demonstrated that the refractory period of the so-called "N" cells in the center of the AV node, greatly outlasts the action potential duration (postrepolarization refractoriness), thus supporting Rosenblueth's conjecture (Rosenblueth, 1958a) that the FRP of the AV conducting system is determined by the time of recovery of the less excitable elements in that system (see Figure 17B above). Sixteen years later, Levy and colleagues (1974) used Mobitz's idea to derive their "positive feedback" model of AV node Wenckebach periodicity. In this model, the gradual shortening of the R–P interval that results from the progressive P–R prolongation can be considered as a gradual increase in the prematurity of impulses crossing the AV node. Thus, as the R–P abbreviates more and more, the AV node is less recovered and the P–R interval must increase with each beat, until failure occurs.

In 1960, the first microelectrode recordings of Wenckebach periodicity in the AV node (Figure 25) revealed no significant changes in the upstroke velocity of the action potential of the AV nodal cell that could explain the gradual increase in the activation time (Paes de Carvalho and de Almeida, 1960). It was later proposed that, at the cellular level, the Wenckebach phenomenon could be explained in terms of electrotonically mediated delays in the excitation of the AV nodal cell (Zipes *et al.*, 1983). In fact, it is clear from the example of 4:3 AV nodal Wenckebach shown by the four superimposed traces in Figure 25, that the time course of the "foot" that precedes each of the superimposed active responses is essentially the same as that of

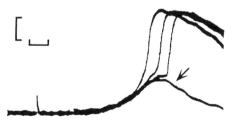

Figure 25 Example of 4:3 Wenckebach recorded from a cell in the NH region of an isolated AV node. Five superimposed traces are shown. Calibrations are: vertical, 20 mV; horizontal, 20 msec. Reproduced from Paes de Carvalho, A. and de Almeida, D.F. (1960) Spread of activity through the atrioventricular node. *Circ. Res.*, **8**, 801–809, by permission of the American Heart Association, Inc.

the subthreshold depolarization (arrow) induced by the atrial impulse during the blocked beat. Because propagation through the N region of the AV node is highly discontinuous, during successful propagation the electrical impulse stops momentarily at that region. Here, the progressive P–R prolongation is seen to result from a progressive decrease in the amplitude and rate of rise of the action potential foot as the relative prematurity of impulses crossing the AV node increases with the decreasing R–P interval. Thus, as the R–P abbreviates more and more, the N region is less recovered which makes it more difficult for the action potential foot to attain threshold for an active NH response. Consequently, the P–R interval must increase with each beat, until failure occurs.

From the foregoing it is clear that Wenckebach periodicity and postrepolarization refractoriness result from a relatively slow recovery of the excitability of cells within a conducting pathway. Slow recovery of excitability is an inherent property of the AV node, as well as other cardiac tissues (Merideth *et al.*, 1968; Jalife, 1983). Since Wenckebach periodicity is demonstrable as a frequency dependent phenomenon, it seems reasonable to suggest that in the setting of discontinuous conduction brought about by complex three-dimensional microanatomy, as well as heterogeneous distribution of intercellular connections, the underlying mechanism of such a cyclic behavior is related to time-dependent changes in the recovery of excitability of individual cardiac cells. In 1989, we tested this hypothesis in single, enzymatically dispersed guinea pig ventricular myocytes maintained in HEPES-Tyrode solution (Delmar *et al.*, 1988; Delmar *et al.*, 1989a, b; Delmar *et al.*, 1990). Whole-cell transmembrane recordings and depolarizing current pulse application were carried out using a single patch pipette. Cells were well polarized, resting potentials were always more negative than −79 mV, and gave rise to action potentials of the expected morphology. However, as shown in Figure 26, under conditions of repetitive stimulation with depolarizing pulses of suprathreshold but relatively low amplitude, it was easy to demonstrate a cyclic behavior in the excitation process of the cell. Such

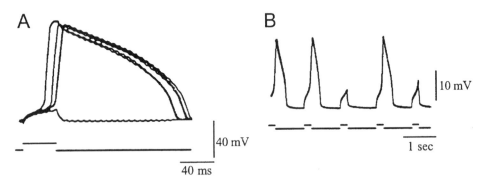

Figure 26 Wenckebach periodicity in single ventricular myocytes. A. Five superimposed microelectrode recordings during repetitive stimulation at a BCL of 1000 msec. Note typical structure of Wenckebach periodicity with increasing delays at decreasing increments. B. Time recording showing a 5:3 pattern of activation in a different cell. In both panels, the bottom trace is a current monitor. Reproduced from Jalife, J. and Delmar, M. (1991) Ionic basis of the Wenckebach phenomenon. In L. Glass, P. Hunter and A. McCulloch (eds.), *Theory of Heart*, Springer Verlag, New York, NY, pp. 359–376 by permission of the publisher.

behavior closely mimicked the Wenckebach phenomenon demonstrated almost 30 years earlier (Paes de Carvalho and de Almeida, 1960) in the rabbit AV node (see Figure 25). Panel A of Figure 26 was obtained from a ventricular myocyte whose resting potential was −81 mV. Five superimposed traces are shown. Depolarizing current pulses, 40 msec in duration and 0.15 nA in strength were applied at a basic cycle length of 1000 msec. A 5 : 4 (stimulus : response) activation pattern was clearly manifest. In fact, the latency between the onset of the current pulse and the action potential upstroke increased in decreasing increments until failure occurred, thus reproducing very closely the typical structure of Wenckebach periodicity (see Figure 24). Panel B of Figure 26 shows another example taken from a different cell. Constant current pulses (amplitude 0.25 nA; duration 200 msec) were applied through the recording microelectrode at a constant cycle length of 1100 msec. Under these conditions, alternations between 3 : 2 and 2 : 1 activation ensued. Note that in both panels, failure occurred always several milliseconds after the repolarization phase of the action potential, thus emphasizing the importance of post-repolarization refractoriness in the development of Wenckebach periodicity.

Mathematical modeling can be used to study excitation block processes because it allows manipulations that would be impossible to carry experimentally in single myocytes. In the 1960's Beeler and Reuter (1977) formulated a model of the cardiac ventricular cell. The model included formulation for four transmembrane ionic currents, including the rapid sodium current, responsible for the action potential upstroke; the calcium current, responsible for the plateau; a time-dependent potassium current (I_K) responsible for repolarization; and a time-independent potassium current (I_{K1}) that maintained the resting potential. I_K was modified to reproduce the experimentally-obtained recovery of deactivation. While the model is somewhat inaccurate and oversimplified in its representation of the electrical activity of the cell (e.g., compare with that in Chapter 8), it is nevertheless a useful tool to study the frequency dependent behavior of the myocyte. Figure 27 shows the simulated action potentials recorded when current pulses were applied repetitively at various cycle lengths. Tracing A shows a 1 : 1 response when the basic cycle length was relatively long. Just as in the ventricular myocyte experiment, progressive abbreviation of the stimulus cycle length yielded patterns of frequency-dependent activation failure, including 5 : 4 (B); 3 : 2 (C) and 2 : 1 (D).

THE RECOVERY CURVE

The tracings shown in Figure 27 suggest that the recovery of excitability after each action potential is indeed a function of the diastolic interval, and that under certain conditions refractoriness can outlast the repolarization phase. Figure 28 shows the results of additional computer simulations in which an S1–S2 protocol was used to study the conditions for recovery of excitability as a function of the diastolic interval. In panels A through C, a test pulse, S2, of relatively long duration and low amplitude was applied at various coupling intervals after the last S1 stimulus in a train of 10 (basic cycle length = 1000 msec). Clearly, the activation delay S2–V2 increased as the coupling interval decreased (compare panel B to panel A), until activation failure

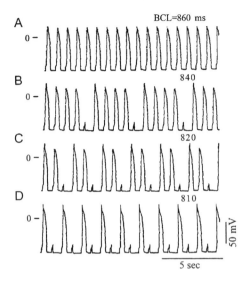

Figure 27 Computer simulations of Wenckebach periodicity using a modified version of the Beeler and Reuter model of a ventricular cell. Action potentials were elicited by repetitive application of depolarizing current pulses (amplitude, $-1.4\,\mu A/cm^2$; duration, 100 msec) at varying cycle lengths. Reproduced from Delmar, M., Michaels, D.C. and Jalife, J. (1989) Slow recovery of excitability and the Wenckebach phenomenon in the single guinea pig ventricular myocyte. *Circ. Res.*, **65**, 761–774, by permission of the American Heart Association, Inc.

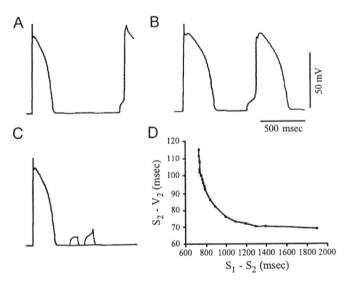

Figure 28 Post-repolarization refractoriness in the Beeler and Reuter model of a ventricular cell. A test pulse (S_2; amplitude, $-1.4\,\mu A/cm^2$; duration, 100 msec) was used to scan the diastolic interval after an action potential induced by S_1. A, at a relatively long S_1-S_2 interval, the S_2-V_2 interval (measured from the onset of the stimulus to 50% of the action potential upstroke) was brief. B, at shorter S_1-S_2 intervals, the S_2-V_2 was prolonged. C, two superimposed tracings show subthreshold responses at two different S_1-S_2 intervals. D, S_2-V_2 as a function of S_1-S_2. Reproduced from Delmar, M., Michaels, D.C., and Jalife, J. (1989). Slow recovery of excitability and the Wenckebach phenomenon in the single guinea pig ventricular myocyte. *Circ. Res.*, **65**, 761–774, by permission of the American Heart Association, Inc.

occurred. Panel C shows two superimposed tracings demonstrating subthreshold responses at two different premature S1–S2 intervals. In panel D, a complete plot of S2–V2 as a function of S1–S2 shows a monotonic recovery curve, which is similar to those described for the AV node (Talajic *et al.*, 1991), and for multicellular preparations of isolated Purkinje fibers and ventricular muscle (Jalife and Moe, 1981; Rozanski *et al.*, 1984).

THE RECOVERY CURVE PREDICTS NONLINEAR DYNAMICS OF RATE DEPENDENT PROPAGATION

In principle, it is expected that any linear system should behave in a simple and totally predictable manner when one of its parameters is changed. For example, if the volume of a closed space is compressed progressively, the resulting pressure within that space will increase proportionately within a given range. Yet, in biology, it is very difficult, if not impossible, to find a completely linear system; nonlinearity is probably the rule and the heart is no exception. Nonlinear dynamical systems, including those which are described by a small number of variables (e.g., action potential duration, latency and excitability) can behave in very complex ways.

From a mechanistic point of view, the common denominator in rate-dependent propagation (excitation) phenomena, such as in Wenckebach periodicity, may be a slow recovery time for membrane excitability after each activation. Such slow recovery is accurately described by the recovery curve, which can be used to make quantitative predictions about the patterns of propagation that emerge when a discontinuous system is forced to conduct at relatively high stimulation rates. For example, in 1987, Shrier *et al.* used the AV nodal recovery curve, obtained with a pacing S1–S2 protocol in patients undergoing electrophysiologic testing, to predict patterns of first- and second-degree AV block induced by rapid pacing. Since the AV nodal recovery curve gives the conduction time through the AV node (i.e., the A2–H2 interval), as a function of the recovery time from the last successful anterograde activation of the His bundle (i.e., the H1–A2 interval), they used a simple numerical iteration of a monotonic function derived from the AV nodal recovery curve to demonstrate that, with increasing stimulation frequency, there was a decrease in the activation ratio, defined as the m/n ratio, where m = number of ventricular responses and n = number of atrial stimuli. Their results provided new insight in our understanding of the dynamics of rate-dependent heart block. Most importantly, they demonstrated that cyclic phenomena such as Wenckebach periodicity, reverse Wenckebach and alternating Wenckebach are demonstrable in very simple discontinuous systems without the need of invoking complex geometrical arrangements in cell bundles or multiple levels of block. In fact our more recent results in single myocytes (see Figure 26) clearly show that Wenckebach-like phenomena are demonstrable in single cells, provided stimuli of appropriately low amplitude and high frequency are used. In the case of Figure 27 above, as the basic cycle length was progressively decreased, the activation ratio, measured as m/n (m = number of cell responses; n = number of stimuli) changed from 1.0 (tracing A), through 0.8 (tracing B), 0.67 (tracing C) and finally 0.5 (tracing D).

As in the case of AV nodal Wenckebach, in single ventricular myocytes, cyclic excitation patterns during repetitive stimulation are predictable using the recovery curve. In Figure 29, we illustrate the dynamics of a 5:4 Wenckebach period in terms of the recovery curve of a normally polarized myocyte driven by repetitive stimuli of constant magnitude and cycle length (Jalife and Delmar, 1991). In this representation, the horizontal boxes represent the excitation and repolarization processes; the white box represent the interval between the onset of the stimulus and the action potential upstroke (time to upstroke); the black box represents the action potential duration (APD) and the dashed box represents the duration of post-repolarization refractoriness (ERP). Recovery time is the interval between the end of the preceding action potential and the occurrence of the next stimulus. The recovery curve is a plot of the time to upstroke as a function of the recovery time. In the middle diagram, the first pulse (labeled 1), which occurs at a relatively long premature interval gives rise to an action potential whose time to upstroke in the recovery curve is relatively short. The second stimulus now occurs at a briefer interval within the recovery curve, and the action potential is further delayed. Since the cycle length is constant, the next recovery time is even briefer, which leads to an even longer delay. After the fifth stimulus, the recovery time is briefer than the refractory phase and failure occurs. Subsequently (not shown) because of a long recovery time, a new cycle ensues, and the 5:4 Wenckebach pattern repeats once again.

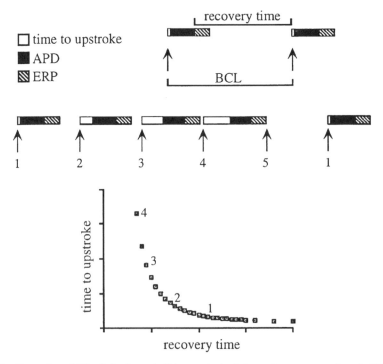

Figure 29 Dynamics of Wenckebach periodicity as derived from the recovery of excitability curve. Reproduced from Jalife, J. and Delmar, M. (1991) Ionic basis of the Wenckebach phenomenon. In L. Glass, P. Hunter and A. McCulloch (eds.), *Theory of Heart*, Springer Verlag, New York, NY, pp. 359–376 by permission of the publisher. See text for details.

IONIC MECHANISM OF WENCKEBACH IN VENTRICULAR AND AV NODAL MYOCYTES

The ionic mechanisms of the Wenckebach-like patterns observed in single ventricular myocytes were studied through a combination of current and voltage clamp techniques (Delmar *et al.*, 1989a, b). Briefly, the results showed that both post-repolarization refractoriness and Wenckebach periodicity, in response to depolarizing pulses of relatively low amplitude, are the result of a slow recovery of cell excitability during diastole, which is determined by the slow deactivation of the delayed rectifier potassium outward current, I_K. This is illustrated graphically in the diagram presented in Figure 30 (and can be tested using the model in Chapter 8). The top tracing represents the membrane potential; an action potential is followed by two subthreshold responses to a depolarizing current pulse of constant amplitude applied at two different intervals. The lower tracing illustrates the time course of change in I_K conductance (G_K) during the cardiac cycle and the bottom arrows represent the time-dependent changes in the magnitude of the effect of I_K opposing the depolarizing current pulse (I_p). The conductance to potassium (G_K) increases gradually in the course of the action potential and becomes maximal during the plateau. Upon repolarization, G_K begins to decrease. Because of the slow time course of deactivation, most of the channel conductance decay occurs after repolarization has been completed. Yet, the diastolic potential remains constant because of the lack of driving force for I_K (i.e., the resting potential is at, or very close to, the potassium equilibrium potential). On the other hand, as shown in Figure 30, when a subthreshold depolarizing pulse is applied early in diastole, the membrane voltage displacement will provide sufficient force for I_K, which would tend to repolarize the membrane. The influence of G_K decreases at the longer diastolic intervals, which allows for an increase in the amplitude of the subthreshold response. Application of a pulse at a later interval should encounter I_K even more deactivated, thus depolarization should be greater and an action potential should ensue (not shown).

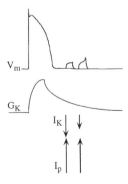

Figure 30 Proposed role of I_K in determining the time course of recovery of excitability in a single myocyte. Top tracing, transmembrane potential (V_m) simulated by the Beeler & Reuter model. Bottom tracing, changes in potassium conductance (G_K) during systolic and diastolic intervals. Arrows, relative magnitudes of I_K and pulse current (I_P) at two different times during I_K deactivation. Reproduced by permission from Jalife, J. and Delmar, M. (1991) Ionic basis of the Wenckebach phenomenon. In L. Glass, P. Hunter and A. McCulloch (eds.), *Theory of Heart*, Springer Verlag, New York, NY, pp. 359–376.

Additional results obtained by Delmar *et al.* (1989a, 1989b) indicated that non-linearities in the current voltage relationship of the inward rectifying current, I_{K1} (see also Tourneur, 1986), played a major role in modulating the amplitude and shape of the foot potentials that precede the progressively more delayed active responses in the Wenckebach cycle, as well as the subthreshold event that ensues when activation fails.

More recent observations in single AV nodal myocytes (Hoshino *et al.*, 1990), obtained by enzymatic dispersion of rabbit hearts, showed somewhat more complex cellular events and ionic mechanisms. As illustrated in panel A of Figure 31, the

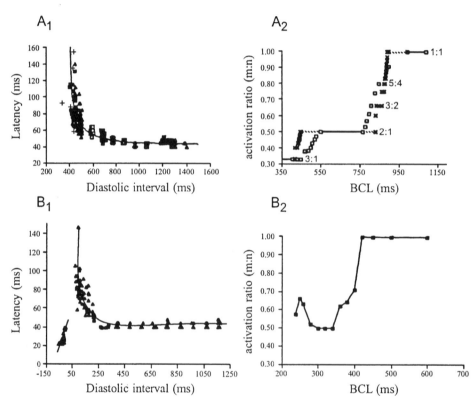

Figure 31 Rate-dependence of activation patterns in relation to the recovery of excitability curve in two different rabbit AV nodal myocytes without (A_1 and A_2) and with (B_1 and B_2) supernormality. A_1, Steady-state recovery of excitability plotted as time to upstroke (latency) versus preceding diastolic interval during repetitive stimulation. Different symbols represent data for stimulation at varying cycle lengths (BCL's). The continuous line represents an empiric monotonic function that considers previous diastolic interval as the sole determinant of latency (Hoshino *et al.*, 1990). A_2, The open symbols show the ranges of stimulus:response ratios observed in the AV nodal myocyte whose recovery was monotonic (A_1). Data are plotted at various basic cycle lengths. The crosses are the stimulus:response ratios predicted by an iterative numerical procedure for the corresponding basic cycle lengths. B_1, Non-monotonic steady-state recovery curve of a single AV nodal myocyte showing supernormal excitability (i.e., shorter than expected latencies at very early diastolic intervals). Lines were fitted by eye. B_2, Activation ratio plotted as a function of basic cycle length. In the presence of supernormality, the dependence of activation ratio on BCL does not decrease monotonically but jumps upward at very short BCL's. Reproduced from Hoshino, K., Anumonwo, J., Delmar, M., and Jalife, J. (1990) Wenckebach periodicity in single atrioventricular nodal cells from the rabbit heart. *Circulation*, **82**, 2201–2216, by permission of the American Heart Association, Inc.

results in some AV nodal cells demonstrated that when depolarizing stimuli of constant but critical magnitude are used to scan the diastolic interval, a monotonic recovery of excitability is clearly observed. However, as seen in panel B1, a few myocytes demonstrated a highly nonlinear time course of recovery after an action potential. Such nonlinear recovery included a period of supernormal excitability where the latency between the stimulus and the action potential upstroke was smaller at very early intervals that at long intervals. This was followed to the right by postrepolarization refractoriness and slow recovery of excitability during diastole. These two different types of time-dependent changes were responsible for the development of two different types of stimulus:response patterns: First, when the myocyte was stimulated by repetitive depolarizing pulses and the recovery curve was monotonic (panel A1), the response patterns were comparable to those observed during first and second degree AV block (panel A2); i.e., as the basic cycle length of the stimulus was shortened, there was a monotonic stepwise change in the excitation pattern, from $1:1$ through $5:4$, $3:2$, $2:1$, and finally $3:1$ (crosses). The latter observation was confirmed using an analytical model (Delmar *et al.*, 1989b; Hoshino *et al.*, 1990) which was devised on the basis of mathematical expressions that simulated the AV nodal recovery curve. Numerical iteration of those equations (open symbols) yielded stimulus:response patterns which were similar to those observed during repetitive stimulation of the single myocyte (panel A2). Second, in the presence of a nonlinear recovery (panel B1), a monotonic change in the stimulus:response patterns was no longer present. As shown in panel B2, nonlinearities in such patterns were observed at stimulus cycle lengths between 200 and 300 ms, where the activation pattern abruptly increased from $2:1$ to $3:2$ and then $6:11$. Such cycle lengths corresponded to very short diastolic intervals in the recovery curve (Panel B1), where supernormality was present. Additional observations using voltage clamp techniques (Hoshino *et al.*, 1990) suggested that at least three different ionic current systems are involved in AV nodal Wenckebach and complex rate-dependent excitation processes: the delayed rectifier potassium outward current, I_K, the anomalous rectifier potassium outward current I_{K1}, and the calcium inward current I_{Ca}. The overall results may have important clinical implications since they provide a direct ionic basis for AV nodal Wenckebach periodicity and other heart rate-dependent AV conduction disturbances.

At first glance, the above results in single AV nodal myocytes seem to contradict the classical microelectrode studies of Merideth and co-workers (1968; see also Moe *et al.*, 1968). These authors studied recovery of excitability in the isolated rabbit AV node but did not demonstrate supernormality during repolarization. Yet, it should be kept in mind that, although Merideth *et al.* (1968) constructed a recovery of excitability curve from the N region of the AV node, they limited their study to scanning the diastolic interval with intracellular stimuli; they did not attempt to determine whether these cells were excitable during the repolarization phase. Single AV node myocyte experiments (Hoshino *et al.*, 1990) clearly showed that even though latency to excitation increased monotonically at progressively earlier intervals until block occurred, a window of supernormal excitability was demonstrable during the repolarization phase (Figure 31B). Merideth *et al.* (1968) failed to demonstrate supernormal AV nodal conduction in response to premature stimuli applied at a distant source. However, it is important to consider that conduction depends not only on the threshold for excitation, but also on the ability of excited cells to depolarize their neighbors; the latter being determined by a number of parameters which include the rate of rise of the action potential, the degree of electrical coupling and the geometrical arrangement of cell-to-cell connections. Thus, the possibility exists that, although present in the single cell, supernormal responses fail to propagate through the AV node.

NONLINEAR RECOVERY AND COMPLEX EXCITATION DYNAMICS

The above results support the idea that, despite their differences, many nonlinear systems with finite recovery time behave in much the same way. Providing that the relevant parameters, which in the case of the myocyte may be excitability, recover monotonically, the sequence of n:m (stimulus:response) patterns that occur as the stimulation frequency is systematically altered can be predicted by the so-called "Farey tree" (Shroeder, 1990; see Figure 32A).

As shown in Figure 32A, for any two n : m and N : M neighboring stimulus : response patterns there is always an intermediate n + N : m + M stimulus:response pattern (Keener, 1981). Therefore, in the case of any given excitable system whose recovery is monotonic, when the stimulus cycle length is changed systematically in extremely small steps and then the resulting activation ratio (m/n) is plotted as a function of that cycle length, the resultant is an infinitely detailed staircase (Shroeder *et al.*, 1990) of m : n steps (Figure 32B), known as the "Devil's staircase".

However, as illustrated above for the single AV nodal myocyte (Figure 31B₁), under certain conditions, cardiac tissues do not have a monotonic recovery of excitability. Similarly, in multicellular Purkinje fibers (Elharrar and Surawicz, 1983; Chialvo *et al.*, 1990a), a relatively supernormal phase of excitability at early diastolic intervals is always present when the fiber is immersed in low-KCl (< 4 mM). Under

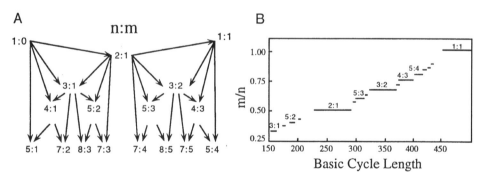

Figure 32 A, "Farey tree" constructed for the first five generations. Starting from seed values 1 : 0, 1 : 1 and 2 : 1 on top line, a new line of activation (n : m) ratios is generated by adding the numerators and denominators of adjacent entries. The ratios in the third line are generated in a similar manner from those in the second line, and so on. B, Devil's staircase obtained by plotting the m/n ratio as a function of basic cycle length. Theoretically, if the basic cycle length is changed in infinitely small steps, there will be an infinite number of n : m steps.

these conditions repetitive stimulation of such fibers may result in very complex patterns of excitation (Chialvo and Jalife, 1987; Chialvo *et al.*, 1990a, b). Careful and systematic experimental and numerical studies of such complex patterns have shown that, under specific sets of circumstances, isolated cardiac cells and tissues can undergo transitions from regular and periodic to highly aperiodic (i.e., chaotic) behavior (Guevara *et al.*, 1981; Chialvo and Jalife, 1987; Chialvo *et al.*, 1990a, b). Chaos theory, if used appropriately, may provide tools and insights into the laws that govern such behavior.

According to its mathematical description, *chaos* is an irregular but non-random behavior that may occur in nonlinear dynamical systems (see Jalife 1993a, b for brief review and further references). A *dynamical system* is any system whose evolution is determined by the interplay of its intrinsic time-dependent variables (e.g., action potential duration, excitability, etc.); when such a time dependence is nonlinear, the system may undergo either ordered or chaotic behavior, depending on the value of the input parameter (e.g., basic cycle length). In the chaotic regime, the system demonstrates irregularity, as well as an exquisite sensitivity to initial conditions (Chialvo and Jalife, 1987), in such a way that it is impossible to make long-term predictions about its behavior. In other words, chaos theory deals with those systems in which periodic and chaotic patterns can emerge. The difference is merely in the value of a single parameter. Very small changes in this parameter can make a huge difference as to the ultimate behavior of the system. Note, however, that chaos is not simply disorder. It is more appropriately described as "order without periodicity". For instance, consider a chaotic sequence of numbers: each number in the sequence must be determined *exactly* and *exclusively* by the number that precedes it. This makes the sequence completely deterministic, as well as completely aperiodic. By contrast in a totally random sequence of numbers, the succession will be governed by the probability distribution, but will not be exactly determined. Based on systematic studies in isolated cardiac Purkinje fibers (Chialvo and Jalife, 1987; Chialvo *et al.*, 1990a, b), we proposed that the mechanism for the chaotic behavior demonstrated by isolated Purkinje fibers during repetitive stimulation was linked to the presence of supernormal excitability. Without going into the details, the main arguments included: 1) the recovery of excitability after an action potential is nonlinear; and 2) during stimulation at a constant cycle length there are negative feedback processes that are established between the action potential duration, the diastolic interval and the latency of excitation, which results in specific patterns of activation.

Clearly, judicious use of nonlinear systems theory and of its mathematical tools allows one to gain insight into the principles that rule the regular and irregular behavior in cardiac tissues. This has been convincingly demonstrated not only in isolated Purkinje fibers (Chialvo and Jalife, 1987; Chialvo *et al.*, 1990a, b) and Purkinje-muscle preparations (Chialvo *et al.*, 1990b) but also in chick embryonic ventricular cell aggregates (Guevara *et al.*, 1981) as well as in the human AV conduction system (Shrier *et al.*, 1987). Although no chaotic patterns of propagation were found in the latter study, the investigators used the appropriate tools to investigate input-output responses of the AV node, and made testable predictions on the basis of such tools. In 1992, a chaos control strategy was used to stabilize arrhythmias induced by digitalis toxicity in isolated cardiac tissues (Garfinkel *et al.*, 1990). By applying electrical stimuli at irregular times determined by chaos theory, the activity recorded locally was converted to periodic beating. Whether such control paradigms are applicable to the treatment of clinical arrhythmias remains speculative.

PROPAGATION AT JUNCTIONAL SITES

Conduction velocity is not only heterogeneous within a tissue, but also across cardiac tissues. Indeed, the heart is a highly complex three-dimensional structure, composed of various regions with drastically different propagation properties. Conduction block can occur at the site in which one region meets another, simply because of the mismatch imposed by the geometrical and/or electrical properties of the tissues. An interesting example is that of the Purkinje-muscle junction (Mendez *et al.*, 1970; Sasyniuk and Mendez, 1971). A Purkinje fiber is a well-organized structure, where most of the current is densely "packed" within a group of cells that are oriented parallel to the fiber direction. The situation therefore arises where a small source of depolarizing current (the end of the Purkinje fiber) has to provide enough excitatory current for a large mass of tissue (the ventricular muscle) that is acting as a current sink (Figure 33).

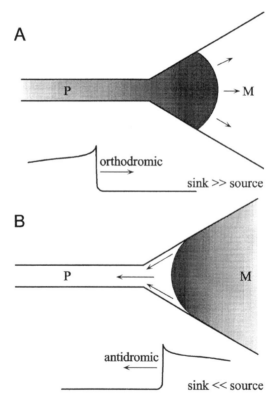

Figure 33   The funnel theory of propagation in an asymmetric sink:source system (e.g., the Purkinje (P)–muscle (M) junction. The safety factor for wave front propagation is larger in the antidromic (M to P; source≫sink) direction than in the orthodromic (P to M; sink≫source) direction.

Studies conducted on this subject have shown that the success of propagation is indeed challenged by this transition (Sasyniuk and Mendez, 1971; Fast and Kleber, 1995b). If the transition is too abrupt (i.e., if the small strand opens abruptly into a large muscle mass), propagation is more likely to fail than if the transition is more graded (e.g., if several Purkinje-muscle junctions exist within a small area). Moreover, propagation in the antidromic direction (i.e., from muscle to Purkinje) is facilitated by the fact that a larger source needs to depolarize a smaller sink (Figure 33B). This mismatch opens the possibility that unidirectional block may occur at the junction. For example, an increase in intercellular resistance at the junction would decrease the amount of excitatory current reaching the muscle during normal propagation. This decrease in the amplitude of the current source may be enough to prevent excitation of the tissue downstream. On the other hand, if propagation is moving in antidromic direction, the excitatory current may still be enough to elicit an action potential. This form of unidirectional block may serve as a source for the development of reentry (Sasyniuk and Moe, 1971). However, as demonstrated by Rohr *et al.* (1997), further uncoupling may paradoxically suppress unidirectional block, as a result of the asymmetry of the effects of uncoupling on source and sink.

The experiments of Spach *et al.* (1982b) demonstrated the conditions for unidirectional block at a branch site formed by the origin of a pectinate muscle from the larger crista terminalis in a superfused canine atrial preparation. When tissue excitability was normal, an impulse that was initiated in the crista, approached the smaller branch from either direction and propagated without block (see Figure 34A). However, when excitability was reduced by elevation of the extracellular potassium concentration, there was unidirectional block at the branch site (Figure 34B). Propagation into the pectinate muscle was still successful from above, a direction in which the branch angle was obtuse. Yet, when the impulse was initiated from below, requiring an abrupt turn of the wave front into the acutely angled branch, block

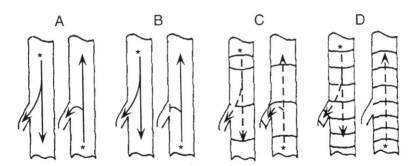

Figure 34 Unidirectional block at a branch site formed by the origin of a pectinate muscle from the larger crista terminalis in a superfused canine right atrium. A and B, behavior according to the interpretation of Spach *et al.* (1982b). A, tissue excitability is normal; an impulse initiated in the crista propagates into the smaller branch from either direction. B, when excitability is reduced by elevation of extracellular K^+ concentration, there is unidirectional block into the branch. According to Spach *et al.* (1982b), the very large anisotropy of the crista terminalis is responsible for such a behavior. C and D, alternative explanation: unidirectional block into the small branch may result from wave front curvature effects. With normal excitability (C), the wave front is able to curl into the branch regardless of its direction of propagation. Under conditions of low excitability (D), the wave front moving from the bottom upward detaches from the left border and is unable to make the steep turn into the branch. Consequently, unidirectional block occurs.

occurred. Spach *et al.* (1982b) attributed the phenomenon to the presence of anisotropy. The idea was that in the crista, the impulse traveled longitudinally with
respect to the fiber orientation but, to enter the branch, the impulse must have
changed direction and moved transversely. An alternative explanation, which had
not been considered before, is that unidirectional block was the result of a critical
curvature of the wave front (Cabo *et al.*, 1994) produced by its interaction with the
sharply angled branch site as it moved into the pectinate muscle (Cabo *et al.*, 1996).
In other words, we speculate that when propagation occurred from below, the wave
front needed to abruptly curve into the branch. When the excitability was normal,
the curved wave front remained attached to the edge of the branch site, and propagation proceeded upward, as well as into the branch (Figure 34C). However, it is
possible that, at a reduced excitability, the curved wave front first detached (Cabo
et al., 1996) from the lower branch border and then propagated up toward the upper
border without exciting the smaller branch (Figure 34D). Whether the phenomenon
of unidirectional block at branch sites depends on curvature effects or results from
nonuniform anisotropy, or from a combination of both, remains to be determined.

Stockbridge and Stockbridge (1988; see also Stockbridge, 1988) have provided
theoretical predictions and experimental demonstration that frequency-dependent
conduction patterns can be induced in bifurcating nerve axons with daughter branches
of disparate length. Indeed, short daughter branches conduct at higher rates of
stimulation than do long branches (Stockbridge, 1988). The mechanism proposed
for such phenomena is that differences in the lengths of the daughter branches
introduce different loads and threshold characteristics and, consequently, frequency-
dependence in the action potentials propagating into them (see Figure 35). Unpublished experiments from our laboratory, done several years ago by Dante Chialvo,
now at the University of Arizona, demonstrated similar frequency-dependent patterns
in branched Purkinje fibers. An example is illustrated in Figure 35A. The preparation
consisted of a main bundle of canine Purkinje cells, approximately 18 mm long and
2 mm in diameter, and a single branch, approximately 6 mm long and 1 mm in diameter, that bifurcated from the main bundle near its midpoint. During superfusion
with Tyrode solution containing 2.7 mM KCl, the fiber was stimulated at a basic cycle
length of 310 msec using current pulses (20 msec duration, 120 nA intensity; current
threshold = 100 nA) injected intracellularly via a microelectrode located near the
end of the main bundle (ME_1). The upper trace (ME_3) was obtained from a cell in
the small branch, the bottom trace (ME_2) was recorded from a cell in the distal end
of the main bundle, opposite from the stimulating electrode. Initially (left) a 4:2
activation pattern occurred at the site of current injection and at the two recording
sites (there are two responses for every four stimulus artifacts). After four repetitions
of the 4:2 pattern, 4:1 block developed at ME_2, whereas 4:2 persisted at the site of
current injection (not shown) and at the small branch. Following Stockbridge's line
of thought (Stockbridge, 1988), the difference in branch thickness and length leads
to slightly different latencies of activation at the recording sites in the two branches,
which results in slightly different times of arrival of the first stimulus after the action
potential and subsequent conduction block.

These data suggest that branching in cardiac tissues can undergo different dynamics
which may be the result of intrinsic differences in geometrical arrangements of cell
to cell connections (see also Fast and Kleber, 1995b; Rohr *et al.*, 1997).

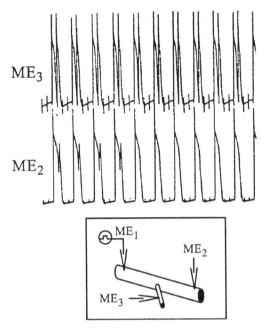

Figure 35 Complex dynamics of propagation at a branch site in an isolated dog Purkinje fiber. Top panel, transmembrane potential recordings; bottom panel, diagram of the preparation. ME_1, microelectrode used to apply repetitive intracellular current pulses at a basic cycle length of 310 msec. ME_2 microelectrode recording from the main trunk, distal to the branch site. ME_3, microelectrode recording from the short branch. Note that loading conditions were such that 4:2 activation occurred at the short branch but only 4:1 activation occurred at ME_3. Chialvo, D. and Jalife, J., unpublished observations.

ROLE OF GROSS ANATOMICAL STRUCTURE IN DISCONTINUOUS PROPAGATION

While there are many studies demonstrating the effects of structural abnormalities on propagation in the atria and ventricles (Fenoglio *et al.*, 1983; Ursell *et al.*, 1985; De Bakker *et al.*, 1988), the role of naturally occurring heterogeneities in the three-dimensional structure of cardiac tissues on propagation has been the aim of study of a small group of investigators (Spach *et al.*, 1981; Spach *et al.*, 1982a, b; Spach *et al.*, 1988; Schuessler *et al.*, 1992; Schuessler *et al.*, 1993; Gray *et al.*, 1996). Most such studies have focused on the importance of atrial structure in clinical arrhythmias such as atrial flutter (Olgin *et al.*, 1995) and fibrillation (Schuessler *et al.*, 1992; Gray *et al.*, 1996). However, while previous studies have demonstrated the importance of the atrial structure in the initiation of reentry (Spach *et al.*, 1989; Schuessler *et al.*, 1992), the question of whether reentrant arrhythmias may be the result of preferential propagation through the complicated network of pectinate muscles in the atrial subendocardium, with discordant activation of the subepicardium has only recently begun to be addressed (Gray *et al.*, 1996).

Spach *et al.* (1981; 1982a, b; 1988; 1989) have greatly advanced our understanding of the role of structural complexities in wave propagation in the atrial subendocardium.

These investigators showed that "macroscopic" discontinuities (i.e., at size scale of 1 mm or greater) in the muscle structure play an important role in the establishment of unidirectional block and the initiation of reentry. Their experiments demonstrated the role of anisotropy in unidirectional block at branch sites of the crista terminalis and pectinate muscles, and at the junction between the crista terminalis and the limbus (Spach *et al.*, 1982b). In those experiments, the safety factor for propagation was highly dependent on clearly visible changes in the gross geometry of the muscular bundles involved. The size of such structural changes (> 1 mm) is similar to that which is relevant to curvature effects leading to wavelet formation in isolated cardiac muscle (Cabo *et al.*, 1994; 1996), and may be the mechanism underlying multiple wavelet formation during reentrant arrhythmias. Schuessler *et al.* (1993) demonstrated discordant activation of the epicardium and endocardium, particularly in those areas of the atrium in which the wall thickness was greater than 0.5 mm. Discordance increased with increases in the excitation frequency, which suggested that, during high frequency excitation, discordant epicardial vs endocardial activation may lead to transmural reentry, particularly in those regions in which the three-dimensional anatomy of the atrium is most heterogeneous. More recently, we used video imaging and a voltage sensitive dye to study the role of atrial structure on activation patterns and reentry (Gray *et al.*, 1996). The results showed that the crista terminalis and pectinate muscles were sites of preferential propagation whose frequency dependence enabled disparity between endocardial and epicardial activation as well as reentry, with appearance of local block at junctional and branching points and epicardial breakthroughs. In addition, computer simulations using a model of a piece of atrial free wall connected to a single pectinate muscle bridging the wall suggested that preferential propagation through the sub-endocardial atrial muscle bundles may destabilize reentry. Those initial results indicated that preferred propagation along the pectinate muscles contributes to complexity in cardiac arrhythmias.

SUMMARY

The focus of this chapter is the study of continuous and discontinuous action potential propagation in the heart. It introduces the reader to basic concepts of electrotonic propagation and local circuit currents, and their role in active one-dimensional propagation. Based on those principles, some of the possible mechanisms by which active propagation may fail are discussed. In addition, the text brings attention to the fact that, although the unidimensional cable equations provide a good analytical tool to characterize the various electrical elements involved in the propagation process, the heart is a highly complex three-dimensional structure and its behavior commonly departs from that predicted by simple cable models. The curvature of the wave front, with its potential to lead to self-organization of the electrical activity into vortices; the property of anisotropic propagation; and the case of propagation across the Purkinje-muscle junction, all serve to illustrate the fact that cardiac impulse transmission does depart from simple unidimensional models. The chapter also discusses the dynamics and ionic mechanisms of complex patterns of propagation, such as Wenckebach periodicity, which provides a framework for the understanding of cellular and tissue behavior during high frequency excitation and arrhythmias. Given the structural complexities of the various cardiac tissues, and the complex nonlinear dynamics of cardiac cell excitation, it seems reasonable to expect that any event leading to very rapid activation of atria or ventricles may result in exceedingly complex rhythms, including fibrillation.

5 Neurohumoral Modulation of Cardiac Electrophysiologic Properties

Michael R. Rosen, Judith M.B. Pinto and Penelope A. Boyden

This chapter focuses on the sympathetic and parasympathetic innervation of the heart, the effects of autonomic neurohumors and peptides on cardiac electrical activity, and the receptor-effector pathways essential to the expression of autonomic modulation.

PARASYMPATHETIC INNERVATION AND RECEPTOR-EFFECTOR COUPLING

Vagal pathways destined to innervate the heart originate in the nucleus ambiguous or the dorsal vagal nucleus of the brain (Spyer, 1981; Machado and Brody, 1988). Preganglionic vagal fibers travel from these medullary sites via a common vago-sympathetic trunk (as in the dog) or via separate trunks (as in the human) to the cardiac neural plexus, which is a repository for preganglionic vagal and post-ganglionic sympathetic efferent fibers (Levy and Martin, 1995). Pre- and post-ganglionic vagal neurons synapse in epicardial fat pads. There is much variability of right and left cardiac innervation (Mizeres, 1958; Janes *et al.*, 1986), such that localized distribution of individual nerve bundles to specific regions of myocardium is demonstrable. However, significant overlap occurs (Randall, 1984; Ardell and Randall, 1986) and there is also crossover of right and left vagal innervation respectively to the left and right sides of the heart. Nonetheless, right vagal dominance is clearly manifested at the sinoatrial node, and vagal innervation is far more dense in the sinoatrial node, atria and atrioventricular junction, than in the ventricles. In the ventricles, innervation is greatest in the septal region, and is far less pronounced distally, in the free walls (Randall and Armour, 1977).

Effects of Vagal Stimulation and of Acetylcholine on Impulse Initiation, Refractoriness and Conduction

Sinoatrial node and atrium
Vagal stimulation decreases sinus rate, the magnitude of effect increasing with the intensity of the vagal stimulus (Löeffelholz and Pappano, 1985). Atrial effective

Certain of the studies referred to were supported by USPHS-NHLBI grants HL-28958 and HL-30557 and a grant from the Wild Wings Foundation

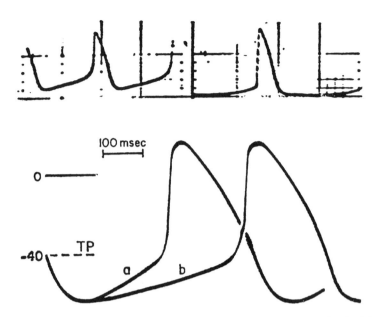

Figure 1 Effects of acetylcholine on sinus node impulse initiation. Upper panel: On the left is a rabbit sinus node action potential firing at a regular rate, with a steep slope of phase 4 depolarization and a smooth transition from phase 4 to phase 0 of the action potential. On the right are demonstrated the effects of acetylcholine. There is a more negative membrane potential, the slope of phase 4 is more shallow, there is a sharp transition from phase 4 to phase 0 (reflecting the fact that this particular cell is no longer the primary pacemaker) and the rate of impulse initiation is slower than on the left. Bottom panel: an idealized sinus node action potential showing the effects of decreasing the slope of phase 4 on the rate of impulse initiation. In "a" the slope is steep and threshold potential (TP) is reached rapidly. In "b" the slope of phase 4 has decreased (as would occur with acetylcholine superfusion) and threshold potential is reached more slowly. In this setting, rate would slow. (Modified after Hoffman and Cranefield, 1960).

refractory periods are decreased but conduction is little affected (Hoffman and Cranefield, 1960). These actions are readily understandable in light of acetylcholine effects on the action potentials and ion channels of nodal and atrial myocytes. In sinoatrial node, the vagal neurohumor, acetylcholine, decreases the slope of phase 4 depolarization, hyperpolarizes the resting membrane potential and shortens the duration of the action potential (Figure 1) (Hoffman and Cranefield, 1960). Acetylcholine effects to accelerate repolarization, shorten refractory periods, and hyperpolarize the membrane occur in atrial myocytes as well (Hoffman and Cranefield, 1960). The decrease in phase 4 depolarization is such that acetylcholine increases the time required for threshold potential to be reached; hence, the slowing of impulse initiation in sinoatrial node and atrial pacemaker fibers.

In settings where atrial repolarization is accelerated a decrease in refractory periods occurs. As a result, tachyarrhythmias such as atrial fibrillation are more readily induced (Kirchhof *et al.*, 1994). That vagal actions actually are important to the initiation of atrial fibrillation clinically has been shown in a small subset of patients (Coumel *et al.*, 1978). Moreover, it is clear that vagally-induced acceleration of repolarization and refractoriness in atrium does predispose to atrial fibrillation in the experimental laboratory (Kirchhof *et al.*, 1994), and in some patients (Coumel *et al.*, 1978); and that fibrillation, itself (or rapid pacing) further shortens repolarization, thereby facilitating both initiation and sustenance of the arrhythmia (Kirchhof *et al.*, 1994).

The ionic basis for acetylcholine's actions on the atria has been studied extensively. Early reports indicated that acetylcholine hyperpolarized the membrane by increasing its potassium permeability (Burgen and Terroux, 1953). The resultant generalized increase in outward potassium current was also thought to contribute to the hyperpolarization of the membrane, the decrease in slope of phase 4 depolarization and the acceleration of repolarization (Brown, 1982). More recent studies have shown that at least two effects of acetylcholine on ionic conductance contribute to the decreased slope of phase 4 depolarization: (1) low acetylcholine concentrations ($\sim 10^{-8}$ M) decrease the amplitude of the hyperpolarization-activated inward sodium current, I_f (DiFrancesco *et al.*, 1989). As a result, there is a reduction in inward pacemaker current during the early portion of phase 4 depolarization, a decrease the slope of phase 4 depolarization and slowing of the pacemaker rate. (2) High concentrations of acetylcholine (in the 10^{-6} M range) also increase potassium conductance (DiFrancesco *et al.*, 1989). Hence, over a wide range of concentrations, acetylcholine decreases the slope of phase 4 depolarization and rate of spontaneous impulse initiation; the effect on I_f occurs at low agonist concentrations, and that on K conductance at high concentrations.

Acetylcholine's effect to increase I_K has recently been shown to occur via an increase in $I_{K, ACh}$, an acetylcholine-activated potassium current, thereby increasing outward current flow across the membrane (Hartzell, 1988). The result is acceleration of repolarization. Acetylcholine also decreases the L type Ca^{2+} current ($I_{ca, L}$) (Löffelholz and Pappano, 1985), although much of this action is attributable to the accentuated antagonism of β-adrenergic actions on this current (see below). This effect on $I_{Ca, L}$ diminishes both the amplitude and upstroke velocity of the sinus node action potential and the plateau of atrial action potentials, and can decrease the slope of the terminal portion of phase 4 depolarization. Furthermore a decrease in inward calcium current exerts a negative inotropic effect on atrial tissues as this current is an important determinant of contractility (Löffelholz and Pappano, 1985).

Atrioventricular node
The atrioventricular nodal action potential is largely calcium-dependent. The major actions of acetylcholine on the atrioventricular node are to decrease the L-type calcium current and, to increase potassium conductance (Nishimura *et al.*, 1988). Reduction in $I_{Ca, L}$, in turn, decreases amplitude and upstroke velocity of the action potential, actions that are associated with slowing of conduction (Figure 2). The increased potassium conductance results in a decrease in action potential duration (Imaizumi *et al.*, 1990). Importantly, despite the reduction in duration of the AV nodal action potential, the effective refractory period of the node is prolonged, with refractoriness at times exceeding the duration of the action potential. This latter effect reflects the delay in recovery of $I_{Ca, L}$ from inactivation.

Ventricle
The effects of acetylcholine on the mammalian ventricle are relatively small in comparison to those on supraventricular tissues. This is determined in part by the limited vagal innervation of the ventricle (Randall and Armour, 1977) and the lesser

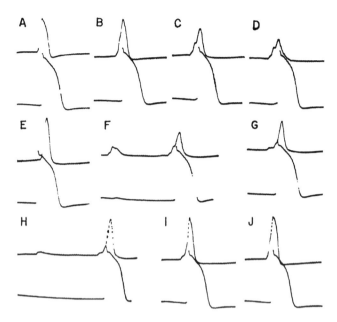

Figure 2 Effects of acetylcholine on atrioventricular nodal action potentials and conduction. Upper traces are from an atrioventricular nodal cell, lower traces from a His bundle cell of the same rabbit heart. A is a control recording with the conduction time from node to His measured between the upstrokes of the two action potentials. Panels B-I show the effects of acetylcholine. Note the progressive fragmentation and decrease in the upstroke velocity and amplitude of the AV nodal action potential, with slowing of conduction to the His bundle, while the action potential of the latter remains normal (Panels B through D). In Panel E, an infra-Hisian pacemaker has fired, and propagation still can occur retrogradely, with a high amplitude AV nodal action potential being demonstrated. In Panels F–H, with antegrade activation occurring there is intermittent conduction block between the node and the His bundle. Panels I and J are an acetylcholine washout, with normalization of both the nodal action potential and propagation. (Reprinted from Hoffman and Cranefield, p. 150, by permission).

density of acetylcholine receptors in mammalian ventricle than atrium (Fields *et al.*, 1978; Wei and Sulakhe, 1978). Hence, acetylcholine only minimally accelerates repolarization in ventricular specialized conducting fibers (and only at concentrations approximating 10^{-4} M or higher) (Danilo *et al.*, 1978). However, in the specialized conducting system of the ventricle, acetylcholine $\geq 10^{-7}$ M decreases the slope of phase 4 depolarization and rate of automaticity (Danilo *et al.*, 1978), presumably via mechanisms similar to those in atria.

Muscarinic Receptor-Effector Coupling

The discussion thus far has focussed on agonist and outcome: i.e., the actions of acetylcholine to elicit an electrophysiologic response. In this section we will consider the processes that couple the acetylcholine-bound muscarinic receptor to its physiologic expression. Three muscarinic receptors (M_1, M_2 and M_3) have been associated with a role in the heart, the dominant receptor being M_2. It appears that M_1 receptors are largely distributed in the cholinergic nerves (Jeck *et al.*, 1988) and the M_3 in vascular endothelium (Pappano, 1995). In contrast, M_2 receptors are found in the myocardium (Pappano, 1995). The result of agonist binding to the M_2 receptor is most markedly expressed with respect to pacemaker current, repolarizing potassium currents, and L type calcium current, as described above.

The immediate downstream linkage of the M_2 receptor is to G_i, a member of the 4l kD family of GTP regulatory proteins. The general role of G proteins is to couple receptors to membrane-associated enzymes and/or to an ion channel or channels. As depicted in Figure 3, G proteins consist of guanine nucleotide-binding α subunits, and smaller β and γ subunits. In the resting or unoccupied state of a receptor, the α, β and γ subunits comprise a heterotrimer, lying in close apposition to the receptor, with GDP being tightly bound to the α subunit (Quarmby and Hartzell, 1995). On binding of agonist to receptor, the latter undergoes a conformational change, linking it more tightly to the G protein whose affinity for GDP markedly decreases (Figure 3). With dissociation of GDP, the binding site is occupied by GTP, bringing about a conformational change in the α subunit, such that its affinity for the β-γ subunits and for the receptor decreases. The α and the β-γ subunits (the latter, now, a dimer) dissociate and then can regulate the activity of targets such as second messengers and ion channels. During this process, the GTP is hydrolyzed to GDP, after which there is reassociation of α and β-γ subunits into a trimer and termination of the signaling process.

Considerable disagreement has been expressed over the relative roles of α and β-γ subunits in molecular signaling. Nonetheless it is clear that the acetylcholine-activated potassium current ($I_{K, ACh}$) increases its conductance state as a result of activation by either α or β-γ subunits (Brown and Birnbaumer, 1988; Ito *et al.*, 1992; Logothetis *et al*, 1988). The unique aspect of this particular type of activation is that it reflects interaction of a G protein subunit with a site on the channel such that open time and/or gating are modified. Whether the α or β-γ subunits are the

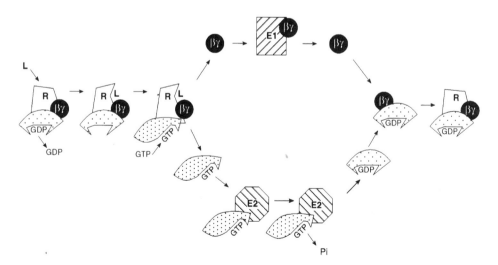

Figure 3   Model of receptor and G protein association. This schematic depicts the relationships between a receptor (R), its GTP regulatory protein, and downstream effector processes before and after ligand (L) binding. The β-γ subunit of the G protein is depicted as a black circle, the α subunit is dotted. The two effector processes are labeled E1 and E2. See text for description. (Reprinted from Quarmby and Hartzell, by permission).

physiologically more important transduction elements still is a matter of some controversy, although the weight of recent evidence appears to favor the latter (Quarmby and Hartzell, 1995; Ito *et al.*, 1992; Logothetis *et al.*, 1988).

The other functional level at which the effects of acetylcholine are expressed is via its actions on the adenylyl cyclase-cAMP second messenger system. Binding to M_2 receptors by acetylcholine and resultant activation of G_i inhibits adenylyl cyclase, resulting in a decrease in intracellular cAMP levels. This action, too, impacts on ion channels. For example, acetylcholine has no effect on basal $I_{Ca, L}$ (Fischmeister and Hartzell, 1986; Hartzell and Simmons, 1987; Hescheler *et al.*, 1986) but does decrease the $I_{Ca, L}$ that has been stimulated by adenylyl cyclase (Fischmeister and Hartzell, 1986; Hartzell and Simmons, 1987; Hescheler *et al.*, 1986). Moreover, in the setting of reduced cAMP, calcium channels are still subject to dephosphorylation by specific phosphatases (Hescheler *et al.*, 1987; Hescheler, 1988). In addition to the expression of acetylcholine effect in its own right, there is another set of effects, referred to as "accentuated antagonism" that antagonize β-adrenergic actions on the heart. These actions will be detailed subsequently.

Few studies have focussed on changes in muscarinic receptor effector pathways in diseased hearts. In patients with terminal heart failure no alterations have been seen in muscarinic receptor properties or receptor-linked G protein regulation of $I_{K, ACh}$ in isolated ventricular myocytes (Koumi *et al.*, 1997; Gruver *et al.*, 1993). However, $I_{K, ACh}$ response to acetylcholine is blunted in myocytes dispersed from diseased human atria (Koumi *et al.*, 1994).

Vagal Release of Neuropeptide

The vagus releases vasoactive intestinal peptide (VIP) from vesicles that are distinct from those which house acetylcholine in the parasympathetic terminals (Lundberg and Hökfelt, 1983). Studies of salivary gland have suggested that whereas acetylcholine release occurs under conditions of low frequency stimulation, VIP release occurs only under conditions of high frequency stimulation (DiFrancesco *et al.*, 1989; Shvilkin *et al.*, 1994; Unverferth *et al.*, 1985; Lundberg and Hökfelt, 1986) indicating that physiologic effects of VIP might be expected only on intense vagal activity.

The magnitude of VIP effect is augmented by atropine administration, consistent with an inhibitory effect of acetylcholine on VIP release at the level of presynaptic muscarinic receptors (Lundberg and Hökfelt, 1986). The mechanism of VIP action has been attributed to its binding to cardiac VIP receptors, and activation of the adenylyl cyclase-cAMP second messenger system (Christophe *et al.*, 1984; Taton *et al.*, 1982). This is the same second messenger pathway that is involved in the effects of β-adrenergic amines and that is inhibited by acetylcholine. Given that β-adrenergic agonists increase the pacemaker current, I_f, (see below) it is of note that VIP, too, increases the I_f current (Chang *et al.*, 1994). In light of this, one might expect VIP to increase heart rate. This effect has, in fact, been demonstrated in human heart (Frase *et al.*, 1987). Moreover, studies in animal models (Shvilkin *et al.*, 1994), have shown that VIP can attenuate the decrease in heart rate induced by high frequency vagal stimulation. Hence there appears to be physiological importance of VIP release as an endogenous control mechanism preventing excess bradycardia. There also may be a pathological action of VIP: i.e., excess tachycardia either following or during vagal stimulation, as has been demonstrated in animal models (Donald *et al.*, 1967; Alter *et al.*, 1973; Riegel *et al.*, 1986). This is most readily elicited following atropine administration (Henning, 1992). Whether unexpected tachycardias in response to vagal stimulation in human subjects reflect the enhanced release of VIP as a result of intense vagal stimulation (Shvilkin *et al.*, 1994; Unverferth *et al.*, 1985) is speculative at present, but worthy of consideration.

SYMPATHETIC INNERVATION AND RECEPTOR-EFFECTOR COUPLING

The origin and the determinants of distribution of cardiac sympathetic innervation are not fully understood. There is evidence for the existence of an intrinsic cardiac neural plexus during development of the embryonic and fetal heart (Ursell *et al.*, 1991a; Ursell *et al.*, 1991b). This plexus is neither cholinergic (i.e., it stains negatively for acetylcholinesterase) nor adrenergic (it stains negatively for tyrosine hydroxylase (Ursell *et al.*, 1991a; Ursell *et al.*, 1991b). However, it manifests positive staining for calcitonin gene related peptide (cGRP) (Ursell *et al.*, 1991a; Ursell *et al.*, 1991b) which is consistent with a non-adrenergic, non-cholinergic neural network.

To a great extent, sympathetic innervation of the heart occurs postnatally, via the stellate ganglia and the thoracic sympathetic trunks. As this process proceeds, the intrinsic cardiac plexus loses its characteristic cGRP staining and acquires, instead, the tyrosine hydroxylase positive staining pattern characteristic of sympathetic neural terminals (Ursell *et al.*, 1991a; Ursell *et al.*, 1991b). This has been interpreted as indicating that the ultimate distribution of sympathetic innervation results from the integration of an extrinsic source of sympathetic neurons with an intrinsic, cardiac neural plexus.

Sympathetic neural distribution is throughout the heart; i.e., at the level of the atria, atrioventricular node and ventricles. Nerve fibers travel along the epicardium and then branch transmurally to reach the midmyocardial and endocardial musculature (Inoue and Zipes, 1987). The sympathetic neurohumor, norepinephrine, binds to the receptors of two major receptor-effector coupling systems, the α- and the β-adrenergic. These will be discussed independently of one another, with the β-adrenergic first because of its more prominent role in sympathetic modulation.

Effects of β-Adrenergic Receptor Stimulation on Impulse Initiation, Refractoriness, and Conduction

Sinus node, atrium and ventricle
Because it is uniquely a β-adrenergic agonist, rather than having the β- and α-adrenergic agonist properties of norepinephrine, isoproterenol is often used to study the effects of β-adrenergic stimulation. Isoproterenol increases sinus rate, decreases atrial and ventricular effective refractory periods and either has no effect on or increases the velocity of conduction. In the sinus node, atrium and ventricle, β-adrenergic agonists induce significant hyperpolarization of membrane potential. This has been attributed to stimulation of the sodium/potassium pump, thereby increasing net outward current (Wasserstrom *et al.*, 1982), and to an increase in

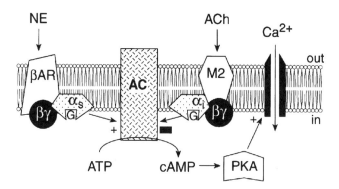

Figure 4 Accentuated antagonism of the β-adrenergic effect of norepinephrine by acetylcholine. Norepinephrine (NE) binds to the β-adrenergic receptor (BAR). Resultant signal transduction by the G protein, G_s (whose α and β-γ subunits are depicted) activates adenylyl cyclase (AC) converting ATP to cyclic AMP. Resultant protein kinase A (PKA) activation increases inward current through the calcium channel. Acetylcholine (ACh) binds to the M_2 muscarinic receptor. Resultant signal transduction by the G protein, G_i, has a braking effect on adenylyl cyclase activation. It has been noted that the effect of acetylcholine increases in the setting of increased β-adrenergic stimulation (see text). The result is a reduction in the magnitude of the inward calcium current. (Reprinted from Quarmby and Hartzell, by permission).

potassium conductance (Gadsby, 1983). There is, as well, an increase in the slope of phase 4 depolarization, that results from displacement of the current activation curve of I_f to more positive voltages (DiFrancesco, 1985). The increased slope of phase 4 depolarization brings the membrane potential to threshold more rapidly, resulting in an increase in cardiac rate. This effect on phase 4 depolarization holds true not only for sinus node, but for other pacemakers as well.

   β-adrenergic agonists also accelerate repolarization (and with this, shorten refractoriness) via actions on potassium currents. The main effect of β-adrenergic agonists on repolarization is via stimulation of the delayed rectifier current, I_{Ks} (Sanguinetti *et al.*, 1991). The resultant increase in outward current decreases the duration of the action potential. β-adrenergic agonist stimulation also increases the L-type Ca current (Figure 4) (Osaka and Joyner, 1992), thereby elevating the plateau and tending to prolong the action potential. The net effect of agonist, then, will depend upon the balance of effects between the increased inward calcium and outward potassium currents.

The atrioventricular node
The atrioventricular nodal action potential is primarily determined by the inward calcium current, $I_{Ca, L}$. β-adrenergic agonists increase $I_{Ca, L}$ density, thereby increasing the amplitude and upstroke velocity of the nodal action potential, and concurrently increasing its velocity of propagation (Billette and Shrier, 1995). Atrioventricular nodal refractoriness tends to be decreased, as well (Billette and Shrier, 1995).

Beta-Adrenergic Receptor Subtypes

Thus far we have described β-adrenergic actions in light of agonist effect on action potentials and on ion channels. However, there are at least two functional β-adrenergic receptor systems in heart, the β_1 and β_2 (Steinberg *et al.*, 1998). A third receptor, β_3, has been described in heart but its transduction pathway and physiology are in the early stages of study (Gauthier *et al.*, 1996). In this section we shall relate the actions of β adrenergic stimulation, described above, to specific subtype pathways. Major electrophysiologic effects occur as a result of β_1 and β_2 adrenergic receptor stimulation. β_1- and β_2-adrenoceptors have been demonstrated in hearts of many species via autoradiographic and functional techniques (Akahane *et al.*, 1989). β_1 and β_2 receptor ratios vary widely, depending on tissues, species, and techniques, from 10/90 in guinea pig ventricle (e.g., Molenaar *et al.*, 1990) to $\sim$30/70 in human atrium (Brodde, 1991) and $\sim$40/60 in guinea pig His bundle (Molenaar *et al.*, 1990).

In the canine ventricle, β_1-adrenergic receptor-effector coupling is the major sympathetic determinant of electrical activity. However, a β_2-adrenergic pathway contributes importantly in normal supraventricular tissues to increase heart rate, atrioventricular conduction velocity, and atrial contractility, and to decrease atrial refractory periods (Akahane *et al.*, 1989; Motomura and Hashimoto, 1992; Takei *et al.*, 1992). Species differences are seen in β_2-adrenergic actions. For example, in sheep, β_2-adrenoceptor stimulation does not increase automaticity in Purkinje fibers, is important to the acceleration of repolarization in Purkinje fibers, and has no effect on repolarization in ventricular muscle (Borea *et al.*, 1992). These observations also emphasize that stimulation of the same receptor subtype in different tissues of any one species may have different effects. Finally, in rabbit, β_2-adrenergic receptor stimulation increases sinus node automaticity and accelerates repolarization in both Purkinje fibers and papillary muscles (Dukes and Vaughan-Williams, 1984), a marked contrast to sheep and dog, further emphasizing the importance of species variations.

In human heart, β_2-adrenergic agonists induce tachycardia by stimulating β_2-adrenergic receptors in the sinoatrial node (Hall *et al.*, 1989) and induce a positive inotropic response by stimulating β_2-adrenergic receptors in ventricular myocytes (Bristow *et al.*, 1986; Altschuld *et al.*, 1995). Moreover, there appears to be a change in function of β_2-receptor pathways in the setting of disease. For example, β_2-receptors assume increased importance as a mechanism for the inotropic support of the failing or aging heart, where there is a selective down-regulation of β_1-adrenergic receptors (Bristow *et al.*, 1986; Bristow *et al.*, 1989; Marzo *et al.*, 1991; White *et al.*, 1994). There is also evidence for upregulation of β_2-receptors in denervated, transplanted human hearts (Farrukh *et al.*, 1993; Brodde *et al.*, 1991). Finally, recent clinical trials have shown that nonselective β-blockers reduce sudden cardiac death in the post-myocardial infarction period, whereas β_1-receptor-selective blockers do not (BEST, 1995). All these studies suggest that β_2-receptors have been underestimated as clinically important mediators of arrhythmias in the setting of myocardial dysfunction.

Beta-Adrenergic Receptor-Effector Coupling

The positive chronotropic, inotropic, and relaxant effects of cardiac β_1-adrenergic receptor stimulation are transduced via coupling to the GTP regulatory protein, G_s. The downstream pathway involves activation of adenylyl cyclase, accumulation of intracellular cAMP, and stimulation of cAMP-dependent protein kinase (PKA), which phosphorylates cellular target proteins (Figure 4). Despite the fact that β_1- and β_2-adrenergic receptors are coupled via G_s to adenylyl cyclase, there are important differences in the coupling mechanism (Levy *et al.*, 1993) that reflect the molecular diversity of the β-adrenergic receptor subtypes, the G protein subunits and/or adenylyl cyclase. As for G_i, described above, activation of G_s leads to the liberation of α subunits as well as β-γ dimers which appear to possess independent functions in β-receptor signaling. In addition, cardiac myocytes express several molecular forms of the G protein γ subunit, adding further complexity to the system, as γ subunits appear to influence the ability of individual G proteins to discriminate between receptors and effector mechanisms (Kleuss *et al.*, 1993; Kisselev *et al.*, 1993). Finally, diversity of G protein function need not be confined to the G_s protein, alone, as β_2-receptors reportedly activate G_i in adult rat ventricular myocytes (Xiao *et al.*, 1995).

There is also diversity of adenylyl cyclase, for which several forms identified in cardiac tissue have been cloned. The regulation of adenylyl cyclase activity depends on the isoform composition in any cell system, since all membrane-bound forms of adenylyl cyclase are activated by $G_{s\alpha}$, yet they exhibit markedly different patterns of regulation by other cofactors (Taussig *et al.*, 1995). In sum, individual cell populations may possess unique capabilities to receive and integrate signals via the cAMP pathway as a result of differences in the ratio of individual adenylyl cyclase isoforms, while individual isoforms may mediate specialized functions in cell signaling.

As a result of adenylyl cyclase activity, cAMP is formed and then binds to the regulatory subunits of protein kinase A, resulting in release of its catalytic subunits and the phosphorylation of target proteins. However, there is important evidence that cAMP release may be compartmentalized. For example, in frog ventricular myocytes (Jurevicius and Fischmeister, 1996), β-adrenergic receptor activation induces localized elevations in intracellular cAMP which activates only the L-type calcium channels in the immediate vicinity of the β-adrenergic receptor. This compartmentalized elevation of cAMP provides a potential mechanism for hormone-specific activation of protein kinase A, suggesting that different initiating hormonal signals may induce spatially restricted elevations in cAMP, thereby activating specific pools of protein kinase A in cardiac myocytes.

Beta-Adrenergic Receptor-Effector Coupling in Hypertrophy and in Failure

Ventricular hypertrophy is associated with a downregulation and desensitization of myocardial β-adrenergic receptors, especially β_1, (Schumacher *et al.*, 1995); hence, the positive inotropic effect of isoproterenol is reduced (Meszaros *et al.*, 1992). There may be an uncoupling of β-adrenergic receptors from calcium channels through damage of the catalytic subunit of adenylyl cyclase, and a decrease in intracellular cAMP concentration (Schumacher *et al.*, 1995), although in some studies, inotropic effects of isoproterenol are reduced but the effect on $I_{Ca, L}$ remains unchanged (Legssyer *et al.*, 1997).

Only one study shows an enhancement of β adrenergic responsiveness as assessed by an increased frequency of isoproterenol-induced automaticity in hypertension-induced hypertrophy (Barbieri *et al.*, 1994). In spite of this enhanced response, the levels of cAMP before and after isoproterenol in hypertensive animals were significantly lower than those in age matched controls.

Like hypertrophy, heart failure is associated with changes in the β-adrenergic pathways that reduce the degree of inotropic stimulation produced by β adrenergic agonists. These changes include downregulation of β_1 adrenergic receptors (Bristow *et al.*, 1990; Bristow *et al.*, 1989; Bohm *et al.*, 1989; Fowler *et al.*, 1986), increase in the ratio of β_2 to β_1 adrenoreceptors (Gengo *et al.*, 1992), uncoupling of β_2 adrenergic receptors (Bristow *et al.*, 1990), change in the number of calcium channels (Gruver *et al.*, 1993; Gengo *et al.*, 1992), and increase in the functional activity of the inhibitory G protein (Feldman *et al.*, 1988).

Whereas some studies have reported that some ionic current responses to isoproterenol and PKA are reduced in heart failure (Koumi *et al.*, 1995), others have reported that β adrenergic or forskolin stimulation of $I_{Ca, L}$ in myocytes from hearts of patients with heart failure remains qualitatively intact (Beuckelmann *et al.*, 1991; Mewes and Ravens, 1994). Finally, in two mouse models, one of hypertrophy and the other of heart failure (Gomez *et al.*, 1997), it has been suggested that defective excitation-contraction coupling is restored in hypertrophied cells with β-adrenergic stimulation (where isoproterenol can still increase $I_{Ca, L}$ but cannot be restored in failing myocytes where the β-adrenergic $I_{Ca, L}$ response is poor (Gomez *et al.*, 1997).

Interestingly, it appears that positive inotropic responses to the β_2 adrenergic stimulation are upregulated in myocytes from pacing-induced failed hearts. The stimulation is not mediated by increases in cAMP or cAMP-dependent phosphorylation of phospholamban (Altschuld *et al.*, 1995) consistent with an increase in β_2 receptor function.

Beta-Adrenergic Receptor-Effector Coupling in Myocardial Infarction

During sympathetic stimulation, shortening of action potentials is minimal in the areas overlying the infarct and in the border zone, compared to areas remote from the infarct (Gaide *et al.*, 1983). Catecholamine-induced increase of the plateau phase of action potentials is absent in the fibers of the epicardial border zone of the 5-day and 14 day infarcted heart (Boyden *et al.*, 1988). Similar abbreviated responses to catecholamines have been documented in ischemic human ventricle (Mubagwa *et al.*, 1994). Furthermore, the inotropic response to isoproterenol is severely blunted in infarction despite a large increase in the amplitude of the Ca^{2+} transient (Litwin *et al.*, 1992). Compared to normal cells, isoproterenol produces a smaller increase in $I_{Ca, L}$ in cells from the 5 day and 2 month old infarct, independent of calcium-dependent inactivation (Pinto *et al.*, 1997; Aggarwal *et al.*, 1996). This is consistent with multiple defects in components of the β-adrenergic receptor complex in epicardial border zone cells of the 5 day old infarct, including decreases in β-adrenergic receptor density; diminished basal, guanine nucleotide-, isoproterenol-, forskolin- and manganese-dependent adenylyl cyclase activities, increases in the EC_{50} for isoproterenol-dependent activation of adenylate cyclase, diminished levels of the α-subunit of the G_s protein and elevated levels of the α-subunit of the G_i protein (Steinberg *et al.*, 1995).

In the areas remote from the infarct, isoproterenol increases $I_{Ca, L}$ to a lesser extent than in control myocytes (Pinto *et al.*, 1997). Another study of right ventricular hypertrophied muscle from rats with myocardial infarction shows that responsiveness to the β adrenergic agonist dobutamine remains unchanged at 1 or 4 weeks after infarction (Itaya *et al.*, 1990).

Alpha-Adrenergic Receptor Stimulation

The heterogeneity of α_1-adrenergic receptors across different types of tissues and species of animals represents a situation analogous to, albeit more diverse, than that of the β-adrenergic receptors. Three α_1-adrenergic and 3 α_2-adrenergic receptor subtypes have been identified. This discussion will concentrate on the α_1 as there is only limited information concerning α_2-adrenergic actions on cardiac muscle (see Jurevicius and Fischmeister, 1996 for review).

Alpha$_1$-adrenergic receptor-effector coupling
There are three cloned α_1-adrenergic receptors: α_{1a} (formerly α_{1c}), α_{1b} and α_{1d} (formerly $\alpha_{1a/d}$) (Hieble *et al.*, 1995) . These correspond to the three native, and pharmacologically identified receptor subtypes, α_{1A}, α_{1B} and α_{1D} (Hieble *et al.*, 1995). Although $\alpha_{1a, b \text{ and } d}$ receptors all have been cloned in heart, pharmacologic and physiologic evidence of a functional α_{1d} receptor is uncertain. The pharmacologic α_{1A} subtype is blocked by the relatively selective drugs, WB4101 and 5 methylurapidil (Bylund *et al.*, 1994). The α_{1A}-adrenergic receptor pathway is transduced by a GTP-dependent process (perhaps via the G protein G_q) and induces an increase in phosphoinositide metabolism (Molina-Viamonte *et al.*, 1990; Steinberg *et al.*, 1987) to activate protein kinase C. Because the increase in automaticity of normal Purkinje fibers by α agonist is attenuated by ryanodine, it has been suggested that sarcoplasmic reticulum calcium release may be an important component of this pathway (Anyukhovsky *et al.*, 1992). However, most studies of α agonist have described at best a modest (<10%) increment in intracellular calcium (see Terzic *et al.*, 1993 for review). Therefore, it has been hypothesized that, in contrast to β-adrenergic agonists, the effect of α agonists to increase contractility derives more from sensitization of myofibrillar elements to existing intracellular calcium levels than from an actual increase in intracellular calcium (Terzic *et al.*, 1993).

Effects of α-Adrenergic Stimulation on Impulse Initiation, Refractoriness and Conduction

Intravenous infusion of α_1-adrenergic agonists has a profound effect to slow sinus rate. However, rather than reflecting a major action on sinus node pacemaker current, this reflects the peripheral vasoconstriction and increase in blood pressure induced by α_1-adrenergic agonists, resulting in a vagal baroreceptor response that increases acetylcholine release to slow sinus rate via the M_2 muscarinic receptor pathway. Diverse effects of α-adrenergic receptor stimulation are found in different tissues and in different species, as follows: in atrial myocytes of rabbit (Dukes and Vaughan-Williams, 1984), rat (Ertl *et al.*, 1991) and guinea pig (Pappano, 1971); in ventricular epicardial myocytes of dog (Lee *et al.*, 1991), rabbit (Dukes and Vaughan Williams, 1984) and rat (Apkon and Nerbonne, 1988); and in Purkinje fibers of dog (Lee *et al.*, 1991), sheep (Ledda *et al.*, 1971) and rabbit (Dukes and Vaughan Williams, 1984), α agonists prolong repolarization. This prolongation of repolarization is of greater magnitude in specialized conducting than myocardial tissues (Lee *et al.*, 1991). Prolongation of action potential duration in the canine heart appears to result from stimulation of the α_{1A}-adrenergic receptor, in that the effect is blocked by the

α_{1A}-adrenergic blocker WB4101 but not the α_{1B}-adrenergic blocker, chloroethyl-clonidine (CEC) (Lee *et al.*, 1991; Lee and Rosen, 1994). The prolongation of repolarization appears to have different receptor-effector linkages in different species: in rat (Apkon and Nerbonne, 1988) and rabbit (Fedida *et al.*, 1990) the transient outward potassium current, I_{to1}, is blocked by α_1-adrenergic agonist. I_{to1} is a major repolarizing current in these species. In contrast, in the dog, α_1-adrenergic stimulation appears to have no effect on I_{to1}; rather it is I_{Ks} that is blocked to prolong action potential duration (Liu *et al.*, 1997). It should be noted, as well, that prolongation of repolarization does not occur in all species; in guinea pig ventricle α-adrenergic agonist decreases action potential duration, an effect that appears to derive from activation of I_{K1} (Dirksen and Sheu, 1990).

The other major effect of α-adrenergic agonist is on impulse initiation. In normal adult canine Purkinje fiber, and sympathetically-innervated neonatal rat ventricle, α-adrenergic agonist decreases automaticity (Rosen *et al.*, 1977). This results from stimulation of the sodium/potassium pump, generating a net outward current that is opposite to the pacemaker current (Shah *et al.*, 1988; Zaza *et al.*, 1990). The pathway here is blocked by CEC and not WB4101, indicating that it is α_{1B}-adrenergic (Del Balzo *et al.*, 1990). Moreover, it depends on signal transduction by a G protein of the 41 kD family (to which G_i belongs, as well) (Steinberg *et al.*, 1985). It appears that sympathetic innervation must be present for this G protein to express its function and for the decrease in automaticity to occur. In fact, in young dogs (Rosen *et al.*, 1977) as well as in non-innervated neonatal rat myocytes in tissue culture (Drugge and Robinson, 1987) in which there is minimal (dog) or no (neonatal rat culture) sympathetic innervation and little demonstrable 41 kD G protein, α-adrenergic agonists increase automaticity, an effect blocked by WB4101 but not CEC (Del Balzo *et al.*, 1990). That the G protein is a critical factor here is seen in the fact that α_{1B}-adrenergic receptor density in the neonate is equivalent to that in the adult; it is the functional signal transduction protein that is lacking (Del Balzo *et al.*, 1990).

Finally, α-adrenergic agonists have a role in the setting of myocardial ischemia and infarction. In ischemic settings, depolarized canine Purkinje fibers manifesting abnormal automaticity show an α-adrenergic agonist-induced increase in automatic rate that is blocked by WB4101, but not CEC (Anyukhovsky *et al.*, 1992, 1997). In addition, in an intact feline model, ischemic arrhythmias induced by coronary artery occlusion are reduced in incidence by α_1-adrenergic blockade (Sheridan *et al.*, 1980).

In infarcted regions of myocardium membrane-bound α adrenergic receptors appear to be functionally intact, in that phenylephrine increases $I_{Ca,L}$ in the healed infarct to the same extent as in control cells (Pinto *et al.*, 1997). Similarly, no change in the sensitivity to the α adrenergic agonist phenylephrine in stimulating $I_{Ca,L}$ is seen in cells remote from the infarct site in feline hearts 2 months after infarction (Pinto *et al.*, 1997).

Sympathetic Release of Neuropeptides

Neuropeptide Y (NPY) is ubiquitous in mammalian heart, where it usually co-localizes with norepinephrine in sympathetic nerve terminals (reviewed in Walker *et al.*, 1991) and can be released with catecholamines during sympathetic neural activation (Gu *et al.*, 1984; Haas *et al.*, 1989). NPY affects the heart in three major ways: through a postjunctional vasoconstrictor action; through prejunctional inhibition of mediator release from sympathetic and parasympathetic nerve endings (reviewed in Walker *et al.*, 1991; Edvinsson *et al.*, 1987; Potter, 1988) and via postjunctional effects on myocardium (McDermott *et al.*, 1993).

Surface membranes of cardiomyocytes have binding sites for NPY with an affinity in the nanomolar range (Balasubramaniam *et al.*, 1990). In concentrations of 10^{-9} to 10^{-5} M NPY suppresses contractile activity (Millar *et al.*, 1991; Piper *et al.*, 1989) and decreases the transient outward current I_{to}, the L-type calcium current, and the delayed rectifier current I_K (Millar *et al.*, 1991; Bryant *et al.*, 1991) in isolated ventricular myocytes. However, the physiologic significance of NPY's postjunctional effects on cardiomyocytes remains controversial. For example, reports on inotropic effects of NPY on isolated cardiac muscle are contradictory (McDermott *et al.*, 1993), and the effective concentrations of NPY in vitro are substantially higher than those measured in human plasma (Lundberg *et al.*, 1985; Pernow *et al.*, 1986). Hence, they are meaningful only on the additional assumption that an increased local concentration of NPY exists in the immediate vicinity of target cells (Potter, 1988).

NPY decreases heart rate by inhibiting mediator release from sympathetic and parasympathetic nerve terminals (reviewed in Potter, 1988). Postjunctionally, NPY does not affect cardiac rhythm in situ (McDermott *et al.*, 1993) nor does it change the beating rates of isolated hearts consistently (Allen *et al.*, 1986; Allen *et al*, 1983; Rioux *et al.*, 1985; Warner and Levy, 1989). In various animal experiments, exogenous NPY does not or only minimally modifies atrial automaticity (Allen *et al.*, 1986; Sosunov *et al.*, 1996). However, NPY has been shown to decrease the pacemaker current I_f in isolated preparations of canine Purkinje fibers (Chang *et al.*, 1994). This implies a negative chronotropic effect on the pacemaker tissue and raises the possibility of direct postjunctional effects of NPY on cardiac pacemakers. However, no counterpart to these actions has been seen in intact hearts.

PARASYMPATHETIC-SYMPATHETIC INTERACTIONS

Thus far, this presentation of cardiac electrophysiologic effects of the autonomic nervous system has focused on each system in isolation. Yet a major aspect of autonomic input to the heart is seen in the interaction of the vagal and sympathetic nervous systems. Specifically, there is a β-adrenergic-muscarinic interaction referred to as "accentuated antagonism" (Levy, 1971) that strongly influences the expression of heart rate and rhythm. This interaction centers on the M_2 muscarinic receptor and β_1-adrenergic receptor linkage to adenylyl cyclase via their respective G proteins, G_i and G_s. Using automaticity as an example, the effect of vagal stimulation, alone, would be to decrease I_f and increase potassium conductance (DiFrancesco *et al.*, 1989), possibly via G protein subunit occupancy of channels, and definitely by decreasing cAMP synthesis and reducing PKA activation. In contrast, the effect of β-adrenergic stimulation, alone, is to activate adenylyl cyclase via G_s, to increase cAMP synthesis, and – via PKA – to increase phase 4 depolarization and automatic rate.

Of note is that in the setting of increased sympathetic tone, there is an ever greater effect of M_2 receptor stimulation to counteract the β-adrenergic (Fleming *et al.*, 1987):

hence, the term, "accentuated antagonism." This is demonstrated with respect to calcium current in Figure 4. In essence, as adenylyl cyclase activation and cAMP synthesis are increased by β_1-adrenergic receptor activation, there is increasing expression of acetylcholine's suppressant effect, via the M_2 receptor and G_i. In this way, the parasympathetic system operates as a "brake" to modulate the sympathetic, thus determining the ultimate expression of autonomic effects on the heart. To some extent these actions may be further influenced by the neuropeptides (see preceding sections on VIP and NPY).

Finally, it should be noted that acetylcholine – α_1-adrenergic interactions occur as well, but detail is as yet insufficient to understand the relative importance of this interaction and the signal transduction that is operative. Experiments in guinea pig heart suggest that activation of an α_{1B}-adrenergic receptor induces a decrease in heart rate, and that this decrease is augmented by M_2 muscarinic stimulation (Chevalier *et al.*, 1998) . Whether such interactions occur in other species and whether they are limited uniquely to the α_{1B} and M_2 receptors remains to be tested.

CONCLUSIONS

The autonomic modulation of cardiac electrical activity is a richly complex subject. It depends on innervation by the two limbs of the autonomic nervous system, and the expression of diverse neurohumoral receptor-effector coupling pathways. Each of these pathways not only is internally consistent in its own right, but interacts importantly with other pathways to determine the ultimate end-organ response. Autonomic modulation is determined as well by neurally-released peptides which have effects of their own, as well as interactions with the autonomic neurohumors.

ACKNOWLEDGMENT

The authors expresses their gratitude to Ms. Eileen Franey for her careful attention to the preparation of the manuscript.

6 Pharmacological Modulation of Cardiac Electrophysiologic Properties

Walter Spinelli

MECHANISM OF ION CHANNEL BLOCKADE

The mechanism of block of ion channels was first explored by Armstrong (1971) in the squid giant axon employing derivatives of tetraethylammonium (TEA), a class of compounds that block the delayed rectifier K^+ channel. These and other studies showed that the receptor for TEA is within the channel pore and that the blocker enters the channel from the cytoplasm (axoplasm). TEA and its derivatives block the channels by interacting with a specific receptor/binding site located inside the pore, so that ion conductance falls to zero while the blocker is inside the channel (See Figure 1). Further studies indicated that the access to the pore is restricted by an activation gate: TEA and other permanently charged analogs can only enter when the channel is in the open state, i.e., when the gate is open, and, conversely, closure of the gate can trap the blocker inside the pore.

Voltage clamp studies showed that if the blocked channels were held, between pulses, at a negative holding potential, then, with time, all channels become unblocked. Using two-pulse activating protocols, it was found that blockers can leave from the channel in two kinetically distinct phases, an initial rapid phase followed by a slower phase. In the first phase, immediately following the activating step that opens the channels, some of the molecules can leave the pore before the activation gates closes upon repolarization, accounting for the initial rapid unblocking. However, a large percentage of the molecules cannot leave before the activation gates close and remain trapped in the rested channels. This fraction of the molecules can only leave when the channels reopen randomly from the closed state, accounting for the slow phase of unblock (Armstrong, 1975).

From these and other findings, it is possible to build the following model of the channel (Figure 1). From the cytoplasmic site, the blocker first encounters an activation gate, which must be open to let the blocker enter a vestibule ($> 10\,\text{Å}$ wide), where the receptor and hydrophobic residues are located. The presence of the hydrophobic regions is required in order to accommodate the hydrophobic moieties present in many blocker molecules. Studies with a variety of blockers have indicated that the binding site is rather close to the cytoplasmic side of the membrane, approximately 15–20% of the way across the transmembrane electric field. The vestibule is connected to the external side by a narrow selectivity filter ($3.3\,\text{Å}$ wide)

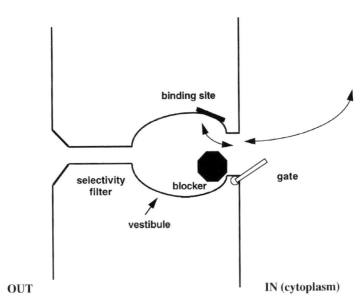

Figure 1   Simplified model of a delayed rectifier potassium channel showing the receptor site for TEA.

that restricts the blocker molecule in the vestibule when the cytoplasmic gate is closed. Hydrophilic blockers can reach and leave the receptor site only via the pore. This simple yet robust model of the channel and of the mechanism of block is over 20 years old and has provided the basis of our understanding of how small organic molecules block ion channels.

Na^+ Channel Blockade

The block of Na^+ channels by local anesthetic antiarrhythmic agents (Na^+ channel blockers) was extensively characterized by Hille (1977). Most local anesthetics share a basic pharmacophore consisting of an aromatic moiety linked by a carbon chain of variable length to a tertiary or secondary nitrogen group. In some compounds, the substituents R_2 and R_3 can be linked and form a heterocyclic moiety (e.g., flecainide). The linker can be a benzamide (e.g., flecainide), an anilino amide (e.g., lidocaine), or an ether (e.g., mexiletine) (Figure 2). These molecules can exist either as tertiary, secondary, or primary amines, or as positively charged ammonium cations. The dissociation constant of the molecule (pK_a) and the pH of the solution regulate the degree of ionization. As most blockers are weak acids with pK_a ranging from 8 to 9, only a small fraction of the molecules are in the uncharged form at physiological pH (Figure 2).

The uncharged form is more lipid-soluble and can diffuse from the extracellular space into the cytoplasm across the lipid bilayer. Once in the cytoplasm, after the molecule has achieved the ionization state dictated by its pK_a and by the intracellular pH, the charged cationic form seems to be the active blocking form. This was shown by altering the medium pH, and thus the ratio of uncharged to charged molecules, without changing the total concentration of the blocker (Ritchie and Greengard,

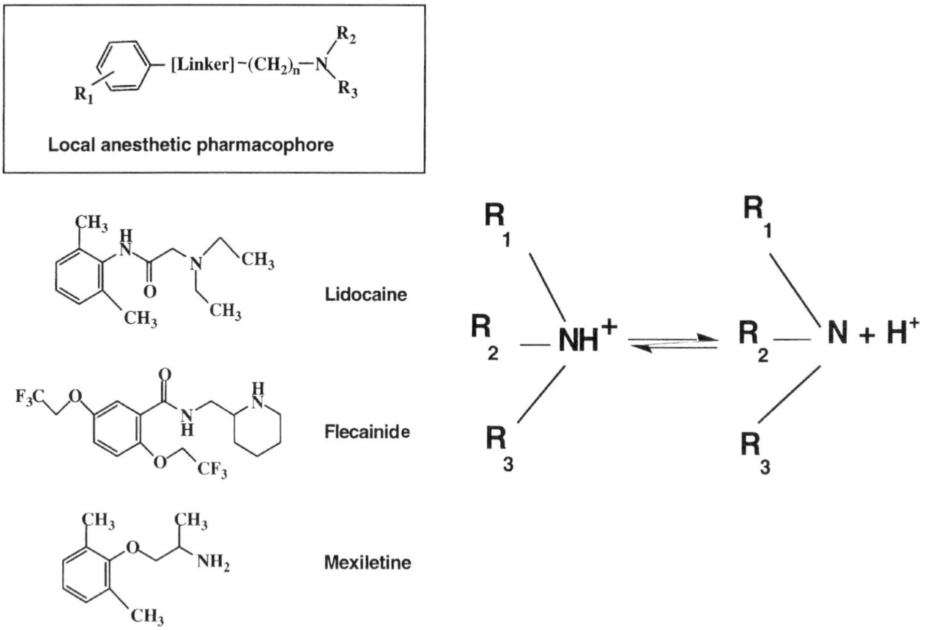

Figure 2 Examples of local anesthetic antiarrhythmic agents. The charge of the amino group is determined by its pKa value and by the environment pH.

1966). The predominant blocking role of the cationic form was also confirmed by the use of permanently charged (quaternary) derivatives of local anesthetics (Narahashi and Frazier, 1971).

Based on studies with permanently charged molecules, we can envision the cationic drug molecule entering and blocking the channel from the cytoplasm. Blocking and unblocking is regulated by activation and inactivation gates and requires open channels. Tertiary and secondary amines behave differently depending on the medium pH. There are at least two pathways to the binding site depending on the charge and physicochemical characteristics of the molecule: there is the "hydrophilic" pathway through the open channel, and the "hydrophobic" pathway through the lipid bilayer of the membrane. At low pH, the molecule is in the charged form and behaves like a permanently charged quaternary derivative entering the channel via a hydrophilic pathway, the open channel pore. When the pH is high, the molecules are in the uncharged and more lipid-soluble form, and can reach the binding site independently of the channel opening via a second hydrophobic pathway. Experimental findings suggest that, even when the blocker is bound inside the channel, the gating of the channel continues to operate and regulates the binding and unbinding of the blocker. However, blockers can significantly affect the gating process. In their presence, the inactivation of the Na^+ channel is intensified and a larger membrane hyperpolarization is needed to remove inactivation and to relieve the channel block (Weidmann, 1955b). Thus, local anesthetic blockers can be thought to bind preferably to the inactivated state of the channel, rather than to the open or rested state.

K⁺ Channel Blockade

The model of the receptor of the local anesthetic blockers resembles that of blockers of the delayed rectifier K^+ channel, albeit with important differences (Figure 3). A gating process restricts the access of the blocker from the cytoplasmic side, but in this case, the model includes two gates, thereby accounting for activation and inactivation properties of the Na^+ channel. Hydrophilic molecules require open gates to enter a vestibule where the receptor and a hydrophobic region are located. The hydrophobic region is thought to provide a binding site for the aromatic moiety of local anesthetic molecules. Electrophysiological evidence examining block at steady state shows that the receptor is located in the middle of the transmembrane electric field, much deeper than in the case of the delayed rectifier K^+ channel. Finally, a selectivity filter restricts passage to the extracellular space. The movement of drug molecules to and from the binding site is governed by the membrane potential and by the state of the channel: open, closed, and, in the case of the Na^+ channel, inactivated (Hille, 1992).

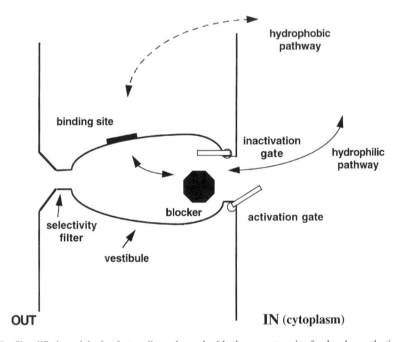

Figure 3 Simplified model of a fast sodium channel with the receptor site for local anesthetic antiarrhythmic agents.

Ca²⁺ Channel Blockade

There are five major chemical classes of Ca^{2+} channel blockers. However, only verapamil, a phenylalkylamine, diltiazem, a benzothiazepine, and bepridil, a diarylaminopropylamine, block cardiac L-type Ca^{2+} channels at clinically relevant concentrations. The block with verapamil and other phenylalkylamines shows similarities to that with local anesthetic antiarrhythmic agents. Studies with a derivative of verapamil indicate that the molecule acts from the inside of the membrane and that block and rapid unblocking require the opening of the channel. Hydrophilic uncharged blockers can only leave slowly when the gates are closed, and quaternary derivatives, like blockers of Na^+ and K^+ channels, can be trapped in the closed channel. However, binding studies with other classes of commonly used Ca^{2+} channel blockers show that these molecules are not competing for a single binding site (Glossman *et al.*, 1984). These and other observations of agonist-antagonistic activity with dihydropyridines (Hess *et al.*, 1984), another class of Ca^{2+} channels blockers, have raised the possibility of the existence of multiple binding sites.

Role of Molecular Biology in Advancing our Understanding of Channel Blockade

Recently, molecular biology techniques have greatly increased our understanding of the structure of the binding sites for Na^+, K^+ and Ca^{2+} channels. Point mutations of the S6 domain of the fourth internal repeat (IVS6) of the α subunit of the brain and heart Na^+ channel have profound effects on the binding of local anesthetic anti-arrhythmic agents and on channel behavior. The binding site for lidocaine in the rat brain Na^+ channel seems to be defined by three amino acids. Phenylalanine (F) 1764 and tyrosine (Y) 1771 are integral componenets of the binding site, while the more external isoleucine (I) 1760 provides a boundary to the receptor (Figure 4). Muta-tion of I1760 to a smaller alanine opens a new pathway allowing access to the receptor from the extracellular side of the membrane. Mutations in the IVS6 region

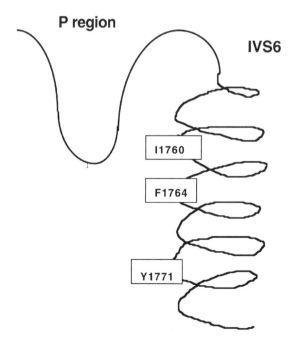

Figure 4   Schematic representation of the binding site of local anesthetic antiarrhythmic agents showing three crucial aminoacid residues.

drastically decrease the block by local anesthetics, alter their frequency dependent effects, and create a new access pathway to the receptor (Qu *et al.*, 1995; Ragsdale *et al.*, 1994). Similar mutations in analogous locations in Ca^{2+} channels also decrease channel block by D888, a phenylalkylamine calcium channel blocker. A different site, however, was responsible for the binding of dihydropyridines, as expected from previous electrophysiological and binding evidence (Hockerman *et al.*, 1995). Thus, these data point to structural determinants that might explain the different specificity of several ion channel blockers. Taken together, these results suggest that the receptor for local anesthetic antiarrhythmic agents is located within the cytoplasmic half of the transmembrane pore and that three specific amino acids in the IVS6 region of the α subunit are required to define high affinity binding and to preserve frequency-dependent block of the channel. Ca^{2+} channel antagonists of the phenylalkylamine, benzothiazepine, and dihydropyridine classes interact with amino acid residues in analogous positions in the IVS6 region of the α_1 region of the L-type Ca^{2+} channel (for a review, see Hockerman *et al.*, 1997).

Recent results have also provided a new understanding of the structural details of the binding site of blockers of cardiac K^+ channels. The binding site for TEA in the drosophila *Shaker* potassium channels is defined by a threonine (T441) in the middle of the P region at the inner mouth of the channel (Choi *et al.*, 1993). This residue, which is highly conserved across different types of K^+ channels, is located proximally to the cytoplasmic side of the channel. This finding is consistent with previous electrophysiological estimates that suggested a location for the TEA receptor 20% of the way across the transmembrane field. Quinidine, a blocker of the Na^+ channel, is also a nonselective blocker of several classes of K^+ channels. The binding of quinidine in the cloned human delayed rectifier channel Kv1.5 is stabilized by hydrophobic interactions deep in the channel pore with amino acid residues that belong to the S6 region (Yeola *et al.*, 1996). Surprisingly, these results show that the S6 domain plays an important role in the open channel block of quinidine, while the equivalent TEA binding site (T477) in the P region seems less important, as mutations that reduced the affinity of TEA in *Shaker* and Kv2.1 K^+ channels by more than one order of magnitude caused only a modest decrease of quinidine's block in hKv1.5. These results show that hydrophobic interactions in S6 have an importance probably equivalent to the ionic interactions that take place at the tertiary (or quaternary) amino group characteristic of many blockers. The study also showed that the most significant increases of affinity for quinidine were seen with mutations that decreased the dissociation rate constant from the receptor, an effect consistent with binding stabilization by hydrophobic interactions in the pore, rather than with mutations that should facilitate access of the blocker to the receptor.

USE-DEPENDENT BLOCK

Use-dependent block (also known as frequency-dependent block) was first studied and has been most extensively characterized for blockers of Na^+ channels. Considerable experimental evidence, some of it briefly summarized in the preceding pages, is consistent with the view that Na^+ channel blockers bind to receptor-like sites in the channel molecule, abolishing conductance while the drug molecule is

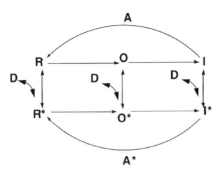

Figure 5 Simplified representation of drug-channel interaction according to the modulated-receptor hypothesis. R, I, O represent the resting, activated and open state of the Na channel; * indicates the drug-blocked (nonconducting) forms of the channel. The A and A* transitions represent the time- and voltage-dependent reactivation process of the channel in presence and absence of drug.

bound to the receptor. According to Hodgkin and Huxley, the Na^+ channel can exist in three different conformations or states: resting (R), open (O), and inactivated (I) (Figure 5). The R state is nonconducting and prevalent at negative membrane potentials, the I state is also a nonconducting state prevalent at depolarized membrane potentials, and the O state, characterized by full conductance, is mostly expressed during depolarization from the R state. In terms of the cardiac action potential, most Na^+ channels are in the R state during diastole, in the O state during the action potential upstroke, and in the I state during the plateau and a large part of the repolarization phase. According to the Modulated Receptor Model, the affinity of the receptor for the blockers is modulated by the state of the channel (Hondehem and Katzung, 1984). The interaction between drug and channel can be represented by the simplified diagram in Figure 5.

Here, R, O, and I represent the states of the channel: resting, open, and inactivated, and R^*, O^*, and I^* are the nonconducting forms of the channels, to which the drug, D, can bind with different affinity. The A and A* transitions represent the time- and voltage-dependent reactivation process of the channel in the presence and absence of drug. Considerable experimental evidence shows that the transition of the channel from I to R is affected by the presence of bound drug and requires a relatively negative membrane potential. As a result, drug-blocked channels tend to accumulate in the I state. However, at more negative membrane potentials, despite the altered voltage-dependence caused by the drug binding, recovery from block can still occur via the I^* to R^* pathway. As a consequence of this transition, two more pathways of recovery can become operative at negative membrane potentials: the R^* to R during diastole, and the O^* to O during the upstroke of the following action potential. The R^* to R pathway is probably most important for lipid-soluble uncharged molecules (e.g., benzocaine), and it might explain the rapid recovery from block observed with these molecules, especially at negative membrane potentials. On the other hand, the O^* to O pathway seems to be the primary pathway of recovery available for hydrophilic or charged molecules, e.g., quaternary derivatives.

Most local anesthetic antiarrhythmic agents seem to bind preferentially to one or two of the possible channel states, for example, to the O state (e.g., quinidine) or I state (e.g., amiodarone) or to both states (e.g., lidocaine). Also, the affinity for the I state of each blocker increases at more depolarized potentials. Affinity for the R state is generally quite low. Binding to the rested state would block conduction preferentially in normal well-polarized tissue and would be proarrhythmic (Hondeghem, 1987). Such preferential binding to the R state is frequently referred to as "tonic block". However, tonic block should more properly refer to the decreased availability of I_{Na} observed after a long period without stimulation. Under these conditions, the decrease of I_{Na} is due not only to block of rested but also of open and inactivated channels. For example, very rapid block of open channels during the first upstroke after the rest period might appear as block of rested channels. In addition, even a moderate membrane depolarization might cause a significant increase in the fraction of channels trapped in the I state. Block of these channels would also appear as tonic block. As a consequence of both the different affinity shown by local anesthetic antiarrhythmic drugs for the states of the Na^+ channel and the drug-induced changes in the voltage- and time-dependence of gating, antiarrhythmic agents show use-dependent electrophysiological effects.

In summary, use dependence defines the reduction of availability of I_{Na} in excess of tonic block, as can be observed during a sequence of action potentials (Hondeghem and Katzung, 1984). The block accumulates during successive cycles when the affinity of the drug is higher for the O and I states and when the drug slows down the transition from I^* to R^* (or I^* to R). Thus, I_{Na} is progressively reduced during successive action potentials until steady state is achieved.

The "modulated receptor hypothesis" (Hondeghem and Katzung, 1984) proposes that each channel state has a different affinity for the drug molecule, as characterized by different rate constants of blocking and unblocking, without proposing any explanation to account for these differences. Starmer *et al.* (1984) have advanced a different hypothesis to account for this state-dependent interaction. According to this hypothesis, referred to as the "guarded receptor hypothesis", the affinity of the channel binding site is constant, while its access is controlled by the state of the channel, more specifically by the state of the activation and inactivation gates. Thus, the guarded receptor hypothesis is a direct extension of the Hodgkin-Huxley model. Hydrophilic and permanently charged molecules can access the receptor when both gates are open, whereas lipophilic molecules only need an open activation gate to reach and leave the receptor.

In considering frequency-dependent block and its electrophysiological implications, it is important to consider the two related processes of block onset and block recovery (Grant *et al.*, 1984). The rate of block onset increases with increasing drug concentration, in agreement with the law of mass action. In addition, block onset seems to be correlated with the molecular weight of the local anesthetic antiarrhythmic agent, such that the lower the molecular weight, the faster the block. In contrast, the correlation of block onset with lipid solubility is poor.

Recovery from block has been studied more extensively than onset. Several factors have been shown to modulate recovery, including physicochemical properties of the drug. Most important among them are molecular size, lipid solubility, and the pK_a (Courtney, 1980; Courtney, 1987). Although most blockers of Na^+ channels share a similar pharmacophore, various substituent groups generate important physico-chemical differences that can influence the electrophysiological profile of each molecule. The following three factors are crucial in determining the kinetic properties of block recovery and, to a large extent, of use-dependent block. High lipid solubility favors rapid recovery. Recovery is also correlated with molecular weight, such that low molecular weight molecules with high lipid solubility can leave the channel very rapidly. When the pK_a of the drug and the pH of the environment are used to calculate Q, the lipid distribution coefficient at a physiological pH, the correlation coefficient further improves. A fourth crucial factor governing recovery from block is the membrane potential. Several studies have shown that even a modest degree of depolarization can produce a significant increase of the time constant of recovery from block (τ_r). This phenomenon has an important clinical implication, as the membrane depolarization occurring during myocardial ischemia contributes to prolongation of τ_r and can cause a significant potentiation of the frequency-dependent block. The acidosis that develops in tissues during ischemia increases the proportion of blocker molecules in the charged cationic form that dissociate more slowly from the receptor. Thus, during ischemia, membrane depolarization and acidosis further increases the blocking effect of local anesthetic antiarrhythmic drugs.

As summarized by Hondeghem (1987), block develops during the upstroke (for drugs that block the open state of the channel) and during the plateau phase of the action potential (for drugs that block inactivated channels). The block decreases during diastole according to the time constant of recovery of the molecule. Thus, action potential duration can be an important determinant of the extent of block. With lidocaine ($\tau_r = 100-200$ msec.), a molecule that shows high affinity for I state, even if most of the channels are blocked at the beginning of diastole, recovery may be almost complete by the end of diastole. In tissues where the action potential is short , i.e., the atria, little block remains by the end of diastole, and this may explain the low efficacy of lidocaine against atrial arrhythmias. On the other hand, with flecainide ($\tau_r > 10$ sec), most channels will be blocked at the end of diastole. The acidosis occurring during ischemia increases the proportion of blocker molecules in the charged cationic form that dissociate more slowly from the receptor. Thus, because of membrane depolarization and acidosis, ischemia can further increase the blocking effects of local anesthetic antiarrhythmic drugs.

There is experimental evidence that the block induced by Ca^{2+} channel antagonists, particularly verapamil and its derivatives, is modulated by voltage and channel state, resulting in frequency-dependent and/or voltage-dependent depression of contraction. However, the clinical relevance of these phenomena is still unclear. Potassium channel blockers show a distinct form of frequency dependence known as "reverse use dependence". This topic is discussed below.

PHARMACOLOGICAL MODULATION OF CONDUCTION

The fast Na^+ current (I_{Na}) generates the rapid upstroke (phase 0) of the action potential and is a major determinant of its conduction, as it provides the predominant source of depolarizing current for propagation. I_{Na} is very large but lasts for a very short time (approximately one msec. in normal cardiac tissue) and is terminated by the transition of Na^+ channels to the inactivated state. After inactivation, the Na^+ channel cannot reopen until reactivation takes place during the repolarization of the action potential. As the measurement of I_{Na} is technically

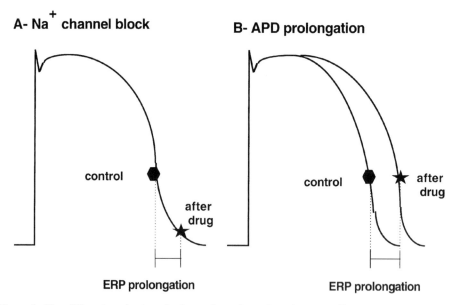

A- Na$^+$ channel block

B- APD prolongation

control

after drug

ERP prolongation

control

after drug

ERP prolongation

Figure 6 Two different mechanisms for increasing refractoriness in myocardium.

difficult, the maximum rate of depolarization ($\dot{V}_{max}$ or dV/dt_{max}) during the upstroke of the action potential (phase 0) is often used as an indicator of the availability of the Na$^+$ channel in many pharmacological studies (Grant *et al.*, 1984). In atrial, ventricular, and His-Purkinje cells, the time constant of the recovery from inactivation is much shorter than the duration of repolarization, so that the recovery of $\dot{V}_{max}$ is a function of the membrane potential during repolarization. As the membrane repolarizes, more and more channels reactivate and become available to be reexcited and to generate a new action potential. The effective refractory period (ERP) is defined as the shortest interval between two propagating action potentials elicited by a suprathreshold stimulus. Antiarrhythmic agents that block the Na$^+$ current produce, for every level of membrane potential, a significant decrease of the availability of I_{Na} by shifting the voltage-dependence of inactivation to more negative potentials, thus prolonging ERP (Figure 6A).

This action can be visualized as a shift of the relationship between $\dot{V}_{max}$ and the transmembrane potential as shown in Figure 7. A "typical" blocker of the Na$^+$ channel shifts the relationship toward more negative membrane potentials, so that $\dot{V}_{max}$ is lower at every level of membrane potential. Also, as shown in Figure 7, the maximum value of $\dot{V}_{max}$ is reduced, independently of the negative value of membrane potential. Na$^+$ channel blockers may also prolong the time course of recovery from inactivation. As mentioned above, in normal tissues, recovery from inactivation is determined by membrane potential. However, after treatment with many Na$^+$ channel blockers, channels take longer to recover such that the myocardium may remain refractory even after full repolarization. This phenomenon is known as post-repolarization refractoriness.

By decreasing the magnitude of I_{Na} available to generate the upstroke of the propagating action potential, local anesthetic antiarrhythmic agents decrease the

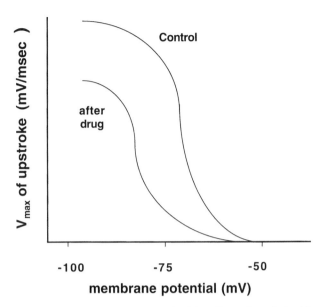

Figure 7 Membrane responsiveness curve and example of the effects of a typical soidum channel blocker (e.g., quinidine).

conduction velocity of the cardiac impulse. It is important to consider that conduction of the action potential in normal cardiac muscle shows a considerable "safety factor": in general, $\dot{V}_{max}$ must be reduced by more than 50% before a significant decrease of conduction velocity is measured. The exceptions are the sinus node and the A-V node. In these tissues, propagation depends on "slow responses" (Cranefield *et al.*, 1972). These are action potentials initiated at depolarized membrane potentials and characterized by very slowly raising upstrokes generated by I_{Ca-L}. Such action potentials propagate slowly and have a low "safety factor". Because the major factor controlling the recovery of excitability of "slow responses" is not voltage, but time, slow responses show post-repolarization refractoriness. However, it is important to consider that even in tissues where the upstroke of the action potential depends on a large and rapidly activating Na^+ current, the availability of I_{Na} is decreased and its reactivation prolonged at depolarized levels of membrane potential and in diseased tissues. Thus, concentrations of antiarrhythmic agents that minimally affect $\dot{V}_{max}$ in normal tissues can easily decrease $\dot{V}_{max}$ in diseased and depolarized tissues to such an extent that the cardiac impulse conducts decrementally, i.e., the impulse becomes progressively less effective in depolarizing the tissue in its pathway of propagation and eventually conduction fails.

Depression of conduction can terminate a reentrant arrhythmia, probably by a selective action in a segment of the reentry pathway where conduction is already depressed, thus transforming a unidirectional block in a bidirectional block. However, generalized depression of conduction in normal and diseased myocardium might create conditions that are favorable for the initiation and maintenance of reentrant arrhythmias. For example, depression of conduction over the entire pathway might simply decrease the wavelength of a reentrant impulse (the product of its conduction velocity times the refractory period) and thus provide new pathways for reentry rather than terminating it.

The electrophysiological effects of antiarrhythmic agents that block the fast Na^+ channel is defined, to a significant extent, by their frequency-dependent profile. If drug binding and unbinding from the channel is fast, as in the case of lidocaine, the block will reach steady state in a few beats, but the extent of block will be significant only at very fast heart rates. At slower heart rates, because of the fast recovery ($\tau_r = 100-200$ ms), lidocaine will unbind rapidly and a low level of block will remain at the end of the diastolic interval before the following upstroke. When drug dissociation from the channel is slow, a significant fraction of channels will still be blocked at the end of the diastolic interval, and this fraction of blocked channels will be added to those blocked during the subsequent action potential. With a drug like flecainide ($\tau_r > 10$ sec), block will increase progressively with each beat and, following a sudden increase of heart rate, a new steady state will be reached after several beats. The difference in use-dependent profile of flecainide and lidocaine is apparent considering their effects on the ECG. Therapeutic concentrations of flecainide frequently prolong QRS duration by more than 20% at a normal heart rate, while lidocaine has no effect at normal rates and causes a modest increase of QRS duration at very rapid rates (Nattel, 1991).

The time constant of recovery is also voltage- and pH-dependent. Acidosis and depolarized membrane potentials can produce a significant increase of τ_r. These factors might be important in determining selectivity of action for Na^+ channel blocking antiarrhythmic agents. However, this possible mechanism of selectivity is likely to be less important for agents with a very long τ_r. One may argue that making a long time constant of recovery even longer will not increase selectivity in diseased tissues and might cause unwanted block of conduction in marginally depolarized and ischemic tissues. This concept seems to be supported by clinical and experimental evidence, as drugs with slow recovery kinetics (e.g., flecainide and encainide) have shown marked proarrhythmic effects (Kuo *et al.*, 1987; CAST investigators, 1989; CAST investigators, 1992).

Blockade of Na^+ channels produces two additional clinically significant effects. First, the threshold strength of the stimulus necessary to excite the heart is increased. This effect accounts, in part, for the increase of pacing threshold and of the energy required to defibrillate the heart after treatment with by Na^+ channel blockers (Echt *et al.*, 1989). In addition, most Na^+ channel blockers decrease, albeit to different extents, cardiac contractility, and this action is particularly important in patients with a depressed ejection fraction. Many different mechanisms probably contribute to this effect, including depression of E-C coupling due to block of impulse propagation, shortening of the plateau phase of the action potential, an effect seen with a subset of Na^+ channel blockers, and a direct blocking action on I_{Ca-L} (Scamps *et al.*, 1989).

Despite the discouraging results with ventricular arrhythmia, potent Na^+ channel blockers, e.g., flecainide, are useful in the treatment of atrial arrhythmias, in particular for the maintenance of sinus rhythm in patients with atrial fibrillation in absence of significant damage to the ventricular myocardium. It may seem puzzling that Na^+ channel blockers characterized by slow on and off rates of block should be useful in the treatment of arrhythmias characterized by very rapid rates of excitation in a tissue where APD is short. Although it is clear that block of I_{Na} contributes to slowing the rate of the arrhythmia and to its termination, it is likely that other mechanisms are instrumental for the therapeutic action. It has been observed, both *in vitro* (Wang *et al.*, 1990) and *in vivo* (O'Hara *et al.*, 1992), that flecainide can increase atrial APD. At normal heart rates flecainide has no effects on the duration of the atrial action potential. However, at the fast rates characteristic of atrial tachyarrhythmias, flecainide causes a significant prolongation of the action potential (Wang *et al.*, 1990). It has been proposed that flecainide produces this effect by blocking the transient outward K^+ (I_{to}), a major atrial repolarizing current (Wang *et al.*, 1995). Alternatively, it has been argued that the frequency-dependent effect of flecainide on the atrial APD is not due to a block of outward K^+ currents but it is the result of Na^+ channel blockade. The very rapid rates characteristic of atrial fibrillation can produce sodium loading. The resulting increase of intracellular $[Na^+]$ stimulates the Na^+/K^+ pump current, which provides a large repolarizing current and shortens the APD. Flecainide, by decreasing sodium loading, counteracts the increase of outward pump current and thus increases APD (Wang *et al.*, 1993).

In summary, the CAST trials not only showed that potent Na^+ channel blockers (flecainide, encainide, moricizine) did not improve survival over placebo in patients with ischemic heart disease or postinfarction arrhythmias, but also changed drug discovery paradigms. Until then, most antiarrhythmic agents, either available or in development, abolished arrhythmias by blocking conduction and, in some cases, prolonging refractoriness. The negative results with drugs endowed with this profile of action focused drug development toward agents that increase refractoriness by prolonging the duration of the action potential without blocking Na^+ channels and depressing conduction.

PHARMACOLOGICAL MODULATION OF REPOLARIZATION AND REFRACTORINESS

Prolongation of refractoriness is considered a useful antiarrhythmic effect, especially when it decreases the dispersion of refractoriness in the myocardium. Differences in the timing of repolarization are particularly evident in the diseased heart and are one of the important factors that favor the initiation and maintenance of reentrant arrhythmias.

Refractoriness can be prolonged by two major pharmacological interventions. The first is to delay the recovery of the Na^+ channels from inactivation during the repolarization of the action potential without altering APD. Na^+ channel blockers shift the voltage-dependent recovery to a more negative potential and, by this action, prolong refractoriness (Figure 6A). Furthermore, Na^+ channel blockers that dissociate slowly from the channel can extend refractoriness beyond full repolarization (post-repolarization refractoriness). Thus, blockers that have little effect on refractoriness at a long cycle length might significantly prolong ERP after premature beats at faster rates of stimulation.

Prolongation of APD is the second basic mechanism to increase refractoriness: as recovery of Na^+ channels is voltage-dependent and closely parallels repolarization, delaying repolarization also prolongs refractoriness, independently of any effect on

I_{Na} (Figure 6B). In broad terms, any decrease of outward repolarizing current or increase of inward depolarizing current can prolong APD. Unlike those local anesthetic antiarrhythmic agents, which increase refractoriness by acting on a single defined target, the Na^+ channel, agents that prolong APD can act on many different targets. For example, it is possible to prolong APD by activating or by delaying the inactivation of components of I_{Na} flowing during the plateau of the action potential (Lee *et al.*, 1990; Buddish *et al.*, 1985), by increasing I_{Ca-L} (Thomas *et al.*, 1985) or by interfering with Cl^- currents that are activated under specific circumstances (Hume and Harvey, 1991). However, most of the clinically available agents, as well as most of the compounds in late development stage, prolong APD by depressing one or more outward K^+ currents, as detailed in the next section.

RECENT APPROACHES TO ANTIARRHYTHMIC DRUG DEVELOPMENT

Selection of Individual Targets

Several agents have been developed that appear to block selectively different repolarizing currents, including the rapidly activating delayed rectifier current, I_{Kr}, the slowly activating delayed rectifier, I_{Ks}, the inward rectifier, I_{K1} and the transient outward current, I_{to}. Despite the variety of currents that contribute to the repolarization of the action potential, until recently, the most common target has been the rapidly activating delayed rectifier current, I_{Kr} (Sanguinetti and Jurkiewicz, 1990a). The channel, named *HERG*, shows the structure of other voltage-activated K^+ channels, characterized by 6 transmembrane domains and a conserved pore region (Curran *et al.*, 1995; Sanguinetti *et al.*, 1995). In contrast, the I_{Ks} channel is constituted by two different membrane proteins, KvLQT1 and minK (Sanguinetti *et al.*, 1996b). KvLQT1 is structurally similar to other voltage-activated K^+ channels and is encoded by the LQT1 locus, while minK is a small protein with a single putative membrane-spanning domain and no structural homology to cloned channels (Takumi *et al.*, 1988). Coassembly of the two proteins reconstitutes the I_{Ks} current (Sanguinetti *et al.*, 1996b).

Several electrophysiologic characteristics distinguish the two components: for example, only I_{Kr} is blocked by methanesulfonamide class III drugs, e.g., dofetilide. I_{Kr} is modulated by divalent cations: it is blocked by La^{2+} (Sanguinetti and Jurkiewicz, 1990b) and increased by Cd^{2+} (Follmer *et al.*, 1992). I_{Kr}, but not I_{Ks}, shows a strong inward rectification at positive potentials and it is activated at potentials more negative than I_{Ks}. I_{Kr} is not affected by β-adrenergic stimulation, while I_{Ks} is significantly increased. The distribution of the two components and the relative abundance shows considerable variability among species: in some, e.g., the guinea pig, I_{Ks} is very large and plays a prominent role in the process of repolarization. Despite species-specific differences, it is likely that both components of the delayed rectifier play an important role in terminating the plateau and in initiating the repolarization phase of the cardiac action potential. Because of the different kinetics and voltage-dependence of activation, I_{Kr}, the rapidly activating component, has a predominant role after short depolarizations, while I_{Ks}, the generally larger but slowly activating component, becomes predominant after longer depolarizations to more positive potentials.

Despite the fact that both components seem to have a significant role in repolarization, I_{Kr} became the preferred target for prolonging repolarization. Several factors had a role in this choice (Colatsky, 1995). First, there are historical reasons: most I_{Kr} blockers are derived from initial lead structures with I_{Kr} blocking activity, such as sotalol (Strauss *et al.*, 1970) and N-acetylprocainamide (Dangman and Hoffman, 1981). Indeed, it was the development of a selective I_{Kr} blocker, E-4031 (Oiunuma *et al.*, 1990), that allowed the identification of the two distinct component of the cardiac delayed rectifier in isolation from one another (Sanguinetti and Jurkiewicz, 1990). Second, the optimization of the initial leads was based on a structure-activity relationship (SAR) with a bias toward the block of I_{Kr}, e.g., introduction of the methanesulfonamide moiety, or one of its bioisosteres, to the para position of the terminal aromatic ring (Lumma *et al.*, 1987). Third, several characteristics of I_{Kr} help to explain why this current has been a preferential target. Because of a well developed SAR, blockers of I_{Kr} are generally highly selective for the heart and very potent. I_{Kr} seems to be distributed homogeneously in the atria and ventricles, unlike I_{to}. Thus, block of I_{Kr} should result in a more uniform prolongation of refractoriness throughout the heart. The conductance of the I_{Kr} channel is increased by an elevation of $[K]_o$ as occurs during myocardial ischemia. Finally, the role of I_{Kr}, as defined by its time- and voltage-dependence and its inward rectifier properties, is to terminate the plateau of the action potential and to initiate repolarization. Thus, its action should be self-limiting and it should not have large effects on other phases of the action potential.

The general pharmacology of "selective" I_{Kr} blockers is quite consistent among various compounds despite the large variety of structures (Colatsky and Argentieri, 1994). These agents prolong repolarization and refractoriness in a uniform manner and show no significant effects on automaticity or conduction, thus indicating minimal effects on I_{Na} and pacemaker currents. On the ECG, the only remarkable effect is a prolongation of the QT and QT_c intervals. Because of these electrophysiological properties, the arrhythmias most vulnerable to these compounds are those that depend on reentry mechanisms (Anderson, 1990). It is generally thought that these compounds, by prolonging refractoriness without affecting conduction, increase the wavelength of reentrant beats, thus reducing the "excitable gap" in the reentry circuit. In most cases, the termination of the reentrant arrhythmias occurs with minimal prolongation of the cycle length, in marked contrast with the effects of Na^+ channel blockers, which cause a significant prolongation of the cycle length before arrhythmia termination (Spinelli and Hoffman, 1989). It has also been proposed that agents that prolong refractoriness might terminate an arrhythmia by altering the boundaries of the reentrant pathway and thus destabilizing the arrhythmia. Agents that block I_{Kr} are not effective against arrhythmias due to enhanced or abnormal automaticity (i.e., arrhythmias induced after myocardial infarction or by toxic doses of digitalis), while they show good efficacy against arrhythmias induced by programmed electrical stimulation. Clinical trials also show that I_{Kr} blockers have good efficacy against atrial flutter and fibrillation. These agents increase the threshold current necessary for induction of ventricular fibrillation (VF) by electrical stimulation and, conversely, minimize the reduction of threshold during myocardial ischemia (Kowey *et al.*, 1991). Spontaneous reversion of VF to sinus rhythm has been reported in several experimental studies with selective I_{Kr} blockers (Black *et al.*, 1991; Spinelli *et al.*, 1992). Clinical data suggest that these agents can improve the performance of implantable cardioverter-defibrillators by reducing both the frequency of discharge, as a result of their antiarrhythmic action, and the energy required to produce cardioversion. With the exception of a limited bradycardic action, they have modest hemodynamic effects, again in contradistinction with Na^+ channel blockers, which can produce a very significant depression of contractility. Most I_{Kr} blockers have been shown to cause a small positive inotropic effect, both *in vitro* and *in vivo*, which is thought to depend on an increased entry of Ca^{2+} during the prolonged repolarization (Wallace, 1991).

Despite the potential advantages of I_{Kr} as a target and the encouraging clinical and preclinical results obtained with many selective I_{Kr} blockers (Colatsky and Argentieri, 1994), large clinical trials with two of these compounds have failed to demonstrate a positive effect on patient survival. In the SWORD trial (Waldo *et al.*, 1996), *d*-sotalol, the dextro enantiomer of racemic sotalol (Figure 8) with significantly lower β-blocking activity and comparable efficacy in prolonging action potential duration (Advani and Singh, 1995), increased mortality in survivors of myocardial infarction. Initial results from the DIAMOND trial showed that dofetilide (Figure 8), a very potent and selective I_{Kr} blocker (Rasmussen *et al.*, 1992), did not improve survival in patients with heart failure or myocardial infarction. The reason for the decrease or lack of improvement in patient survival is not clear, and it may vary depending on the specific compound and the characteristics of each trial. However, a common concern

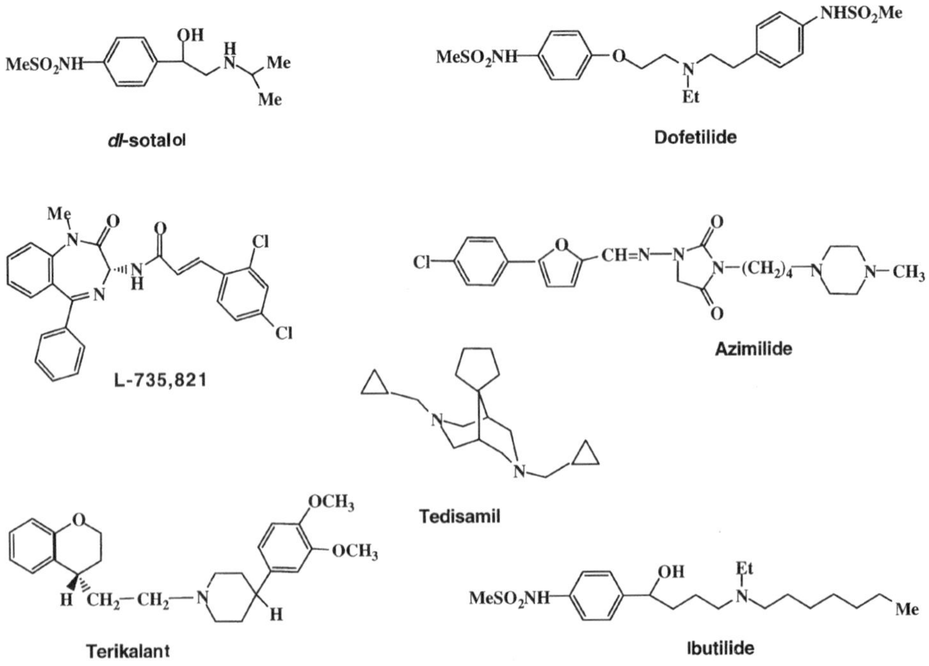

Figure 8 Examples of class III antiarrhythmic agents.

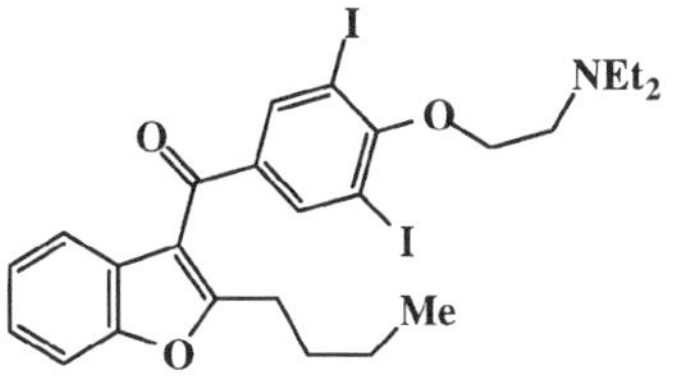

Amiodarone

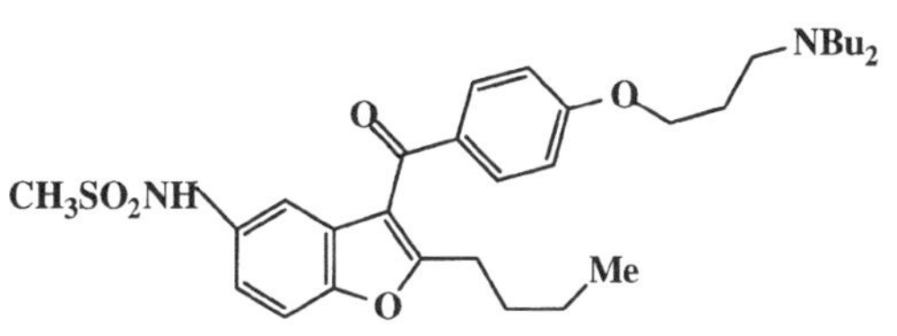

Dronedarone (SR 33589)

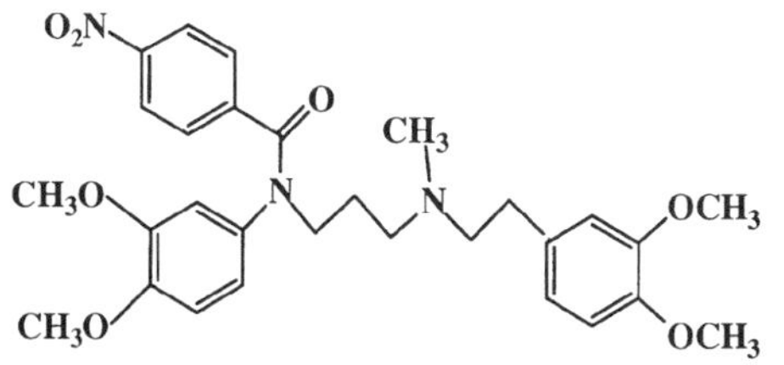

BRL 32872

Figure 9   Examples of compounds with multiple mechanisms of action.

is that the proarrhythmic potential of I_{Kr} blockers might negate any benefit resulting from their pharmacological action.

A concern with agents that selectively block I_{Kr} is that these molecules show unfavorable use-dependent properties that might be proarrhythmic. Microelectrode studies have clearly shown that the increase of APD produced by these agents is highest at low rates of stimulation and diminishes progressively as the rate of stimulation becomes faster. This use-dependent effect is opposite to that of Na^+ channel blockers, which depress conduction more profoundly at faster rates of stimulation. Not only can "reverse" use dependency reduce antiarrhythmic efficacy at faster heart rates (for example during an episode of tachycardia) but, conversely, it can produce excessive prolongation of APD during episodes of bradycardia. Excessive or inappropriate prolongation of the APD might produce distortion of repolarization (EADs, early afterdepolarizations), and trigger premature action potentials that could initiate an arrhythmia (Figure 10).

The mechanism of the "reverse" use-dependent action on the APD is not clear. It has been proposed that the effect of selective I_{Kr} blockers is relieved by depolarization and augmented by hyperpolarization, which would decrease the amount of block during frequent stimulation, as channels spend more time at depolarized potentials (Hondeghem and Snyders, 1990). It has also been proposed that a drug blocking the open K^+ channel would produce a favorable profile of use dependence, as it would increase block at faster rates of stimulation. However, studies with several blockers of I_{Kr} of different structure have shown that the voltage dependence of block resembles that of the Na^+ channel blockers (Furukawa *et al.*, 1989; Follmer, 1990). The on-rate of block and the magnitude of block are both increased when the membrane is depolarized to more positive potentials. In addition, the block requires open channels, and, finally, repolarization to more negative potentials causes the drug to leave the blocking site, resulting in unblock. Other studies have shown that quinidine (Snyders *et al.*, 1992) and terfenidine (Rampe *et al.*, 1993) produce an open channel block of hKv1.5, a human cardiac delayed rectifier potassium channel clone. Similarly, block of I_{Kr} by dofetilide and by ibutilide in a mammalian atrial cell line has been shown to require open channels (Yang *et al.*, 1995).

In summary, these results suggest that the reverse use-dependence observed in action potential studies is not the result of a frequency-dependent interaction of the drug with the channel. Evidence from several studies also suggests that the receptor site is inside the channel, and that the blocker reaches the receptor when the activation gate of the channel opens following depolarization. On repolarization to membrane potentials comparable to physiological diastolic resting potentials, the activation gate closes very rapidly trapping the blocker in the closed channel. At more depolarized potentials, the rates of channel deactivation and drug unbinding are similar; this allows the blocker to leave the channel before the activation gate closes, thus decreasing the degree of block (Nair and Grant, 1997). In general, it has been difficult to demonstrate use-dependent block with I_{Kr} blockers in voltage-clamp studies, unless the myocytes were held at negative potentials, or the channel was kept closed during drug exposure (Carmeliet, 1992; Carmeliet, 1993). While many studies, both preclinical and clinical, show that the effect of I_{Kr} blockers on APD is strongly dependent on heart rate, most of the same studies have also shown that a significant prolongation of APD is still observed even at very rapid rates of stimulation (Colatsky and Argentieri, 1994).

It is thought that the incomplete deactivation of the delayed rectifier current during diastole leaves a residual outward current at the beginning of the following action potential. This repolarizing current can accumulate and grow in amplitude over successive action potentials, especially at rapid heart rates, and this accumulation of outward current is thought to be one of the mechanisms that account for the frequency-dependent shortening of the cardiac action potential (Hauswirth *et al.*, 1972). As discussed above, the effect of selective blockers of I_{Kr} in prolonging APD is attenuated at faster heart rates, which is the opposite of what could be expected from the hypothesis of the role of accumulating outward current. This finding suggests that other plateau currents might have a larger role in defining APD during tachycardia. The slowly activating delayed rectifier (I_{Ks}) is one of the possible candidates among plateau currents. Its slow activation kinetics should result in current summation at fast heart rate, and one might envision that, under these conditions, I_{Ks} will grow much larger than I_{Kr}, overwhelming its contribution and any consequence of its block on APD (Jurkiewicz and Sanguinetti, 1993). Because of its possible role in determining APD, I_{Ks} has been considered as a possible target. Furthermore, I_{Ks} is increased by adrenergic stimulation, thus a blocker of I_{Ks} should maintain its efficacy and prolong APD, even in presence of high adrenergic stimulation, as, for example, during ischemia. Blockers with various degrees of selectivity for I_{Ks} and I_{Kr} have been developed. Azimilide (NE-10064), a chlorophenylfuranyl compound (Figure 8), is structurally different from other methanesulfonamide class III drugs (Busch *et al.*, 1993). Azimilide blocks both I_{Kr} and I_{Ks} but shows higher potency toward I_{Kr}. This lack of selectivity creates problems in interpreting some of the published preclinical data (Salata and Brooks, 1997). L-735,821 (Merck), a

1,4 benzodiazepine (Figure 8), is a potent and selective blocker of I_{Ks} (Salata *et al.*, 1996). No information is available regarding the frequency-dependent effects of this compound or its antiarrhythmic effects in animal models. It is at this time unclear whether I_{Ks} blockers show a therapeutic advantage over selective I_{Kr} blockers. In general, it is unclear whether I_{Ks} is a suitable target, as its abundance and kinetics vary in different species (Gintant, 1996). Recent studies have also shown that the I_{Ks} channel is constituted by two different membrane proteins, KvLQT1 and minK, and that their coassembly reconstitutes the I_{Ks} current (Sanguinetti *et al.*, 1996). As mutations of the KvLQT1 gene are responsible for the most common form of congenital long-QT syndrome (Editorial, 1996), these findings underscore the likely proarrhythmic potential of selective blockade of I_{Ks}.

Other cardiac potassium channels have been considered as possible targets to induce prolongation of APD and refractoriness, although none of these currents has yet shown a significant advantage as a target.

The transient outward K^+ current (I_{to}) is prominent in the atrium where it may be the major source of repolarizing current. In most species, there are two types of transient outward current: one is a voltage-gated current (I_{to1}), while the other is activated by intracellular Ca^{2+} (I_{to2}) (Siegelbaum and Tsien, 1980). The relative magnitude of the two components differs from species to species, although in most species I_{to1} is predominant. Therefore, one might speculate that a selective blocker of I_{to1} should be effective against supraventricular arrhythmias and show some degree of selectivity due to the predominance of I_{to1} in the atrium. However, I_{to1} is also present in the ventricle, where its distribution is not homogeneous; I_{to1} is prominent in epicardial cells but very modest in endocardial cells. Action potentials from myocytes with very large I_{to} show a prominent phase 1, with a "spike and dome" profile, while myocytes with little I_{to} do not show a clear phase 1 and their plateau lies at more positive potentials. Because of a rather slow reactivation, the magnitude of I_{to1} is very dependent on cycle length and this might limit its importance during fast heart rates or after premature stimulation. The slow reactivation kinetics of I_{to1} accounts for the attenuation or disappearance of phase 1 (i.e., the notch) of the action potential and the transition of phase 2 (i.e., the plateau) to more positive potentials as the rate of stimulation increases. No selective blockers of I_{to1} are available. Tedisamil, a heterocyclic compound related to spartein (Figure 8), blocks both I_{to1} and I_{Kr} and can produce bradycardia (Dukes *et al.*, 1990; Wallace *et al.*, 1995). Tedisamil can increase APD and refractoriness and shows antiarrhythmic effects (Friedrichs *et al.*, 1998). However, as the block of I_{Kr} occurs at concentrations equivalent or lower than those needed to block I_{to1} (Ohler *et al.*, 1994), it is unclear to what extent the block of I_{to1} contributes to the increases of APD and refractoriness. In humans, the increase of refractoriness and APD produced by tedisamil shows reverse use dependence (Bargheer *et al.*, 1994). This, in conjunction with the bradycardic effect, might increase the risk of producing excessive prolongation of repolarization and of inducing proarrhythmic effects. In summary, I_{to} does not look like a promising target for ventricular arrhythmias, although it might have potential for the treatment of atrial arrhythmias.

The inward rectifier current, I_{K1}, has an important role in determining the resting membrane potential and the final phase of the repolarization (late phase 3 of the action potential). RP-62719 (terikalant), a benzopyran derivative (Figure 8), has been reported to inhibit I_{K1} in guinea pig ventricular myocytes without affecting the delayed rectifier or the K_{ATP} current (Escande *et al.*, 1992). Several studies showed that terikalant has a clear class III activity and significant antiarrhythmic properties (Rees and Curtis, 1993). However, later studies have also shown that terikalant has significant inhibitory effects on I_{Kr} at concentrations lower than those needed to inhibit I_{K1} (Jurkiewicz *et al.*, 1996; Bridal *et al.*, 1996). In general, one might speculate that a dual block of I_{K1} and I_{Kr}, by altering at the same time the resting membrane potential and the entire phase of repolarization, might have a significant proarrhythmic potential, as it might produce abnormalities of both repolarization and conduction.

The ATP-sensitive K^+ channel (K_{ATP}) has also been proposed as a target for antiarrhythmic agents. In addition, experimental evidence suggests that K_{ATP} channels modulate myocardial recovery after ischemia. As these channels have very high conductance and are expressed in high density in myocytes, few channels need to be activated to generate a large repolarizing current and to produce a significant shortening of APD (Faivre and Findlay, 1990). Opening of K_{ATP} channels mediates the shortening of APD during ischemia and contributes to the loss of intracellular K^+. By increasing repolarizing current, openers of K_{ATP} channels (KCOs) could produce an antiarrhythmic effect by restoring normal repolarization in cells developing early and delayed afterdepolarizations (EADs and DADs) (Spinelli *et al.*, 1991). Glyburide, a sulfonylurea hypoglycemic drug and a blocker of K_{ATP} channels, can reduce the rate of K^+ loss (Wilde *et al.*, 1990) and reverse the APD shortening during ischemia (Smallwood *et al.*, 1990). However, glyburide has also been shown to worsen the recovery of contractility after ischemia (Grover *et al.*, 1989), while KCOs have been shown to have a cardioprotective effect (Grover *et al.*, 1990), although the experimental data are conflicting (Kitzen *et al.*, 1992). Independently from the possible cardioprotective action, there is concern that the K_{ATP} channel is not a promising target for new antiarrhythmic agents for the following reasons. First, opening these channels in vascular smooth muscle will cause vasorelaxation and decrease arterial pressure. Second, as the cardiac ATP-sensitive K^+ current is time-independent and its intensity depends on the intracellular ATP concentration, there is the possibility of excessive shortening of APD and consequent weakening of the cardiac contraction. In addition, an excessive shortening of APD will cause a proportional decrease of refractoriness and this might increase the likelihood of certain types of arrhythmias (Chi *et al.*, 1990; Spinelli *et al.*, 1990).

Ibutilide (Figure 8), an analog of sotalol, is thought to prolong APD by activating a slow inward Na^+ current during the plateau and by blocking I_{Kr} at low concentrations (10^{-9} M). At higher concentrations (10^{-7} M), ibutilide activates an outward K^+ current and shortens APD (Lee, 1992; Lee *et al.*, 1993). Thus, APD increases at low concentrations and shortens at higher concentrations, resulting in a bell-shaped concentration-response curve, which is said to provide a higher margin of safety against excessive APD prolongation. However, a later study in an atrial tumor cell line showed that ibutilide is a potent blocker of I_{Kr} and that its mechanism of action resembles that of dofetilide (Yang *et al.*, 1995). Despite the bell-shaped concentration-response curve for APD prolongation, ibutilide induced torsades de pointes in 12.5% of a series of patients treated for atrial flutter (Stambler *et al.*, 1996). Ibutilide was recently approved by the FDA for the treatment of atrial fibrillation and flutter.

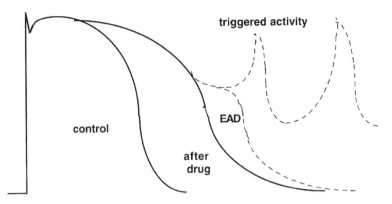

Figure 10 Excessive prolongation of APD can induce a defect of repolarization (EAD) that can trigger extrasystoles.

Finally, β-adrenergic agonists acting via the c-AMP and protein kinase A pathway can activate a large, time-independent chloride current in the heart. This current is blocked by nonselective anion channel blockers (anthracene-9-carboxylic acid or 4-4′dinitrostilbene-2,2′-disulfonic acid) (Harvey and Hume, 1989; Bahniski *et al.*, 1989). As the reversal potential for Cl$^-$ in cardiac myocytes is in the range of -30 to -40 mV under most conditions, the cAMP-activated chloride current will be an inward depolarizing current at the normal resting membrane potentials and an outward repolarizing current at plateau potentials. Thus, activation of this chloride current can result in both membrane depolarization and shortening of APD. Both of these actions have been observed *in vitro* and in isolated tissues (Hume and Harvey, 1991). No selective blockers of this current are presently available.

Selection of Multiple Targets

Recently, the principle of selectivity of drug action against a particular target has been abandoned and molecules have been designed to have additional blocking effects at Na$^+$ and Ca^{2+} channels and/or β-adrenergic receptors. This approach is based, in part, on the appreciation of the action of amiodarone (Figure 9). Amiodarone, first developed as an antianginal agent, was later found to block Na$^+$, K$^+$, and Ca^{2+} channels, to exert significant antiadrenergic actions, and to block the effects of thyroid hormones by antagonizing their receptor binding in cardiac myocytes (Singh and Vaughan Williams, 1970; Latham *et al.*, 1987). It has been speculated that the serendipitous balance of these multiple actions might account for the lack of reverse use dependence observed with amiodarone (Hondeghem and Snyders, 1990; Sager *et al.*, 1993), and for the extremely low incidence of torsades de pointes arrhythmias, despite a significant prolongation of the QT interval (Breithardt, 1995; Amiodarone Trials Meta-Analysis Investigators, 1997). Several new agents under development attempt to combine actions at different molecular targets to mimic amiodarone's efficacy while avoiding some of that drug's potential liabilities. Unlike previous selective I_{Kr} blockers, these newer drugs have significant blocking effects against Na$^+$ and Ca^{2+} channels, albeit with lower efficacy or at higher concentrations than for the inhibition of I_{Kr}. The purpose of blocking Na^+ and Ca^{2+} channels is to limit APD prolongation at high drug concentrations and to decrease the likelihood of inducing early afterdepolarizations, thus diminishing the risk of torsade de pointes. Furthermore, block of inward currents contributes to APD prolongation at shorter cycle lengths, when the inward currents have a more significant role in determining the duration of the plateau. Finally, the β-blocking action of these molecules is expected to produce cardioprotective effects, including a decrease of heart rate, a decrease of Ca^{2+} overload, an inhibition of abnormal automaticity, and an increase of the energy required to fibrillate the heart.

Dronedarone (SR 33589; Sanofi) (Manning *et al.*, 1995) and BRL-32872 (SKB) (Bril *et al.*, 1995) are two examples of this approach. Dronedarone is an analog of amiodarone, and its preclinical profile of pharmacological activity is comparable to that of the parent compound. However, unlike amiodarone, dronedarone does not contain iodine and thus it is expected to lack the characteristic adverse effects related to the alteration of the thyroid function. BRL-32872 exerts a dual blocking action on I_{Kr} and I_{Ca-L} channels. Preliminary data showed that BRL-32872 suppressed the early afterdepolarizations produced by other action potential-prolonging agents, suggesting that the compound might have an appropriate balance of potassium and calcium channel block (Bril *et al.*, 1994).

As with other drugs with multiple pharmacological activities, there are uncertainties regarding the correct balance of effects against the various targets and concerns that this approach will also increase the risk of adverse effects, including cardiac depression, bradycardia, and hypotension. Thus, it seems reasonable to speculate that the remarkable efficacy of amiodarone is not due to any specific action but rather to the fine balance of many actions. From the point of view of drug discovery, developing molecules with multiple pharmacological activities presents a number of formidable difficulties as their rational design requires the combination of different structure-activity relationships in the same molecule and the adoption of screening paradigms against multiple molecular targets. As an added difficulty, it is also reasonable to expect that the ideal balance of action will vary from molecule to molecule and that its definition will require extensive *in vitro* and *in vivo* studies.

PROARRHYTHMIA

In addition to suppressing arrhythmias, both of Na^+ and K^+ channel blockers can aggravate existing arrhythmias or induce new arrhythmias, an undesirable effect known as proarrhythmia. There are two major mechanisms responsible for proarrhythmia. The first consists of excessive depression of conduction without a simultaneous prolongation of refractoriness. These actions, observed with Na^+ channel blockers, favor the initiation and maintenance of reentrant arrhythmias. While it is possible that depression of conduction can terminate the arrhythmia, for example by converting unidirectional to bidirectional block, it is also true that excessive depression of conduction creates conditions favoring reentry. For example, depressed conduction may cause the impulse to block in a "weak link" of the reentry pathway, causing a unidirectional block, or it may allow the reentrant impulse to fractionate and propagate in smaller reentry circuits. This action can shorten the cycle length of a tachycardia and increases the likelihood of its conversion to fibrillation. The ventricular tachycardias resulting from reentry are generally monomorphic or, if polymorphic, lack the characteristic repeated alternation of the major vector typical of torsades de pointes. The QT interval is not prolonged excessively and the arrhythmias tend to be resistant to conversion to sinus rhythm (Nattel, 1991).

The results of the CAST trial have clearly indicated that the potent Na^+ channel blockers flecainide and encainide increased mortality over the placebo group, despite their efficacy in suppressing ventricular premature depolarizations (CAST Investigators, 1989). As discussed previously, excessive depression of conduction is observed much more frequently in diseased myocardium, where conduction is already impaired, and where ischemia and depolarization can further potentiate the depressant effect of Na^+ channel blockers. Evidence from experimental studies and supportive clinical data suggest that transient myocardial ischemia might be an important factor in triggering lethal arrhythmias in the presence of potent blockers of the Na^+ channels. Several experimental studies show that induction of acute myocardial ischemia produces ventricular fibrillation more frequently in animals treated with class I agents than in controls (Nattel *et al.*, 1981; Kou *et al.*, 1987). Analysis of the results of the CAST trial also suggests that the risk of death was increased 1.7-fold in patients with transmural (Q-wave) infarction and 8.7-fold in patients with non-transmural infarction (non-Q-wave), where the risk of recurrent ischemic episodes is known to be elevated (Akiyama *et al.*, 1991). This hypothesis is supported by a different analysis of the same data showing that an episode of myocardial ischemia is more likely to result in a fatal event in patients treated with encainide or flecainide than with placebo (Echt *et al.*, 1991).

A different proarrhythmic effect of Na^+ channel blockers is observed in patients with atrial flutter or fibrillation. Here, depression of conduction can decrease the rate of the atrial arrhythmia, but ventricular rate might increase abruptly to tachy-cardia levels before final conversion to sinus rhythm occurs. This paradoxical effect results from the following mechanism: as the frequency of atrial impulses entering and blocking in the A-V node (concealed conduction) decreases, the refractoriness of the nodal tissue similarly decreases, allowing 1:1 A-V nodal conduction. Thus, a higher proportion of atrial impulses reaches the ventricle producing a tachycardia. This proarrhythmic effect is common in patients treated with quinidine, whose vagolytic effects contribute to the proarrhythmic response by enhancing A-V conduction, but it is also observed with other Na channel blocking agents.

The second major mechanism of proarrhythmia consists of excessive prolongation of repolarization and is observed with agents that prolong refractoriness such as I_{Kr} blockers. Excessive prolongation of repolarization is accompanied by a significant increase of the QT interval and is associated with a form of ventricular arrhythmia, known as torsades de pointes, with a characteristic ECG appearance. Major additional risk factors for this form of arrhythmia are bradycardia and low serum K^+, conditions known to prolong APD. These factors have been shown in *in vitro* experiments to produce abnormalities of repolarization (early afterdepolarizations) that can trigger premature upstrokes and are thought to contribute to the initiation of torsades de pointes (Roden and Hoffman, 1985).

Although it is clear that early afterdepolarizations are associated with excessive prolongation of APD, the cellular mechanism responsible for their generation is still unclear. It is known that the inward current generating the afterdepolarization mostly depends on I_{Ca-L} (January and Riddle, 1989). However, because excessive prolongation of APD increases intracellular Ca^{2+}, it also seems possible that the current produced by the $Na^+ - Ca^{2+}$ exchanger contributes to the afterdepolarization (Szabo *et al.*, 1994).

CONCLUSION

Before the results of the Cardiac Arrhythmia Suppression Trials (CAST Investigators, 1989 and 1992), most antiarrhythmic agents in use or in development blocked cardiac Na^+ channels and depressed conduction. There is now a consensus that long-term treatment with these agents does not improve survival in patients with ischemic heart disease or previous myocardial infarction, although these agents may still be useful for the treatment of atrial fibrillation in selected patients. The results of the CAST trials have stressed the need of improving the benefit/risk ratio for any new antiarrhythmic agent and have redirected drug development toward agents that increase refractoriness by prolonging repolarization without depressing conduction. Over the past few years there has been speculation that the newly acquired understanding of the molecular mechanism of action of Na^+ channel blockers, together with the definition of their voltage- and frequency-dependent effects, could facilitate the discovery of more selective, effective and safer Na^+ channel blockers (Hondegem, 1987). However, no new Na^+ channel blockers has yet been developed with an improved profile of efficacy and safety.

Most of the newer agents designed to increase APD achieve this effect by specifically blocking one or more cardiac K currents, with the primary target being the rapidly activating component of delayed rectification (I_{Kr}). The initial analysis of the results of the DIAMOND trial show that dofetilide, a potent and selective I_{Kr} blocker, had a neutral effect on survival in patients with heart failure ($n = 1518$) or myocardial infarction ($n = 1510$), but decreased the incidence of atrial fibrillation in these patient populations. These findings are at variance with the results from the Survival With Oral D-Sotalol (SWORD trial) (Waldo *et al.*, 1996). This trial was terminated prematurely ($n = 3121$) because patients receiving *d*-sotalol appeared nearly twice as likely to die as patients receiving placebo. It is possible that the difference in outcome may be explained by the fact that more high-risk patients were enrolled in the DIAMOND trial, thus altering the risk/benefit ratio in this trial. A long-standing concern for drugs that prolong APD has been proarrhythmia, particularly torsades de pointes. Overall, the risk of torsades appears to be $< 3-5\%$ for I_{Kr} blockers, and is considerably more predictable than the type of proarrhythmia seen during treatment with I_{Na} blockers. At this time, it is not known whether specific block of a certain type of potassium channel is intrinsically more or less proarrhythmic, whether non-selective block of multiple potassium channel types predisposes the heart to proarrhythmia, or whether in some patients there is a congenital or idiosyncratic predisposition to torsades de pointes.

Current mid- to late-stage development activity in the antiarrhythmic area remains largely focused either on modulators of specific K channels or on more complex agents that attempt to mimic the pharmacologic profile of amiodarone. To date, the only antiarrhythmic drug (apart from β-blockers) shown to reduce mortality and cardiac events in patients with ischemic heart disease has been amiodarone, a compound with complex electrophysiological and anti-sympathetic effects. A recent meta-analysis of data from 6500 patients from eight post-MI and five CHF trials showed that amiodarone treatment produced a 13% reduction in all-cause mortality, and a 29% reduction in arrhythmic death (Amiodarone Trials Meta-Analysis Investigators, 1997). This analysis included results from both EMIAT ($n = 1456$) (Julian *et al.*, 1997) and CAMIAT ($n = 1202$) trials (Cairns *et al.*, 1997), which individually found significant reductions in the number of resuscitated ventricular fibrillation episodes and arrhythmic death but no effect on overall survival.

Early stage discovery efforts are seeking new ion channel targets that may show relative specificity for atrium *vs.* ventricle, for exclusive use in supraventricular arrhythmias. An obvious difficulty is the need to identify an atrial-selective target. There has been speculation that hKv1.5, a cloned K^+ channel highly expressed in human atrial myocytes might represent such a target. However, the identity of the native atrial current expressed by this channel is still controversial and its atrial-selectivity questionable. At this time, no atrium-specific compounds have as yet been disclosed. There also appears to be growth in the number of compounds under study for their cardioprotective or anti-ischemic effects, as an alternative to a more classic electropharmacologic antiarrhythmic approach. Prominent among these are compounds acting on ATP-sensitive K^+ channels. Previously discussed results obtained from preclinical models raise questions about both safety and efficacy of either K_{ATP} channel openers and blockers. Whether modulating K_{ATP} channels in either direction can provide consistent benefit in patients with ischemic heart disease and arrhythmia remains to be proven.

7 Electrophysiologic Abnormalities in Hypertrophied, Failed or Infarcted Hearts

Judith M.B. Pinto and Penelope A. Boyden

Fibers from diseased and arrhythmic hearts can generate abnormal transmembrane action potentials. Yet, until recently very little has been done to clarify the function and pharmacology of the ion channels that underlie the action potentials of myocytes from chronically diseased hearts. This chapter concentrates on the function and molecular determinants of ion channels that reside in the sarcolemma and that contribute to the distinct phases of the transmembrane action potentials of myocytes from hypertrophied hearts, from failed hearts and from infarcted hearts (Figure 1).

Hypertrophy is an accompaniment of hypertension and certain cardiomyopathies and can be complicated by the occurrence of ventricular arrhythmias. It may be global or regional and is associated with changes in ion channel function. To some extent evolution into cardiac failure can be compensated by increased cellular hypertrophy.

Because there are not clear demarcations between hypertrophy and failure and altered ion channel function per se, discussions of ion channel function in failure and

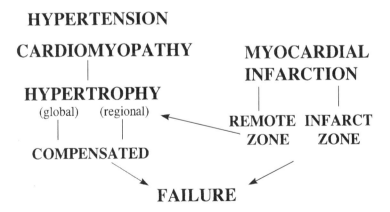

Figure 1 Overview of focus of chapter.

Supported by grants HL-34477 and HL-30557 from the National Heart Lung and Blood Institutes of Health, Bethesda, Maryland

hypertrophy will be combined. We shall also discuss ion channel function in cells surviving after myocardial infarction within two general categories (Figure 1). First, the myocardial substrate in the infarcted regions will be discussed and linked to the occurrence of ion channel changes and subsequent arrhythmias in experimental models of infarction. We shall then discuss the ion channel changes in myocytes remote from the infarcted regions.

HYPERTROPHY (GLOBAL)

Studies in the cat (Bassett and Gelband, 1973; Cameron *et al.*, 1983; Tritthart *et al.*, 1975), guinea pig (Ryder *et al.*, 1993), rabbit (Hamrell and Alpert, 1977), and rat (Capasso *et al.*, 1981; Gulch *et al.*, 1979; Hayashi and Shibata, 1974; Aronson, 1980; Tomita *et al.*, 1994; Coulombe *et al.*, 1994; Benitah *et al.*, 1993; Brooksby *et al.*, 1993a; Brooksby *et al.*, 1993b) have shown that changes in cellular electrical activity associated with experimentally induced global hypertrophy are qualitatively similar. The most consistent and pronounced change is a prolongation of the ventricular myocyte action potential (see Hart, 1994) (Figure 2), such that, in some studies, action potential duration continues to increase as the degree of hypertrophy becomes more severe.

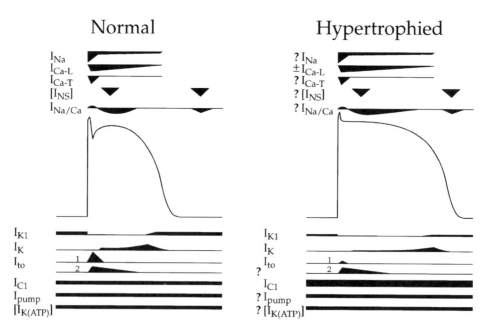

Figure 2 Schematic illustrating action potentials of epicardial ventricular myocytes from normal and hypertrophied hearts. Relative contributions of selected ionic currents are shown. Currents in red are those that have been found to be altered in myocytes from hypertrophied hearts. Question marks indicate there is still incomplete knowledge of ion channel function in these types of myocytes. See text for more detail. Modified after The Sicilian Gambit I (1991). *See* Color Plate 1.

Resting Potential

Transmembrane action potentials have been recorded from atrial fibers in man and in cats with cardiomyopathy or myocardial hypertrophy, and from ventricular muscle and specialized conducting fibers from failed and ischemic human heart (Kleiman and Houser, 1989; Zhang *et al.*, 1991; Beuckelmann *et al.*, 1993; Boyden *et al.*, 1984; TenEick and Singer, 1979). In all instances, resting potentials tend to be less negative than those of normal myocytes or fibers. The reasons for the decrease in resting potential are not totally understood, but several factors may be important. In some instances, ion content of the extracellular environment may be altered. An elevation in extracellular K ($[K]_0$) can lead to a decrease in resting potential since the resting potential of normal myocyte is a function of $[K]_0$. Alternatively, intracellular ion concentrations may be altered secondary to changes in the active Na^+/K^+ pump rate, or changes in the permeability of the cell membrane to K^+, Na^+ or Ca^{2+}. If cardiac disease has caused either a decrease in pump rate or an increased permeability of the membrane to K^+, the results may be a decrease in intracellular K^+ and/or an increase in intracellular Na^+. Either or both alterations can reduce the resting potential of a myocyte.

Another cause for the decline in resting membrane potential can be a decrease in the function of the inwardly rectifying K^+ channel, I_{K1}, resulting from alterations in protein or lipid metabolism. The relatively high resting potential in a normal myocyte not only results from the marked differences in intra and extracellular K^+ concentrations (see Chapter 3) but also from the fact that the resting cardiac membrane is highly permeable to K^+ via I_{K1}. If permeability through this ion channel is decreased, fewer K^+ ions will exit across the membrane and a lower potential may result.

Although activation of I_{K1} does not play a role in repolarization of the normal ventricular action potential during the plateau, it does contribute to the terminal phase of repolarization (Shimoni and Giles, 1992). Therefore, the reduced density of I_{K1} may prolong action potentials as is observed in hypertrophied myocytes. Although an increase in I_{K1} has been reported in a feline model of RV hypertrophy (Kleiman and Houser, 1988), other studies on feline hypertrophic myocardium (Barrington *et al.*, 1988; Zhang *et al.*, 1991) report a decrease in I_{K1} density. The reasons for these differences are not known at this time but they may reflect the heterogeneity of the disease process. In ventricular myocytes from hearts of patients with either dilated or ischemic cardiomyopathy the density of I_{K1} is significantly reduced at hyperpolarized potentials (Beuckelmann *et al.*, 1993). In the pacing-induced canine model of heart failure, there is a significant decrease in I_{K1} reflecting a reduction in channel number, a change in the frequency of substate openings and a decrease in the probability of the channel opening (Kaab *et al.*, 1996). All these changes may contribute to instabilities of resting potential and the APD prolongation in cells from these failing hearts.

Upstroke Velocity of Phase 0 of the Action Potential

In the setting of cardiac disease, the upstroke velocity of the action potential (Phase 0) might be significantly decreased for either or both of two reasons: first, a reduction in resting membrane potential changes the upstroke velocity of the action potential.

This is due to the effect of membrane potential on the availability of the fast inward Na^+ current (Chapter 3). Action potentials elicited in fibers with low resting potentials and reduced upstroke velocities that depend on Na^+ current flowing through partially inactivated channels have been called depressed fast responses. This term underlines the fact that the depolarization phase is still caused by Na^+ current even though the upstroke velocity is low. Second, cardiac disease may directly decrease the number and/or function of the fast Na^+ and the T and L type Ca^{2+} channels through which depolarizing inward currents flow.

Na^+ current

Indirect evidence using hypertrophied rat myocardium (Gulch *et al.*, 1979) and data on voltage clamped feline hypertrophied myocytes (Barrington *et al.*, 1988) support the idea that neither the fast nor slowly inactivating cardiac Na^+ current is altered with hypertrophy. Na^+ current studies using ventricular myocytes from canine hearts with pacing-induced failure (Kaab *et al.*, 1996) agree with the studies of atrial and ventricular myocytes from failing human hearts and show that there are no significant differences in the density or kinetics of I_{Na} among patient groups with different underlying diseases that lead to failure (Sakakibara *et al.*, 1992; Sakakibara *et al.*, 1993).

Ca^{2+} currents

Data on the function of L type Ca^{2+} current ($I_{Ca,L}$) in myocytes from experimentally induced hypertrophied hearts are diverse, perhaps because notable differences in experimental conditions exist in the various studies. Thus there is not as yet a clear understanding of the effects of hypertrophy on $I_{Ca,L}$. Peak $I_{Ca,L}$ density is not different in RV (Kleiman and Houser, 1988) and LV (Furukawa *et al.*, 1994) hypertrophied myocytes, and the slow component of $I_{Ca,L}$ decay is delayed significantly in both. Similar findings of no change in $I_{Ca,L}$ density in myocytes from genetically determined hypertensive rats with or without failure (Brooksby *et al.*, 1993b; Cerbai *et al.*, 1994; Gomez *et al.*, 1997) or in myocytes from canine hearts with pacing-induced failure (Kaab *et al.*, 1996) have been reported. On the other hand, in hypertension induced hypertrophy in the rat (Keung, 1989) or guinea pig myocyte (Ryder *et al.*, 1993), peak $I_{Ca,L}$ density appears to increase. Reexamining the effects of hypertrophy secondary to aortic stenosis in the rat, others have found no change in $I_{Ca,L}$ density or the appearance of T type Ca^{2+} currents (Scamps *et al.*, 1990). Feline myocytes appear to respond differently. Nuss and Houser (Nuss and Houser, 1993) suggest that although the peak density of $I_{Ca,L}$ is reduced, with the additional slowing of Ca^{2+} current kinetics in myocytes from severely, globally hypertrophied hearts, the total Ca^{2+} influx via $I_{Ca,L}$ may not differ from control.

Little information is available regarding the function of Ca^{2+} currents in normal human myocytes (Escande *et al.*, 1986; Ouadid *et al.*, 1991; Benitah *et al.*, 1992a; Cohen and Lederer, 1993) or on the function of Ca^{2+} currents in cells from hypertrophied or failed human hearts. $I_{Ca,L}$ density determined in ventricular myocytes from hearts of patients with end stage failure (Beuckelmann *et al.*, 1991; Mewes and Ravens, 1994; Beuckelmann *et al.*, 1992) is similar to that of myocytes from healthy hearts.

Interestingly, in hypertrophied feline LV myocytes, the T type Ca^{2+} current becomes quite prominent while in the normal feline ventricular cell it is lacking (Nuss and Houser, 1993). Increases in T type Ca^{2+} current amplitude/density have also been seen in other models of hypertrophy (e.g., growth hormone (Xu and Best, 1990) and endothelin induced hypertrophy (Furukawa *et al.*, 1992)). A change in the prominence of a T type Ca^{2+} current in hypertrophied cells may be related to changes in intracellular Ca^{2+} handling in these cells since in normal cells, either a direct increase in Ca_i (Tseng and Boyden, 1991) or superfusion with agents that are known to increase Ca_i (neuraminidase (Yee *et al.*, 1989) and ouabain (Le Grande *et al.*, 1990; Alvarez and Vassort, 1992)) increase the amplitude of T type Ca^{2+} current.

Repolarization and Refractoriness

Another prominent effect of hypertrophy/failure is on the refractoriness of cardiac fibers. Changes in refractoriness can occur for at least two reasons. First, a reduction in resting potential alters the relationship between repolarization of the action potential and recovery of excitability (availability) of the normal fast Na^+ inward current. Second, in hypertrophy, prolongation of the action potential, particularly at slow pacing rates, is observed. Because recovery of excitability tends to vary with the duration of the action potential, refractoriness is prolonged concomitantly.

K^+ *currents*

I_K In hypertrophied RV feline myocytes, the delayed rectifier current (I_K) decreases in density, shows steeper rectification and slower activation with rapid deactivation (Kleiman and Houser, 1989) compared to control. Such findings are consistent with the action potential prolongation accompanying hypertrophy. These changes have been confirmed in feline endocardial myocytes from hypertrophied LV (Furukawa *et al.*, 1994). As yet, there is little information on the function of I_K in human hypertrophy/failure. A small and partially time dependent I_K was recorded in some human ventricular cells from myopathic hearts whereas myocytes from healthy human ventricle showed no such current (Beuckelmann *et al.*, 1993). Thus the role of decreased I_K density in APD changes in human hypertrophy remains unresolved.

I_{to} The voltage dependent (Ca_i-independent) transient outward current (I_{to1}) is important to the early phase of repolarization of transmembrane potentials of myocytes of most species including human. Therefore, a change in its density could significantly alter the time course of repolarization. I_{to} is significantly reduced in myocytes from various models of hypertrophy in the rat; these include hypertrophy induced by increased growth hormone secretion (Xu and Best, 1990), sustained pressure overload secondary to abdominal aortic constriction (Benitah *et al.*, 1993; Tomita *et al.*, 1994), DOCA-salt induced hypertension (Coulombe *et al.*, 1994), and genetically determined hypertension (Cerbai *et al.*, 1994), (Figure 3). In pressure overload, the diminished macroscopic I_{to} is not the result of differences in the unitary single I_{to} channel current amplitude, slope conductance or maximum open state probability (Tomita *et al.*, 1994). Rather, nonstationary fluctuation analysis has

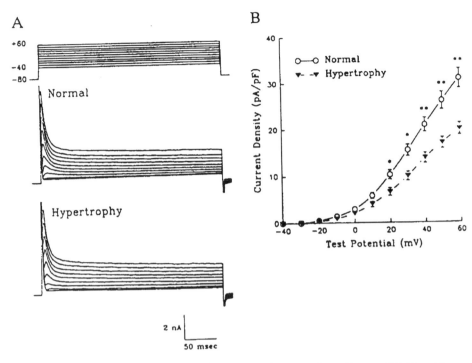

Figure 3 Representative current recordings from a normal myocyte (capacitance = 134pF) and from a myocyte from a heart with left ventricular hypertrophy (capacitance = 201pF) (Panel A). Using the protocol in Panel A, both cells show voltage-dependent activation of transient outward currents (I_{to}) which are similar in amplitude but not density. Panel B: average peak current density-voltage relation for normal (unfilled circles) and hypertrophied (filled triangles) cells Values are mean±SEM. (*P < 0.01 and **P < 0.001). Reproduced from Tomita *et al.* (Tomita *et al.* 1994) with permission.

shown diminished I_{to} to be due to a reduction in the number of functional I_{to} channels in the canine model of pacing induced failure (Kaab *et al.*, 1996a).

In contrast in RV hypertrophied feline myocytes (TenEick *et al.*, 1993) I_{to} is increased in amplitude and density while the number of myocytes exhibiting I_{to} actually increases. These findings are consistent with an observed change in Phase 1 of repolarization in these cells. An enhanced I_{to} in hypertrophied cells can lead to action potential prolongation by resetting the voltage time course of early repolarization (and thus of subsequent activation of inward currents). This is the opposite of what is seen in canine epicardial (Tseng and Hoffman, 1989) or human myocytes (Escande *et al.*, 1985; Shibata *et al.*, 1989) where enhanced I_{to} can be associated with decreased action potential duration.

Studies of hypertrophied myocytes from hearts of adult patients with acquired aortic stenosis (Benitah *et al.*, 1992b) or midmyocardial myocytes from explanted failing human hearts (Beuckelmann *et al.*, 1993) clearly support the idea that at some stage, hypertrophy can result in a diminished I_{to}. Action potential durations of the myocytes from failing hearts show prolongation similar to that of hypertrophy, which is partially explained by a reduction in densities of both the inward rectifier (see above) and transient outward currents.

We now appreciate the heterogeneity in the density of K^+ channel currents among species, between young and old animals, and even across the normal atrial or ventricular wall of the same heart in the same species (Liu *et al.*, 1993) (Chapter 3). This heterogeneity can often cloud our understanding of the effects of disease (e.g., hypertrophy/failure) on the function of specific K^+ channels. A recent study has juxtaposed the density of I_{to} of the endocardial and epicardial human LV myocyte isolated from control nonfailing hearts and hearts from patients with clinical failure (Wettwer *et al.*, 1994). Endocardial cells from failing hearts showed a significant reduction in I_{to} density compared to control, while epicardial myocytes did not (Wettwer *et al.*, 1994). However, in this study, it was not determined whether significant action potential prolongation accompanied the I_{to} changes of the hypertrophied/failed myocytes of endocardial origin.

Cl^- current

Just as a loss in K^+ channel function and thus outward current flow can explain action potential prolongation in hypertrophied/failing myocytes, other current components may gain in function during the disease process, thus partially balancing the effects of decreased K^+ channel function on action potential duration. One such current is a time independent chloride current. Inward movement of Cl^- ions causes an outward current while outward Cl^- movement results in inward current. In the hearts of rats, with global hypertrophy secondary to aortic stenosis, time dependent outward currents are not altered, while semi-selective time independent Cl^- currents are upregulated (Benitah *et al.*, 1997). A variety of Cl^- channels appear to be present in cardiac cells and could be acutely upregulated in response to various stimuli including α and β adrenergic stimuli, ATP, adenosine, cell swelling and stretch.

Pacemaker Current

The nonselective inward cation current (I_f) that is sensitive to extracellular cesium and activated by hyperpolarization is found in sinus node cells of normal hearts (Chapter 3). An I_f current has been recorded at very negative potentials in normal ventricular cells of some species (guinea pigs, dog, rats) but its physiologic role remains uncertain. In hypertrophied cardiac myocytes from genetically determined hypertensive rats, I_f density increases as severity of hypertension increases (Cerbai *et al.*, 1996). As recently reported, in myocytes from failing human hearts, I_f density tended to increase but the increase did not reach significance (Hoppe *et al.*, 1998; Cerbai *et al.*, 1997). It is hypothesized but not yet proven that such an increase in I_f in diseased ventricular cells may be arrhythmogenic.

MYOCARDIAL INFARCTION – ARRHYTHMIA SUBSTRATE FINDINGS

Various phases of arrhythmias occur after the onset of experimentally produced myocardial ischemia and infarction in animal hearts. Over the 24–48 hrs following coronary occlusion (subacute phase of infarction) arrhythmias result from enhanced automaticity of subendocardial Purkinje fibers. These ventricular tachycardias may have counterparts in humans. During the healing (days, weeks) or healed (months) infarct phases, sustained ventricular tachycardias are inducible in both animal and human hearts, thus suggesting that the reentrant substrate is present.

While the true site of origin of these arrhythmias is technically difficult to localize, it can be estimated based on the site of earliest epicardial activation of an arrhythmic impulse and is often found in surviving cells that overlie the infarct. In one canine model in which these arrhythmias have been mapped, they were localized to an area overlying the infarct and on the epicardial surface, referred to as the epicardial border zone (Wit and Janse, 1993).

Numerous studies have described the specific changes in action potential configuration that occur in the canine subendocardial Purkinje fiber and the subepicardial ventricular fiber post coronary artery occlusion. Generally, by 24 to 48 hrs after total coronary artery occlusion the action potentials of the subendocardial Purkinje fibers show reduced resting potentials and $\dot{V}_{max}$, as well as an increase in total time of repolarization. Five days after complete coronary occlusion, cells of the epicardial border zone of the infarct show a reduction in $\dot{V}_{max}$ and a shortening and triangularization of the action potential. Such changes may be responsible for the abnormalities in conduction and refractoriness observed at various times after coronary artery occlusion.

Resting Potential

24–48 hrs post occlusion; subendocardial Purkinje myocytes
The origin of the delayed phase of spontaneous arrhythmias secondary to coronary artery occlusion in canine and porcine hearts is most likely in the depolarized and abnormally automatic subendocardial Purkinje fibers that survive the infarction. The loss of resting potential is significant and dramatic in the multicellular preparations of these fibers. Concomitant with this dramatic loss is a reduction in intracellular K^+ ion concentration $(a_K)^i$. However, a decrease in K^+ equilibrium potential (E_K) (average change 16 mV) cannot fully account for the loss in resting potential (average change 35 mV) (Dresdner *et al.*, 1987).

Reduction in resting potentials of subendocardial Purkinje fibers surviving in the infarcted heart persists even after they are enzymatically disaggregated and studied as single myocytes (Boyden *et al.*, 1989). In the myocyte, a reduction in a_K^i cannot provide the basis for the reduced resting potential. Rather, Purkinje myocytes isolated from the infarcted myocardium show an increase in the ratio of the membrane permeability of Na^+ to K^+ ions (P_{Na}/P_K) as compared to control. The larger value of P_{Na}/P_K in these cells could be due to an increase in P_{Na} or a decrease in P_K or both. Input resistance measurements suggest that total membrane conductance may be decreased in subendocardial Purkinje myocytes from the infarcted myocardium as compared to those of non-infarcted regions; this is in agreement with studies on multicellular preparations (Argentieri *et al.*, 1990). This observation, combined with the P_{Na}/P_K measurements, suggests that a decrease in P_K may contribute to depolarization of diastolic potential. This, in turn, is consistent with a decrease in the density of I_{K1} recently described in these diseased Purkinje myocytes (Pinto and Boyden, 1998).

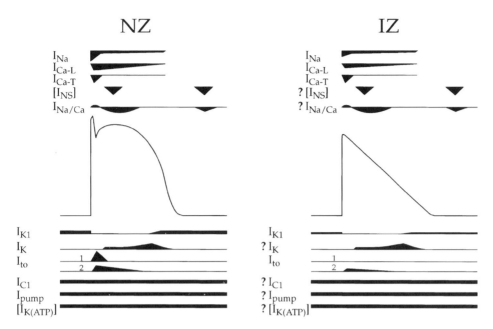

Figure 4 Schematic illustrating action potentials of epicardial ventricular myocyte from a normal heart and from the epicardial border zone of a 5 day infarcted heart. Relative contributions of selected ionic currents are shown. Currents in red are those that have been found to be altered in myocytes from the diseased heart. Question marks indicate there is still incomplete knowledge of ion channel function in these types of myocytes. See text for more detail. Modified after Sicilian Gambit I (1991). *See* Color Plate 2.

5 days post occlusion; Epicardial Border Zone myocytes

In multicellular preparations of myocardium from the epicardial border zone of 5-day old infarcts, the following abnormalities have been described: a decrease in resting potential, total action potential amplitude and $\dot{V}_{max}$, a reduction in action potential duration at both 50 and 90% repolarization and a loss in the plateau potential (e.g., see (Ursell *et al.*, 1985)) (Figure 4). However, when the cells of the epicardial border zone are dispersed and studied as isolated myocytes *in vitro* (Lue and Boyden, 1992), the resting transmembrane potential is not different from control, suggesting that other factors, extrinsic to the myocyte, control resting membrane potential in the multicellular preparation. One likely factor may be extracellular ion accumulation, since in single myocytes electrical activity is studied after the cell is removed from the syncytium and superfused in an environment where immediate extracellular ion accumulation and depletion are not significant.

Healed Myocardial Infarction: ventricle

Investigations of changes in the electrical function in the healing or healed infarct (weeks to months) include studies of cells overlying the infarct scar, known as the central "infarct zone" cells, and those of the surrounding thin rim of cells called the lateral adjacent "border zone" cells. In the feline healed infarct model, fifty percent of the hearts have ectopic activity (Myerburg *et al.*, 1977; Wong *et al.*, 1982). The site of origin of these arrhythmias is not known but it may reside in cells within the healed border zone.

Cells overlying the healed infarct area do not show alterations in transmembrane resting potentials (Wong *et al.*, 1982). However, in the border zone, there are changes in resting potential that vary in different experimental models. Cells from the endocardial border zone of feline healed infarcts show significant reduction in resting potential (-70 mV in border zone cells vs -80 mV in control cells) (Wong *et al.*, 1982); this may be explained by decreased intracellular K^+ activity; a change not observed in tissue overlying the infarct (Kimura *et al.*, 1986). In contrast in rabbit hearts 8 weeks after coronary occlusion, resting membrane potentials of border zone myocytes were significantly more negative than in control myocytes (Litwin and Bridge, 1997). No changes in resting potential were observed in myocytes from 2 month old rat infarcts (Santos *et al.*, 1995), or in epicardial border zone tissue of canine infarcts of similar age (Ursell *et al.*, 1985). There are no studies available on function of I_{K1} in myocytes surviving healed myocardial infarction.

Upstroke Velocity of Phase 0 of the Action Potential

24–48 hrs post coronary artery occlusion; subendocardial Purkinje moycytes

$\dot{V}_{max}$ *and Na^+ current* Reduction in $\dot{V}_{max}$ of the subendocardial Purkinje myocytes that survive in the infarcted myocardium may be accounted for by depolarization of diastolic potential. As yet, there have been no voltage clamp studies that have identified whether the fast Na^+ current density is altered in myocytes dispersed at this time period after coronary artery occlusion.

Ca^{2+} currents Peak $I_{Ca,L}$ density is significantly reduced in subendocardial Purkinje myocytes dispersed from 48 hrs infarcted heart as compared to control and to those from the 24 hrs infarcted heart (Boyden and Pinto, 1994). Current density reduction is not accompanied by a shift in the current–voltage relationship or a change in the time course of $I_{Ca,L}$ current decay. Peak T type Ca^{2+} current density is also decreased in subendocardial Purkinje myocytes that survive in the 24 hrs infarcted heart, and further reduction occurs by 48 hrs. The loss in Ca^{2+} channel function could contribute to the depressed and triangular plateau phase of the action potentials of Purkinje myocytes at this time following coronary occlusion.

5 days post coronary artery occlusion; epicardial border zone myocytes

$\dot{V}_{max}$ *and Na^+ current* Arrhythmias arise in the epicardial border zone region of the 5 day infarcted heart most probably because of abnormalities in impulse conduction (Wit and Janse, 1993). These abnormalities may result from alterations in the fast Na^+ current that is responsible for $\dot{V}_{max}$ of these fibers. While microelectrode recordings from the myocytes of the infarcted heart have shown resting potentials similar to those of control epicardial cells, the mean $\dot{V}_{max}$ of these cells remains significantly reduced when compared to control. Steady-state availability relationships of $\dot{V}_{max}$ (reflecting voltage-dependency of I_{Na} inactivation) in cells from the infarcted heart are shifted by 10 mV along the voltage axis in the hyperpolarizing direction (Lue and Boyden, 1992; Patterson *et al.*, 1993). Lazzara *et al.* (Lazzara and Scherlag, 1984) have suggested that in surviving cells in the 5 day infarcted heart, inexcitability can outlast the repolarization phase of the action potential. The

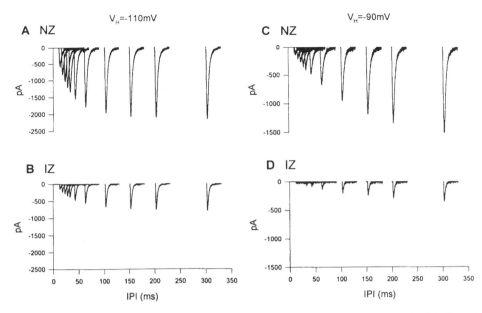

Figure 5 Recovery of peak I_{Na} using a double-pulse protocol in a representative normal cell (NZ) and epicardial border zone cell (IZ). Voltage-clamp protocol consists of a 350 ms prepulse and a test pulse elicited at varying intervals of 2 to 3000 ms every 5s. Original current tracings are superimposed to illustrate recovery of peak I_{Na}. Cell capacitance NZ = 124 pF; IZ = 150 pF (Pu and Boyden, unpublished).

mechanism of this post repolarization refractoriness may reside in changes of the kinetics of I_{Na}. In control noninfarcted cells, the time constant of recovery of $\dot{V}_{max}$ is rapid and voltage dependent while in myocytes from the epicardial border zone of the 5 day infarcted heart, the time course of recovery of $\dot{V}_{max}$, although remaining voltage-dependent, is significantly prolonged (Patterson *et al.*, 1993; Lue and Boyden, 1992). Recent whole cell voltage clamp data have confirmed that the reduced $\dot{V}_{max}$ of cells of the epicardial border zone are secondary to decreases in I_{Na} density and altered Na^+ current kinetics (Pu and Boyden, 1997). In particular, a marked lag in recovery of I_{Na} appears to account, at least in part, for post repolarization refractoriness in these myocytes (Pu and Boyden, 1997) (Figures 5, 6).

Ca^{2+} currents The peak $I_{Ca,L}$ current density of epicardial border zone cells from the 5 day infarcted heart is significantly reduced compared to control (Aggarwal and Boyden, 1995). This reduction is not associated with changes in either steady-state availability or time course of recovery from inactivation. However, the time course of decay of $I_{Ca,L}$ is significantly faster than in control myocytes. These findings may be related to a decrease in the number of functioning channels as well as an acceleration of inactivation of the remaining ones. Unlike findings in the subendocardial Purkinje myocytes studies (see above), no significant differences were found between peak density of T type Ca^{2+} currents in epicardial border zone myocytes surviving in the 5 day infarcted heart.

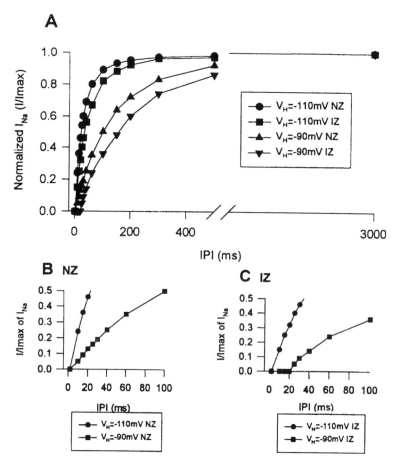

Figure 6 Time course of recovery of I_{Na} from inactivation in a single myocyte from normal heart (NZ, circles) and from the epicardial border zone of a 5-day infarct (IZ, squares). The amplitude of I_{Na} is normalized to I_{Na} at the interpulse interval (IPI) = 3000 ms. Panel A illustrates recovery in a typical NZ and IZ at two $V_h (V_h = -110$ mV, unfilled; $V_h = -90$ mV, filled symbols). Inset shows average data obtained for short IPIs for $V_h = -90$ mV. Panels B and C illustrate that recovery of I_{Na} depends on V_h. Note the lag in recovery of I_{Na} seen in IZ when $V_h = -90$ mV, suggesting that IZ Na$^+$ channels may deactivate slowly. It is also possible that there are two populations of cells with different recovery kinetics. Slow recovery of I_{Na} in IZs may contribute to slowed conduction or prolongation of refractoriness after repolarization in epicardial border zone fibers of the infarcted heart ((Pu and Boyden, 1997) with permission).

Healed Myocardial Infarction: ventricle

In the feline healed infarct model, the surviving endocardial cells surrounding the 2 month old infarct have characteristics different from those during acute ischemia and early infarction (Wong *et al.*, 1982). Electrophysiological abnormalities in these cells include prolonged action potentials with normal resting membrane potentials and upstroke velocities. In contrast, border zone cells between the scar and normal tissue have short APDs with reduced upstroke amplitudes and upstroke velocities, similar to those observed in acute phase post infarction. The duration of the AP shortens to a greater extent in healed infarct myocytes as stimulation frequency increases (Litwin and Bridge, 1997; Wong *et al.*, 1982). Thus, the initial ischemic insult together with subsequent chronic healing can differentially affect membrane functions and/or cell-to-cell coupling of border and central infarct zone cells (Wong *et al.*, 1982).

Na$^+$ currents   Whole cell Na$^+$ currents have not been measured in cells surviving in the healed infarcted heart. Intracellular sodium activity in the infarct zone does not differ from that in normal zone tissues (Kimura *et al.*, 1986). Increased Na$_i$ activity in border zone tissue of infarcted feline hearts suggests a depressed Na$^+$ – K$^+$ pump activity and/or increased Na$^+$ leak. These latter changes could indirectly affect $\dot{V}_{max}$ of action potentials of these myocytes.

Ca^{2+} currents   Myocytes adjacent to the 8 week infarct in the rabbit heart show a significant decrease in peak $I_{Ca, L}$ density without a change in current-voltage relations or voltage-dependent and steady-state inactivation kinetics (Litwin and Bridge, 1997). In the 2 month feline infarct model, myocytes from the area underlying or immediately adjacent to the infarct scar also have reduced calcium current amplitudes at most test voltages (Pinto *et al.*, 1997). These values differ from those in cells from normal hearts and those from remote, non-infarcted regions of the infarcted heart. Reduced current density and accelerated current decay persist even when barium is used as the charge carrier, suggesting a decrease in the number of functional Ca^{2+} channels at this time (Figure 7). Furthermore, the voltage at which Ca^{2+} channels are half-maximally available is shifted such that smaller L type Ca^{2+} inward window currents eventuate. Such changes in $I_{Ca, L}$ could contribute to the reduced plateau of the action potential observed at this stage of infarction.

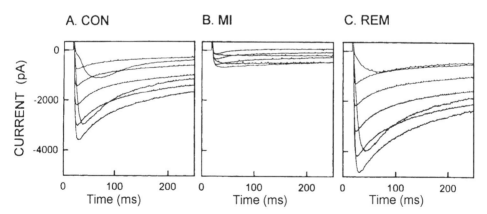

Figure 7   Inward barium current (I_{BaL}) tracings from a representative ventricular myocyte from a control heart (CON) are compared to a myocyte from the area immediately adjacent to (MI) and a myocyte remote from (REM) a 2 month old feline infarct. Replacement of extracellular calcium with equimolar barium caused a 1.8 fold increase from 1736 pA in the CON myocyte, no increase from 780 pA in the infarct myocyte and a 3.3 fold increase in the inward current in the REM myocyte. Attenuation of the inward barium current in MI myocytes may be secondary to a decrease in the number of functional L-type Ca channels. The accentuation of inward current in REM myocytes when barium replaces calcium as a charge carrier may reflect a faster calcium-dependent inactivation and a slower voltage-dependent inactivation (Pinto *et al.*, 1997).

Repolarization and Refractoriness

24–48 hrs post occlusion; subendocardial Purkinje myocytes

I_{to} Action potentials of subendocardial Purkinje fibers that survive 24 to 48 hrs after occlusion have reduced phase 1 repolarization. Whereas pacing at fast rates causes little or no change in phase 1 of repolarization in normal Purkinje fibers, it has a dramatic effect on the time course of repolarization of subendocardial Purkinje myocytes surviving in the infarcted heart. In some cases, with an increase in drive rate, the rapid phase 1 of repolarization of action potentials in these fibers completely disappears (see Figure 3.30 of (Wit and Janse, 1993)). Whole cell voltage clamp experiments have shown that the density of I_{to} in these cells is reduced by 50%. Moreover, I_{to} currents in Purkinje myocytes from the 48 hrs infarcted heart showed specific kinetic changes. Notably, the time course of current decay is accelerated while the time course of reactivation of I_{to} is significantly delayed. This slowing of recovery implies that less outward repolarizing current would be available for action potentials occurring at high pacing rates or during closely spaced voltage clamp steps.

I_K New information is available on the function of K^+ currents (e.g., the delayed rectifying current(s)) in Purkinje myocytes that survive in the infarcted heart. Subendocardial Purkinje myocytes from the 48hr infarcted heart have significantly increased density of I_{Kr} (measured as E4031 sensitive current) compared to those of normal Purkinje myocytes. The current sensitive to E4031 in Purkinje myocytes differs from that recorded from normal or infarcted ventricular myocyted (Pinto and Boyden, 1998). These data suggest that repolarization of surviving Purkinje myocytes might be more sensitive to the action of E4031-like antiarrhythmic drugs (methanesulfonanilides) than control myocytes.

5 days post coronary artery occlusion; epicardial border zone myocytes

I_{to} Action potentials recorded from the epicardial border zone cells usually show no phase 1 or a reduced phase 1 repolarization suggesting a loss in the voltage dependent transient outward current (Lue and Boyden, 1992). Voltage clamp studies confirm that the density of the voltage dependent, (non-Ca$_i$-dependent) transient outward current (I_{to1}) is absent or markedly reduced in the cells demonstrating the loss in the notch (Lue and Boyden, 1992).

Healed Myocardial Infarction: ventricle
Repolarization of normal, lateral border and infarct zone cells in the heart with healed infarct is nonuniform. In some models, APs of different morphologies and varying degrees of prolongation are found in almost all regions of the LV, especially immediately adjacent to the infarct scar (Wong *et al.*, 1982; Santos *et al.*, 1995; Myerburg *et al.*, 1977).

The duration of refractoriness in infarct zone cells is consistent with the variability of APDs. Infarct zone and lateral border cells have functional refractory periods which often outlast the total time course of repolarization in the healed, infarcted heart (Wong *et al.*, 1982). Although the initial damage to lateral border zone cells may be less than that of central ischemic area cells, electrophysiological abnormalities appear to persist in cells from the border zone well beyond the early phase post myocardial infarction (Wong *et al.*, 1982).

Both epicardial and endocardial tissues in hearts with healed infarcts demonstrate marked disparity in refractoriness in the border and infarct areas, especially during sympathetic stimulation (Gaide *et al.*, 1983). The prolongation of refractoriness could be related to a slowed recovery of I_{Na} or delay in deactivation of outward K^+ currents in the infarct substrate. To date however, there have been no direct measurements of these latter currents in cells overlying the healed infarct.

REGIONS REMOTE FROM THE INFARCT – REGIONAL HYPERTROPHY CHANGES

Structural remodeling of the left ventricle after myocardial infarction involves the regions of necrosis and infarct scar, as well as the noninfarcted myocardium remote from the infarcted region. In many models, the myocardium shows gradual morphological changes indicative of hypertrophy. These may reflect adaptation to the increased workload resulting from compromised contractility of the ischemic area. In the long term, persistent elevated myocardial and cellular load may account for the disease progression toward end-stage heart failure.

Regional hypertrophy that accompanies ventricular remodeling is of interest because left ventricular hypertrophy is a strong risk factor for ventricular arrhythmias (Ho *et al.*, 1993). Remote areas include noninfarcted LV or RV tissue. Typically, regional increases in remote area cell size occur as discerned by measurements of cell capacitance, morphometry and flow cytometry (Cox *et al.*, 1991; Kozlovskis *et al.*, 1991; Pinto *et al.*, 1997; Olivetti *et al.*, 1991). Increase in cell size depends on the size of the infarct. Large (40% of LV) infarcts tend to show greater increases in cell size, compared to smaller infarcts (< 15%) (Cox *et al.*, 1991). Non-transmural infarcts show increases in cell diameter adjacent to the infarct, but not in the remote areas; conversely, in transmural infarcts, all cell diameters increase (Cox *et al.*, 1991). In some models increases in myocyte length but not width have been described (Santos *et al.*, 1995).

SUBACUTE AND HEALING (3 DAY, 3–4 WKS) MYOCARDIAL INFARCTION – REMOTE

Resting Potential

I_{K1} is reduced in epicardial but not endocardial LV myocytes of 3 day old infarcted rat heart. Minor changes in I_{K1} density occur in RV myocytes remote from the infarcted region of the 3 day rat heart (Yao *et al.*, 1997). It is unlikely that these changes would be accompanied by a change in resting potential of the myocytes. No change in resting potential is seen in myocytes from the 3 week infarcted rat heart (Qin *et al.*, 1996).

Upstroke Velocity of Phase 0 of the Action Potential

Na$^+$ currents   No definitive data are yet available.

Ca^{2+} currents   Hypertrophied LV myocytes from a 3 week post infarction model show a significant increase in $I_{Ca, L}$ amplitude but when normalized to cell capacitance changes, no significant change in $I_{Ca, L}$ density versus control is observed (Qin *et al.*, 1996). A reemergence of the T type Ca^{2+} current has been reported to occur in myocytes of the hypertrophied rat ventricles (Qin *et al.*, 1995).

Repolarization and Refractoriness

Marked variations in APD configuration can also be seen in single post-infarct cells obtained from the remodeled LV wall (Qin *et al.*, 1996). Outward K$^+$ currents in rat remodeled LV decay with two phases. The characteristics of the fast component are similar to I_{to}, while the slow component resembles I_K. Differences in the relative densities of I_{to} and I_K can explain the differences in action potential characteristics between epicardial and endocardial myocytes. Noninfarcted RV myocytes from the 3 day old rat infarct show no reduction in I_{to} or I_K current density compared to myocytes from sham-operated hearts, however, both K$^+$ channel densities are increased relative to control RV myocytes, possibly as a result of surgical trauma (Yao *et al.*, 1997).

   For the rat LV myocytes not overlying the 3 day infarct but adjacent to it, I_{to} densities are reduced with more severe reductions occurring in myocytes from the epicardial versus the endocardial layers. I_K is reduced in density evenly across the myocardial wall in cells remote from the infarct (Yao *et al.*, 1997). By 3 weeks post MI in the rat, the hypertrophied LV myocytes continue to show reduced I_{to} and I_K densities with little change reported for channel kinetics (Qin *et al.*, 1996). These latter studies are consistent with the persistent action potential prolongation in these myocytes.

HEALED (2–6 MONTHS) MYOCARDIAL INFARCTION – REMOTE

Resting Potential

In general, there are no differences in resting potentials in myocytes from epicardial and endocardial areas that are remote from the 2–6 month old infarcts (Pinto *et al.*, 1997; Yuan *et al.*, 1999; Santos *et al.*, 1995).

Upstroke Velocity of Phase 0 of the Action Potential

Rats with 2 month old infarcts have a significantly reduced $\dot{V}_{max}$ of Phase 0 in cells from the LV free wall (Santos *et al.*, 1995). No studies to date have identified whether there are persistent changes in the density or function of I_{Na} in these cells.

Ca^{2+} currents   Typically, areas remote from the infarct scar show a tendency toward an increase in Ca^{2+} current magnitude (Santos *et al.*, 1995; Pinto *et al.*, 1997), regardless of the holding voltage. Current–voltage curves have a typical bell-shaped configuration, with similar peak potential ranges in both post-infarct and sham-operated or control cells. However, peak $I_{Ca, L}$ density is reduced as a result of an increase in capacitance of the remote area myocytes (Pinto *et al.*, 1997; Santos *et al.*, 1995). When barium is used as the charge carrier, inward current in remote cells is enhanced compared to control cells, suggesting that voltage-dependent inactivation is decreased, but more importantly, that calcium-dependent inactivation may be increased (Figure 7). The time course of decay of calcium currents is unchanged in remote cells (Pinto *et al.*, 1997; Santos *et al.*, 1995). Steady-state availability curves may be unchanged (Santos *et al.*, 1995), or shifted to more negative potentials (Pinto *et al.*, 1997), while restitution of $I_{Ca, L}$ remains normal.

No reemerging T-type Ca^{2+} currents have been recorded in the grossly hyper-trophied myocytes of the 2 month feline healed infarct model (Pinto *et al.*, unpub-lished data).

Repolarization and Refractoriness

APD is typically prolonged in remote areas. The extent of AP prolongation appears to depend on the age of the infarct; myocytes from older infarcts (6–11 month) show greater prolongation compared to younger infarcts (1–2 month)(Santos *et al.*, 1995). Action potential durations at all phases of repolarization appear to be increased to a greater extent than in the infarct zone (Santos *et al.*, 1995); this may vary depending on whether cells are epicardial or endocardial in origin. There are no data on function or density of I_{to} in myocytes from areas remote to the healed infarct. In non-infarcted subendocardial myocytes adjacent to the healed infarct, I_K density (but not its amplitude) is significantly decreased. This is similar to the change observed in global left ventricular hypertrophy (Yuan *et al.*, 1999; Kleiman and Houser, 1989; Furukawa *et al.*, 1994), and reflects cell enlargement that is unac-companied by an increase in K^+ channel expression.

MOLECULAR MECHANISMS UNDERLYING THE CHANGE IN ION CHANNEL FUNCTION IN CARDIAC DISEASE

It is obvious, from the examples cited above, that disease states can and do alter ion channel function. Observed changes in macroscopic currents can be the result of a change in structure and function of normally expressed channels, or a change in the number of functional channels, or a combination of both.

A change in the number of functional channels can be determined at both the single channel and molecular levels. From a molecular standpoint, a change in the number of functional channels could be due to changes in the levels of expressed protein or to alterations in channel protein incorporation into the membrane.

A change in expression of functional channel proteins is most likely due to a change in gene transcription, translation, or post translational modification. Tran-scription, the initial step in protein expression, involves the production of an mRNA copy from a DNA template.

Changes in intracellular Ca^{2+} and hormonally induced changes in cAMP levels have both been linked to altered transcription of mRNAs encoding different ion channel proteins (Sherman and Catterall, 1984; Sherman *et al.*, 1985). In some studies, increases in intracellular Ca^{2+} have been reported to cause a fall in mRNA encoding Na^+ channels and to decrease the density of the fast inward Na^+ current (Chiamvimonvat *et al.*, 1995). On the other hand, forskolin induced changes in cAMP stimulate synthesis of Na^+ channel mRNA. Additionally, cAMP presumably through a protein kinase system, decreases the rate of transcription of a K^+ channel gene (Kv1.5) (Mori *et al.*, 1993). In contrast, neonatal atrial cells depolarized with KCl for 30 mins in primary culture show a dramatic increase in Kv1.5 transcript (Mori *et al.*, 1993).

The presence of catecholamines appears to regulate the level of L type Ca^{2+} channel expression in cardiac cells. In particular, α adrenergic agonists decrease, while β agonists increase, L type Ca^{2+} channel mRNA (Maki *et al.*, 1993). In these latter studies, the change in the level of mRNA is correlated with an increase in functional channel density. More direct contact of sympathetic neurons with cardiocytes increases Ca^{2+} channel expression (Ogawa *et al.*, 1992).

Recent studies suggest that transcription of different ion channel proteins is greatly affected by disease state. For instance, experimental myocardial hypertrophy, and treatments to prolong action potential duration, result in a substantial increase in the K^+ channel Kv1.4 mRNA levels in cultured rat myocytes (Matsubara *et al.*, 1993a). This gene regulation is reversed by normalization of hypertrophy (Matsubara *et al.*, 1993b). There is no report yet, as to whether this enhanced transcription results in an enhancement of functional channel proteins in the hypertrophied cell. In ventricles of renovascular hypertensive rats (global hypertrophy), expression levels of Kv4.2 and Kv4.3 (thought to encode I_{to} proteins) are significantly reduced while Kv1.2, Kv1.4, Kv1.5, Kv2.1 or KvLQT1 mRNAs are unchanged (Takimoto *et al.*, 1997). In the rat model by 3 days post MI there is a significant reduction in Kv4.2 channel protein levels in noninfarcted tissues with no changes in Kv2.1 or Kv1.5 levels (Yao *et al.*, 1997). By 3 to 4 weeks in the same model, mRNAs of Kv1.4, Kv2.1 and Kv4.2 all appear to be significantly decreased with no changes detected in Kv1.2 or Kv1.5 levels (Gidh-Jain *et al.*, 1996). Quantitative analysis of mRNA levels in normal and failing human ventricles show that steady state mRNAs for Kv4.3 and HERG are decreased while no mRNA changes occur for Kv1.2, Kv1.4, 1.5, 2.1 or I_{K1} (Kaab *et al.*, 1996b).

In regional hypertrophied myocardium 3 weeks post MI where L type Ca^{2+} currents are relatively normal, a brief report has suggested that mRNA level of the fetal isoform of the L type Ca^{2+} channel has reemerged suggesting new functioning L type Ca^{2+} channels may be more fetal like in phenotype (Gidh-Jain *et al.*, 1995).

Once the mRNA has been transcribed from the DNA template, it must be translated into the polypeptide product. It is possible that a change could occur in the ability of the cell to translate the mRNA into a polypeptide, perhaps by altering the ability of the mRNA to interact with ribosomes. A breakdown in translation may be a manifestation of a disease state, rather than an adaptation of the cells to disease. As yet, there is no documented evidence of a disease-related breakdown in translation of mRNA into ion channel proteins.

After mRNA has been translated into a polypeptide, it undergoes post translational modifications leading to incorporation into the cell membrane. Post translational modifications include glycosylation, anchoring, and phosphorylation. In the case of potassium channels, posttranslational modifications also include the assembly of channel α subunits into a functional homo- or heterotetramer. For sodium, calcium and some potassium channels, posttranslational aligning with specific subunits is required for appropriate ion channel function (for review see (Isom *et al.*, 1994)). An alteration in subunit availability (due to changes in translation), and/or tetramer assembly could then greatly affect channel function (Babila *et al.*, 1994).

CONCLUSIONS

In summary, it is clear that in even very specific settings (myocardial hypertrophy, myocardial infarction), there is a host of changes in ion channel structures and activities that vary among species, regions of the heart and time after the pathological event. It should be understood that this complex behavior pattern extends to other diseases processes, as well. For example, atrial disease and fibrillation incorporate some similar and some dissimilar changes in both molecular determinants and electrophysiologic expression of ion channels. Only through continuing systematic investigations of the determinants of these changes in electrophysiologic properties of cells of the arrhythmic substrate can we hope to understand fully the dynamic nature of the arrhythmic process and, as a result, devise therapeutic approaches that have the promise of more successful endpoints than has been the case to date.

8 Synthesis of the Cardiac Purkinje-fiber Action Potential Using a Computer Model

Chris Clausen, Michael R. Rosen and Ira S. Cohen

INTRODUCTION

The cardiac action potential results from the flow of ionic currents generated by membrane channels and pumps located in the sarcolemmal membrane. Many of these currents are time and voltage dependent. The voltage-clamp technique has been used to study the properties of each of the individual membrane current components, but how these currents sum to generate the action potential waveform is readily appreciated by computer simulation.

Our overall approach is to describe each of the ionic currents using a set of equations. These equations characterize any time and voltage dependence of the flow of individual currents. In the present model a *membrane* action potential is generated (see Figure 1). With this formulation, all points on the membrane are at the same potential and there is no axial current flow. Under these conditions the

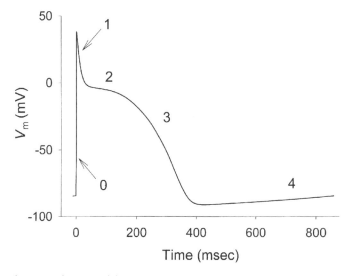

Figure 1 Steady-state action potential computed from the model at a pacing rate of 70/min. Numbered phases of the action potentials are labeled.

sum of all the membrane currents (i_m) is related simply to the rate of change of membrane voltage with time (t) through the following equation

$$i_m = -C_m \frac{dV_m}{dt},$$ (1)

where C_m is the membrane capacitance and V_m is the membrane potential. The current flow through the different channels is gated (see Chapters 2 and 3), and the kinetics of their gating can be described using the so-called Hodgkin-Huxley formalism (Hodgkin and Huxley, 1952a). Namely, for an arbitrary gating variable a (which ranges between 0 and 1) describing activation or inactivation of a given channel type, the differential equation

$$\frac{da}{dt} = \alpha_a(1 - a) - \beta_a a$$ (2)

describes its kinetics, where α_a and β_a are first-order rate constants that are dependent on V_m but not on time.

The entire model consists of 11 differential equations: Equation 1 describes voltage, and there are ten equations of the form of Equation 2, each representing the gating of the different channels. Additional equations describe the rate constants (α_a and β_a) for channel activation and inactivation derived from voltage-clamp studies, as well as 13 separate equations describing each of the different membrane currents. Solution of the model involves specifying appropriate initial conditions for the differential equations, with subsequent integration of the equations as a function of time using a numerical algorithm.

It is important to understand what computer models of the cardiac action potential can and cannot do. First, results of model simulations are only as accurate as the description of the ionic currents measured experimentally. Second, if a model simulation does not reproduce experimental results, it is the model, not the experiment, that must be modified. In fact, the precise purpose of such a model is to try to reproduce experimental studies of the cardiac action potential. Failure of the model is a valuable outcome, because the model can then be refined to more accurately represent the experimental reality.

When a computer model does reproduce experimental results it can provide valuable insights. It can suggest the contribution of each ionic-current component to overall changes in the action-potential waveform. Ideally, if all the ion-current properties are specified, a computer model has direct utility, as in the development and testing of new pharmaceutical agents. For example, model simulations can help the investigator target the specific ionic currents whose alterations by drugs would have clinical efficacy, and in the testing of new drugs, model simulations are useful in the quantitative assessment of their actions by reproducing experimentally observed drug-induced changes in the action potential.

Below, we show simulations performed using a mathematical model of the mammalian Purkinje fiber. We chose to develop a Purkinje-fiber model as opposed to, say, a model for sinus node or ventricle, for two major reasons. First, most of the ionic currents have been well characterized, owing to the specific geometric characteristics of the preparation that facilitate voltage-clamp studies. Second, Purkinje fibers exhibit a wide variety of membrane currents that are also seen in other regions of the heart. For example, they exhibit a transient inward sodium current also observed in ventricle but not sinoatrial node, and they exhibit pacemaker currents similar to those observed in sinoatrial node but not ventricle. Finally, there have been extensive experimental studies of the Purkinje-fiber action potential, so that the model could be tested and refined by examining its ability to reproduce known experimental results.

In three representative examples, we examine (1) the changes in membrane currents that give rise to the differences between an action potential initiated from rest and a steady-state action potential in a paced fiber, (2) the effects of a selective sodium-channel blocker, tetrodotoxin (TTX), on the action potential duration, and (3) how early afterdepolarizations (see Chapter 3) can be generated by increased persistent sodium current. We use these examples to show how a model can increase our understanding of the complex interactions of time- and voltage-dependent ionic currents.

All computer models are simplified compared to experimental reality. As such, the model ignores some properties of a real Purkinje fiber. First, the action potential propagates in a Purkinje fiber due to the generation of axial current flow, yet the model considers the case of a region of the fiber that is isopotential. Second, changes in electrical activity produce changes in intracellular ion concentrations, yet the model lacks equations to account for these changes. Third, besides time- and volt-age-dependent channel gating, second messengers alter channel and pump properties, and these secondary effects are not included in the formulation. Although these determinents of electrical activity could be included in more complex versions of the model, they have been excluded in the interest of simplicity, and to render the model readily solvable using a standard laboratory computer with modest computational capabilities.

Time Dependent Currents Included in the Model

1. The transient TTX-sensitive inward sodium current (i_{Na}) generates the upstroke of the Purkinje-fiber action potential. This current activates rapidly on depolarization (less than a millisecond), and inactivates within a few milliseconds. Both the rate of activation and that of inactivation are voltage dependent as is the probability of the channel being open. The equations we use to describe this current are obtained from the experiments of Ebihara and Johnson (1980). They have been modified to take into account the different conductance and voltage dependence of the sodium current observed in Purkinje fibers. (There is also a rapidly activating TTX-sensitive sodium current that is largely time independent, see below.)

2. An L-type calcium current, i_{Ca} (see Chapter 3), helps sustain the plateau of the Purkinje-fiber action potential. Like the sodium current, it possesses both an activation and an inactivation process. We have employed the equations presented by Wilders *et al.* (1991) for their sinus-node simulations, and modified the equations to best fit experimental calcium currents recorded in Purkinje myocytes by Datyner and Cohen (1993).

3. The transient outward current (i_{to}) contains multiple components whose molecular identity is still being defined. Its function is to repolarize the action

potential rapidly from the peak of the overshoot to plateau levels. We have employed the formulation presented by McAllister, Noble and Tsien (1975). Note that these investigators refer to i_{to} by the name i_{qr}. This current possesses both an activation gate and an inactivation gate.

4. The delayed rectifier potassium currents (i_K equivalent to $i_{Kr} + i_{Ks}$) activate during the plateau of the action potential and lead to ultimate repolarization during phase 3 of the Purkinje-fiber action potential. These delayed rectifier currents were studied initially in Purkinje fibers by Noble and Tsien (1968). Their report of fast and slow components was confirmed at the single myocyte level by Gintant et al. (1985), although the two components of kinetics were ascribed to a single channel with multiple closed states. More recently evidence in favor of two channels has been presented in ventricular myocytes by Sanguinetti and Jurkie-wicz (1990a). We have adopted the two-parallel-conductance formalism as initi-ally presented by McAllister, Noble and Tsien (1975), where one current (i_{Kr}) activates with a time constant of hundreds of milliseconds, while the other slower current (i_{Ks}) activates over a period of seconds. Note that McAllister et al. (1975) refer to i_{Kr} and i_{Ks} as i_{X1} and i_{X2}, respectively.

5. A hyperpolarization activated current (i_f) contributes to pacemaker activity and prevents excessive hyperpolarization. It was first described in Purkinje fibers by DiFrancesco (1981a, b) and was characterized in isolated Purkinje myocytes by Yu et al. (1995). We have employed the equations from the isolated-myocyte study for the present simulation.

6. The slowly deactivating inwardly rectifying current ($i_{K_{dd}}$) is important in gen-erating the pacemaker depolarization. This current was initially described by Noble and Tsien in (1968) in sheep Purkinje fibers and called i_{K_2}. More recent analysis questioned its relevance to pacemaker activity because of the discovery of the inward current activated on hyperpolarization (i_f, see above). However, a recent study in canine Purkinje myocytes has demonstrated its existence in the diastolic range of potentials. The equations we employ were presented by McAllister et al. (1975), which describe an inwardly rectifying potassium current that activates on depolarization in the voltage range of -90 to -60 mV, and has a time constant of activation or deactivation of hundreds of milliseconds to seconds.

Time Independent Membrane Currents Included in the Model

1. Besides the rapidly inactivating component of TTX-sensitive sodium current (i_{Na}, see above), Saint et al. (1992) reported the existence of a persistent component of TTX-sensitive current ($i_{Na, p}$). This current activates but does not inactivate over the time scale of the action potential, and so is modeled as having the same voltage activation dependence, but no inactivation. It is essentially time inde-pendent at plateau potentials and can play a significant role in controlling the action potential duration.

2. The maximum diastolic potential approaches the equilibrium potential for potassium, because of the presence of a large inwardly rectifying background current called i_{K_1}. This current does activate, but the activation process is so rapid (fraction of a millisecond) that it can be considered time independent when compared to the time scale of the action potential. The rectification is due to

block by internal magnesium and polyamines and this is also extremely rapid. The equations used to model the current were developed by Oliva *et al.* (1990) in their study of i_{K_1} in Purkinje myocytes.

3. The Na, K-pump extrudes three sodium ions while importing two potassium ions in each cycle. This electrogenic transport provides a net outward current (i_p) while restoring the ionic gradients dissipated during each cardiac cycle. The current is voltage dependent and we employed an equation used to fit data obtained from guinea pig ventricular myocytes by Gao *et al.* (1996). The half activation voltage is assumed to be -80 mV.

4. Three background leak currents are included. They are assumed to be ohmic and are described in McAllister *et al.* (1975). These include a background sodium current, a chloride current, and a nonspecific leak current. The nonspecific leak current is usually set to zero; nonetheless, its formulation is included to permit simulations where the fiber is in a depolarized state (e.g., owing to ischemic damage).

METHODS

The model is implemented as a FORTRAN program, and is distributed in executable form on the accompanying diskette. A comprehensive user's manual describing the detailed operation of the program is found in the Appendix and also on the diskette. The program and associated documentation can also be downloaded from an Internet web site (`http:/physiology.pnb.sunysb.edu/faculty/clausen/ clausen.htm`). The program will run efficiently on any IBM PC running the Windows 95 or Windows NT operating systems. The program produces no graphical output. Rather, operation of the program consists of the execution of user-entered commands that result in the generation of output files containing all model computations. One can then import these results into standard spreadsheet programs (e.g., Excel, Lotus) for the manipulation of tabular data and the generation of rudimentary graphs, or sophisticated graphics programs (e.g., SigmaPlot) for generation of finished graphs.

The program was compiled and linked using Fortran PowerStation Version 4.0 Professional Edition (Microsoft Corp., Redmond, WA, U.S.A.) running under the Windows NT operating system on a Pentium Pro system. All computations are performed using double precision (64-bit) arithmetic. The relative (local) error during integration of the differential equations is less than 10^{-6}. The algorithm used to integrate the equations is adaptive, and automatically subdivides time intervals in order to attain this accuracy.

Also included on the diskette is the source code (FORTRAN statements) for the model. Although virtually all model parameters can be modified or adjusted while the program is running, distribution of the source code permits detailed verification of the model's formulation, coupled with the ability to change the formulation, if so desired. In addition, the source code permits installation of the program on different computer platforms. The only portion of the program that is not distributed is a proprietary subprogram for the numerical solution of an arbitrary system of differential equations. This subprogram (needed *only* if one intends to make changes to the program) is available from the IMSL library, a commercially available library of mathematical subroutines (Visual Numerics Inc., Houston, TX, U.S.A.); this library is included as a component of Microsoft Fortran Powerstation, as well as this compiler's successor, DIGITAL Visual Fortran (Digital Equipment Corp., Maynard, MA, U.S.A.). Alternatively, one can substitute a different, but functionally equivalent, routine to integrate the equations.

RESULTS

The results of three representative simulations will be presented to illustrate operation of the computer program that implements the Purkinje-fiber model.

Generation of a Steady-state Paced Action Potential

Figure 2 shows console input and output while running the model. When the program is waiting for user commands, it displays the prompt purkinje> seen in the first line. At this point, one can enter a number of different commands to display the state of the model, change all model parameters, control integration of the model equations, and save computed results. For example, the show all command in the first line of Figure 2 directs the program to display all adjustable model parameters, which are shown in the 15 lines that follow. These parameters are the default values built into the program. A detailed description of all the program commands, their arguments, and the model parameters, is discussed in the user's manual (see Appendix).

Before integrating the model equations, one must supply initial conditions for the 11 differential equations comprising the model. One can manually enter arbitrary values for the initial conditions, but it is typically more reasonable to compute values based on a given experimental condition or protocol. For example, in *in vitro* studies of isolated Purkinje fibers, one often finds that upon initial impalement with a microelectrode, V_m is at a stable resting potential. An action potential can subsequently be initiated by passing a brief depolarizing current pulse. If the current pulses are applied repetitively, say once every 600 msec, then the isolated fiber resembles a paced fiber *in vivo* (in this example, one being paced at 100/min). When this experimental protocol is used, one observes the following: the action potential elicited after the first current pulse (where the fiber was initially at rest) is long in duration, and exhibits a rapid transient repolarization to a nearly flat plateau. Upon repetitive stimulation, one attains a steady state where the action potentials are shorter in duration, and exhibit less flat plateau phases (compared to the first). The computer model must be able to reproduce this basic experimental observation.

In Figure 2, the rest −80 command initializes V_m to the resting potential. This command invokes a procedure whereby the user specifies an initial estimate of the resting potential (e.g., −80 mV), and the program subsequently refines this value iteratively until the true resting potential – the membrane potential resulting in zero net membrane current flow – is determined. Under resting conditions, the gating variables are at their equilibrium values. Note that for an arbitrary gating variable a (e.g., sodium activation m, sodium inactivation h, etc.), its equilibrium value at any

```
purkinje>show all
  alpha    .3200         .0000         .5000         .0000      8.0000E-03  2.0800E-05
         1.0000E-03  5.0000E-04   1.2700E-04   7.2930E-06
   beta   5.806         .0000         .5000         .0000      8.0000E-02  2.0000E-02
         5.0000E-05  1.3000E-03   3.0000E-04   2.9130E-03
   ebar  -47.13         .0000       -6.600         .0000        .0000      -26.00
        -52.00         .0000         .0000       -52.00
   gbar   500.0         .8000        5.000         .1050      1.0000E-02   2.430
          2.800        2.200        25.00         .3850      5.000        5.000
        7.5000E-02    .4000         .0000
 hkinet  -7.000      2.9400E-02    -.1395       -68.94       4.8980E-03    .1393
        -73.34         .1876      -9.8570E-03
   erev   40.00        70.00       -70.00       -100.0       -41.00        .0000
        -70.00          .
    cap   10.00
   curr    .0000         .5000       -800.0
purkinje>rest -80
purkinje>init /
purkinje>check
Time:            .0000
Equation values (indices  1 through 11)...
  1.5641E-02    .4316       6.0340E-05    .9995       1.1240E-05    .2374
   .7213      2.1345E-02   5.5911E-06   2.7410E-02  -70.72
Derivatives (indices 12 through 22)...
   .0000         .0000         .0000       6.9389E-18  5.4210E-20    .0000
   .0000         .0000         .0000         .0000       80.00
Currents (indices 23 through 35)...
  -9.1420E-02 -6.7896E-03    2.923         7.160         .2156     -1.2457E-05
  -9.6317E-06   1.759       -11.63       -7.2202E-03 -3.1776E-05  -.3259
   .0000
purkinje>file rest.txt
purkinje>start 2 0.05
t =   5.0000E-02  Vm =  -66.72        dVm/dt =    80.02
                   ↓
t =   2.000       Vm =   28.65        dVm/dt =   -2.323
dVm/dt-max of    332.5     at t =    .5000
purkinje>cont 600 2
t =   4.000       Vm =   22.62        dVm/dt =   -3.429
                   ↓
t =   600.0       Vm =  -90.28        dVm/dt =  1.3557E-02
dVm/dt-max of    332.5     at t =    .5000
purkinje>close
```

Figure 2 Console input and output when running the program to generate an initial action potential. User input (typed at the keyboard) is shown in *italic* typeface. All other text is displayed by the program. A downward arrow ($\downarrow$) denotes one or more lines deleted for brevoty. Exponential notation is used to display small or large numbers (e.g., 2.0800E-05 is equivalent to 2.08×10^{-5}). Consult text for discussion of the commands and resulting output.

value of V_m can be computed as $\alpha_a/(\alpha_a + \beta_a)$. The init/command initializes the gating variables to equilibrium values at the previously determined resting potential. At this point, all initial conditions are specified for a fiber at rest.

The check command displays values for all the model equations, derivatives and membrane currents. The first ten equation values are the gating variables (m, h, etc.), and the last element is V_m, which shows that the resting potential is -70.72 mV. Notice that the corresponding derivatives of the gating variables are all zero (to within computer accuracy), owing to the fact that the initial values of the gating variables are equilibrium values. The initial dV_m/dt is 80 V/sec, because under the default conditions when running the program, a $-800 \, \mu\text{A}$ (depolarizing) current pulse is set to occur during $0 \leq t < 0.5$ msec. Since membrane capacitance (C_m) is specified at $10 \, \mu\text{F}/\text{cm}^2$ (a value appropriate for Purkinje fiber), this accounts for

80 V/sec (see Equation 1). Finally, under resting conditions, one observes that a number of the membrane currents are substantial. Nevertheless, if one were to sum up all of the 13 ionic currents, one would find that the net current is zero.

At this point, the model can be integrated in order to compute the first action potential starting from resting conditions. One first specifies an output file to receive the model computations, notably, all equation values, derivatives and currents. This is done with the `file rest.txt` command (Figure 2), which directs all output to a text file called `rest.txt`. The integration is started using small time steps in order to resolve the rapid inward sodium current; the `start 2 0.05` command directs the program to integrate from 0 to 2 msec using 0.05 msec time increments. As the integration proceeds, time, V_m and its derivative are displayed on the console ($\downarrow$ in Figure 2 denotes console output deleted for brevity). When the integration reaches 2 msec, the program stops and displays the maximum V_m time derivative, 332.5 V/sec, that occurred at $t = 0.5$ msec. Next, the user changes the time increment to 2 msec, and continues the integration to 600 msec using the `cont 600 2` command. The console output shows that at 600 msec, V_m has repolarized to -90.28 mV following the action potential. The user then closes the output file using the `close` command, and the results of the integration can then be imported into a graphics

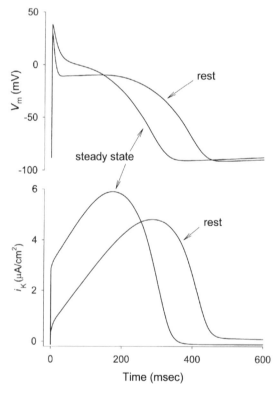

Figure 3 Upper: membrane potential, V_m. Lower: outward delayed-rectifier current (i_K). Rest: first action potential generated with equation values (gating variables and V_m) initialized to their resting values. Steady State: steady-state action potential generated by repetitive pacing at 100/min.

spreadsheet program. The resulting action potential is shown in the upper half of Figure 3 (labeled "rest").

A steady-state action potential in a fiber paced at 100/min can be generated by repeatedly integrating the model from 0 to 600 msec using the 0.5 msec current pulse at the start of each interval to simulate the electrotonic depolarization caused by cells just proximal to the Purkinje fiber. After each 600 msec duration, if one does not alter the equation values, then the values (gating variables and V_m) at 600 msec are used as initial conditions for the subsequent 600 msec interval. This is illustrated in Figure 4. Initially, the program is in the state immediately following generation of the initial action potential (i.e., end of Figure 2). The start 600 600 command integrates the equations from 0 to 600 msec producing no sub-intervals that would normally be needed to produce a smooth graph. After the second action potential, V_m attains a value of -88.60 mV at 600 msec, compared with -90.28 mV after the initial integration. The start 600 600 command is then repeated ten times (not shown, ↓ in Figure 4), until two consecutive periods result in the same 600 msec value for V_m, in this example -88.20 mV. This potential is the diastolic potential just prior to the onset of the action potential in a fiber at steady state paced at 100/min. The check command shows that the equation values are significantly different compared to the values at rest (see Figure 2). Finally, an output file is opened (file steadystate.txt command), the equations are integrated at finely spaced time

```
purkinje>start 600 600
t =    600.0        Vm =  -88.60      dVm/dt =  1.5463E-02
                 ↓
purkinje>start 600 600
t =    600.0        Vm =  -88.20      dVm/dt =  1.5447E-02
dVm/dt-max of  1.5447E-02 at t =   600.0
purkinje>start 600 600
t =    600.0        Vm =  -88.20      dVm/dt =  1.5447E-02
dVm/dt-max of  1.5447E-02 at t =   600.0
purkinje>check
Time:          600.0
Equation values (indices  1 through 11)...
   9.0517E-04    .9903       4.2536E-06   1.000       5.1700E-07  8.0872E-02
    .8312       6.8869E-02  4.3952E-02  3.0349E-02  -88.20
Derivatives (indices 12 through 22)...
   2.1406E-06 -4.0660E-05  9.9292E-09 -6.6003E-08   1.2783E-09  2.2291E-04
  -4.6507E-04 -3.1064E-04 -4.8372E-05  4.3034E-05   1.5449E-02
Currents (indices 23 through 35)...
  -4.7075E-05 -5.3831E-04   2.126       7.561        .2667      -.3936
  -3.8040E-06   4.502     -13.46       -.1820      -7.1305E-09 -.5729
    .0000
purkinje>file steadystate.txt
purkinje>start 2 0.05
t =  5.0000E-02  Vm =  -84.20      dVm/dt =   79.91
                 ↓
t =    2.000        Vm =   37.52      dVm/dt =  -1.174
dVm/dt-max of   476.1      at t =   .7000
purkinje>cont 600 2
t =    4.000        Vm =   34.82      dVm/dt =  -1.486
                 ↓
t =    600.0        Vm =  -88.20      dVm/dt =  1.5449E-02
dVm/dt-max of   476.1      at t =   .7000
purkinje>close
purkinje>save steadystate.prm
```

Figure 4 Console input and output when running the program to generate a steady-state action potential paced at 100/min.

intervals (`start 2 0.05` and `cont 600 2`) in order to produce a smooth graph, and all the model equation values and parameters are saved in a so-called parameter file (`save steadystate.prm` command). In subsequent simulations, this parameter file will be used to initialize all equations with initial conditions appropriate for a steady-state action potential paced at 100/min.

The upper half of Figure 3 (labeled "steady state") shows that the model reproduces the experimental observations noted above. The duration of the steady-state (paced) action potential is about 100 msec less than the first action potential stimulated from resting conditions, and the action potential lacks an extended plateau period. The main reason for these differences becomes apparent if one plots the outward delayed-rectifier current (i_K) shown in the lower half of Figure 3. When stimulated from rest, the delayed-rectifier current increases slowly (over a period of ca. 100 msec), thereby permitting a stable plateau of long duration. Under steady-state paced conditions, the current increases much more rapidly, and is the direct cause for the reduction in action-potential duration. It is also interesting to note the differences in the maximum upstroke velocities in the two action potentials. Under steady-state paced conditions, V_m initially depolarizes at a rate of 476 V/sec (see Figure 4), and rises to a peak amplitude of +38.2 mV. The first action potential stimulated from rest depolarizes at a rate of only 333 V/sec (see Figure 2), and exhibits a peak amplitude of +30.1 mV. This is caused by differences in steady state inactivation of transient sodium channels. The *h*-gate starts off at 0.99 (second equation value, Figure 4) under steady-state conditions, while its initial value under resting conditions is 0.43 (Figure 2) indicating that 57% of the transient sodium channels are initially inactivated. Under steady-state paced conditions, the initial value for h closely approximates h_∞ at −88.2 mV; for the initial action potential, h equals h_∞ at −70.2 mV (the resting potential).

Effects of Open-channel Sodium Blockers Like TTX

A well known experimental finding is that the Purkinje-fiber action-potential duration shortens following the application of open-channel sodium blocking agents like TTX (Coraboeuf *et al.*, 1979). Figure 5 shows the operation of the program to test if it reproduces this important experimental finding.

The `print` command simply disables output to the console during integration of the model. The `load steadystate.prm` command restores all model equation values and parameters to that of a steady-state action potential paced at 100/min (see Figure 4) by interrogating the previously saved parameter file. The `show gbar` displays a number of maximum conductances ($\bar{g}$ values) and current amplitudes ($\bar{i}$ values). The first value of the list is $\bar{g}_{Na}$, the maximum conductance of the fast transient sodium channels; its default value is 500 mS/cm^2. An output file is opened with the `file control.txt` command, and then the model equations are integrated to 600 msec at finely spaced time intervals using the `start` and `cont` commands. Recall that an action potential is triggered at $t = 0$ by a brief depolarizing current pulse. Next, the user enters the `set gbar 250` command, which reduces $\bar{g}_{Na}$ to 250 mS/cm^2 thereby simulating application of a sub-maximal dose of TTX. All other model parameter values are left unchanged from their default values. A new output file is opened and the model is again integrated to 600 msec.

```
purkinje>print
Console print disabled.
purkinje>load steadystate.prm
purkinje>show gbar
    gbar    500.0       .8000       5.000       .1050       1.0000E-02  2.430
            2.800       2.200       25.00       .3850       5.000       5.000
            7.5000E-02  .4000       .0000
purkinje>file control.txt
purkinje>start 2 0.05
dVm/dt-max of   476.2       at t =   .7000
purkinje>cont 600 2
dVm/dt-max of   476.2       at t =   .7000
purkinje>close
purkinje>set gbar 250
purkinje>show gbar
    gbar    250.0       .8000       5.000       .1050       1.0000E-02  2.430
            2.800       2.200       25.00       .3850       5.000       5.000
            7.5000E-02  .4000       .0000
purkinje>file block.txt
purkinje>start 2 0.05
dVm/dt-max of   301.0       at t =   .8000
purkinje>cont 600 2
dVm/dt-max of   301.0       at t =   .8000
purkinje>close
```

Figure 5 Console input and output when running the program to generate a control action potential, and an action potential after 50% blockage of $\bar{g}_{Na}$.

As seen in Figure 5, the reduction in $\bar{g}_{Na}$ caused a dramatic decrease in the maximum upstroke velocity of the action potential: from 476 V/sec under control conditions to 301 V/sec under conditions simulating application of TTX. However, Figure 6 (upper) shows that the two action potentials are virtually identical in shape, and thus a reduction of $\bar{g}_{Na}$ alone does not produce the reduction in action-potential duration observed experimentally. The reason for this is seen in Figure 6 (middle), which plots i_{Na}, the current through the inactivating sodium channels. The reduction in $\bar{g}_{Na}$ causes a large decrease in the peak value of i_{Na} (not shown in the figure, $-4765 \, \mu A/cm^2$ under control conditions and $-3013 \, \mu A/cm^2$ after 50% reduction of $\bar{g}_{Na}$) and this explains the reduction in maximum upstroke velocity. However, i_{Na} rapidly inactivates and the current is essentially zero during the entire plateau phase of the action potential. Thus, the model predicts that the fast transient sodium channels should *not* be a significant determinant of action-potential duration. However when the action potential enters phase 3 (final repolarization) the membrane enters a voltage range where the a small fraction of transient sodium channels have both their activation and inactivation gates open in the steady state (the product of m^3h is non-zero). This small steady state component is called the "window" sodium current. The reduction of window current by the open channel blocker has a small effect to speed this final phase of repolarization.

In 1984, Gintant *et al.* reported a slowly inactivating sodium current, with a time constant of several seconds, resulting in sustained inward current at plateau potentials in Purkinje fibers. More recently, Saint *et al.* (1992) reported the discovery of a small population of sodium channels that rapidly activate, exhibit TTX sensitivity, but fail to inactivate in time periods ranging up to 500 msec in ventricular muscle resulting in a *persistent* sodium current. The maximum conductance, $\bar{g}_{Na,p}$, of this population of channels in the model is 0.075 mS/cm² (thirteenth element in the list

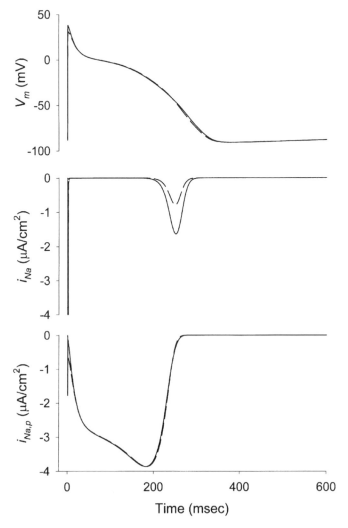

Figure 6 Membrane potential V_m (upper), transient inward sodium current i_{Na} (middle), and persistent sodium current $i_{Na,p}$ (lower). Solid lines: control conditions. Broken lines: after 50% reduction in $\bar{g}_{Na}$.

following the show gbar command, see Figure 4). The current through these persistent sodium channels ($i_{Na,p}$) is shown in Figure 6 (lower), which shows substantial inward sodium current occurring during the plateau phase. Since in creating the simulation we (erroneously) postulated that TTX selectively reduced *only* $\bar{g}_{Na}$, it is not surprising that $i_{Na,p}$ is unaffected by the maneuver.

Figure 7 shows the resulting action potentials (upper) and sodium currents (middle and lower) following a 50% reduction in *both* $\bar{g}_{Na}$ and $\bar{g}_{Na,p}$ (console input and output while running the program not shown). The large reduction in $i_{Na,p}$ reduces the plateau of the action potential, and the action potential repolarizes roughly 60 msec sooner than under control conditions. Thus, the model reproduces the experimental finding that open-channel blockers shorten action-potential

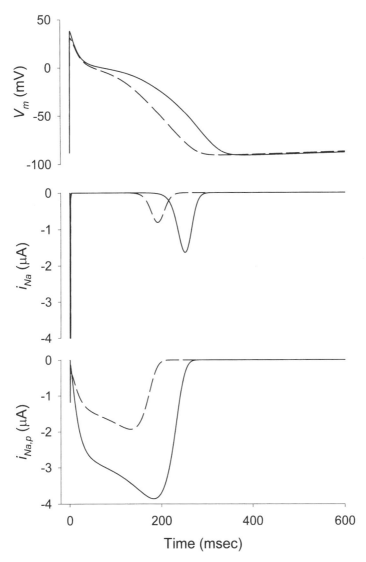

Figure 7 V_m (upper), i_{Na} (middle), and $i_{Na,p}$ (lower). Solid lines: control conditions. Broken lines: after 50% reduction in both $\bar{g}_{na}$ and $\bar{g}_{Na,p}$.

duration. The model predicts, however, that the shortening is caused by a decrease in $i_{Na,p}$ and not a decrease in i_{Na}.

Early Afterdepolarizations Caused by Increased Persistent Current

Recently, it has been proposed that an abnormality in a gene called *SCN5A* is one causative factor for a subset of cases of congenital long Q-T syndrome (Bennett *et al.*, 1995b). This genetically determined (autosomal dominant) disease results in long Q-T intervals on the electrocardiogram and an arrhythmia referred to as *torsades de pointes*, which causes syncope and sudden death. *SCN5A* encodes for a sodium channel, and it has been proposed that an increase in inward sodium current during the plateau phase of the action potential triggers the *torsades de pointes* arrhythmia, secondary to the generation of early afterdepolarizations (EAD). The role of inward sodium current as a contributor to the long Q-T interval has been demonstrated clinically in studies where administration of the i_{Na}-blocking antiarrhythmic drug, mexiletine, has shortened the Q-T interval (Schwartz *et al.*, 1995). The links between a clinical arrhythmia, association with a specific ion channel, and response to a selective antiarrhythmic drug, provide an ideal milieu for demonstrating the value of a computer model to test the interrelationship of physiological variables.

Figure 8 shows console input and output while running the computer program in an attempt to test whether an increase in $i_{Na,p}$ would be capable of generating an EAD. Initially, we knew from experimental data (Damiano and Rosen, 1984) that conditions most conducive to producing an EAD would occur at times of brady-cardia, since this produces the longest action-potential plateau durations even under normal conditions. The setv −80 command specifies an initial diastolic potential of −80 mV, and init/initializes the gating variables as before. The start 1200 1200 integrates the equations to 1200 msec, the time period corresponding to a pacing rate of 50/min. Subsequently, start 1200 1200 was repeated ten times (not shown,

```
purkinje>print
Console print disabled.
purkinje>setv -80
purkinje>init /
purkinje>start 1200 1200
                  ↓
purkinje>start 1200 1200
dVm/dt-max of   6.1045E-02 at t =   1200.
purkinje>file control.txt
purkinje>start 2 0.05
dVm/dt-max of    413.3     at t =    .5000
purkinje>cont 1200 2
dVm/dt-max of    413.3     at t =    .5000
purkinje>close
purkinje>set gbar ,,,,,,,,,,,,0.203
purkinje>show gbar
    gbar   500.0        .8000        5.000       .1050     1.0000E-02   2.430
           2.800       2.200        25.00       .3850        5.000       5.000
            .2030       .4000         .0000
purkinje>file first.txt
purkinje>start 2 0.05
dVm/dt-max of    413.5     at t =    .5000
purkinje>cont 1200 2
dVm/dt-max of    413.5     at t =    .5000
purkinje>file second.txt
purkinje>start 2 0.05
dVm/dt-max of    490.4     at t =    .8000
purkinje>cont 1200 2
dVm/dt-max of    490.4     at t =    .8000
purkinje>file third.txt
purkinje>start 2 0.05
dVm/dt-max of    431.0     at t =    .5500
purkinje>cont 1200 2
dVm/dt-max of    431.0     at t =    .5500
purkinje>close
```

Figure 8 Console input and output when running the program to generate action potentials exhibiting EADs and an alternans, resulting from an increase in $\bar{g}_{Na,p}$.

denoted by ↓) in order to generate a steady-state action potential paced at 50/min. An output file was then opened with the `file control.txt` command, and the equations were integrated once again at small time increments (`start 2 0.05 and cont 1200 2` commands) to produce the control action potential shown in Figure 9 (upper, solid line). Comparison of this action potential (paced at 50/min) with that shown in Figure 6 (paced at 100/min) shows that simulated conditions of bradycardia result in about a 100 msec increase in action-potential duration, a well known experimental observation.

Next, we simulated conditions of increased $i_{Na,p}$ by changing $\bar{g}_{Na,p}$ to 0.203 mS/cm^2, a 2.7-fold increase from its default value of 0.075 mS/cm^2. This was done with the `set gbar` command (n.b., the commas cause the program to skip over the other model parameters leaving them unchanged); the `show gbar` command verifies that only $\bar{g}_{Na,p}$ was changed (thirteenth listed value following the `show gbar` command). Then the equations were integrated at finely spaced time intervals while saving the results of the first (`file first.txt`), second (`file second.txt`) and third (`file

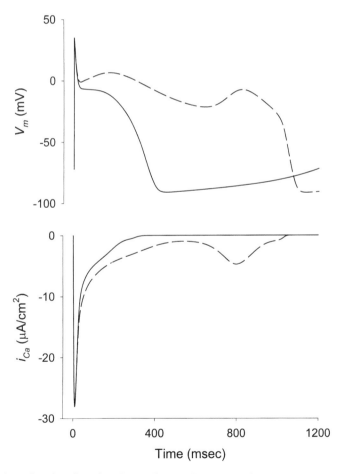

Figure 9 V_m (upper) and i_{Ca} (lower) under conditions of bradycardia (pacing rate of 50/min). Solid lines: control conditions. Broken lines: after 2.7-fold increase in $\bar{g}_{Na,p}$.

`third.txt`) paced action potentials following the increase in $\bar{g}_{Na,p}$. The first action potential is shown in Figure 9 (upper, broken line). This action potential exhibits a dramatically elevated plateau, with duration extended about 400 msec. However, instead of repolarizing normally, V_m again depolarizes producing an EAD. The underlying cause of the EAD becomes apparent when one plots the inward calcium current (i_{Ca}) through the L-type calcium channels. Figure 9 (lower) shows that under control conditions (solid line) i_{Ca} inactivates during the plateau phase, and remains inactivated. However, under conditions of increased $\bar{g}_{Na,p}$ (broken line), i_{Ca} recovers from inactivation and then reactivates, producing the inward current that causes the EAD.

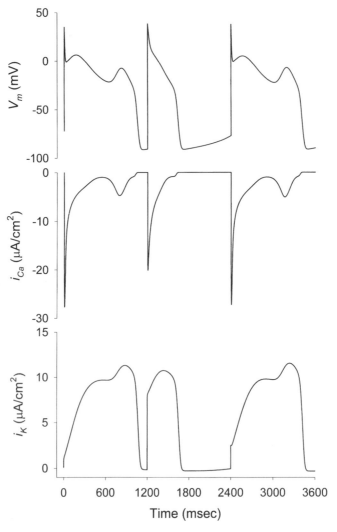

Figure 10 V_m (upper), i_{Ca} (middle) and delayed-rectifier current i_K (lower) during alternans resulting from a 2.7-fold increase in $\bar{g}_{Na,p}$.

Repetitively pacing the model following the increase in $\bar{g}_{Na,p}$ produces a so-called alternans seen in Figure 10 (upper), which plots the first through third action potentials following the increase in $\bar{g}_{Na,p}$. As shown in Figure 10 (middle), the first and third action potentials that show EADs contain a second "hump" of inward calcium current, but the shorter second action potential has only a single phase of inward calcium current that is smaller in amplitude. What generates the alternans? The second action potential is shorter than the first because it follows a shortened diastolic interval. This reduced period at hyperpolarized potentials does not allow for full deactivation of the delayed rectifier, whose outward current (i_K) is shown in Figure 10 (lower). Ultimately this results in more rapid and larger delayed-rectifier currents during the early phase (first few milliseconds) of the second action potential thereby shortening the plateau phase and preventing the EAD.

CONCLUSIONS

The purpose of our presentation is to acquaint the reader with computer modeling of the cardiac action potential in general, and to illustrate the actual operation of the computer program distributed with this volume. The present simulations employed a membrane model and our best estimates of membrane-current parameters in Purkinje fibers. We used the model to simulate three experimental conditions. For the first two, the outcome of the simulations closely approximates known experimental results. The third example illustrates use of the model to demonstrate that an increased persistent sodium current is capable of generating EADs. Recent studies on long-QT syndrome have suggested this hypothesis, and the results of our simulation reaffirm that it is certainly plausible.

The first simulation on going from rest to a steady-state action potential (Figure 3) not only reproduces experimental data, but also provides mechanistic suggestions for the causes of the changes in action potential shape that are observed. The shortening of the action-potential duration on repetitive stimulation (e.g., pacing) can readily be attributed to the more rapid activation of outward delayed-rectifier currents. The elevation of the plateau to more positive potentials is the cause of this more rapid activation. Although not shown, the higher plateau is the direct result of reduced transient outward current (i_{to}), which prevents the rapid repolarization to more negative plateau potentials. The reduced transient-outward current occurs because of the known slow recovery kinetics after this current is inactivated. The changes in action potential duration which occur on initiating pacing demonstrate the complicated voltage-dependent interactions between a change in one ionic current, the change in voltage it induces, and the resultant changes in other ionic currents.

This interaction between changes in one membrane current, its effects on the trajectory of the action potential, and resultant changes in other membrane currents is also illustrated in the third simulation (Figure 9 and 10). An increase in persistent sodium current lengthens the action potential, but in and of itself, does not generate the EAD. Instead, it is the lengthening of the action potential and the change in the trajectory of the action-potential plateau that allows for recovery from inactivation of the calcium current, which generates the secondary depolarization known as an EAD.

The second example (Figure 6 and 7) demonstrates how the computer model can be used to test an hypothesis directly. Prior to discovery of the channels responsible for the persistent sodium current, the hypothesis was that transient sodium channels and their associated "window current" were responsible for the changes in action-potential duration associated with application of open-channel blockers of sodium channels (e.g., TTX, see Colatsky, 1982). The results of the model simulation clearly show that this notion is incorrect, and furthermore suggest the importance of persistent sodium current in controlling action potential duration. One must remember, however, that this result is entirely dependent on the parameters chosen to represent the properties of the sodium currents, which to date are our best estimates of the reality. If subsequent experiments show that our estimates are inaccurate, this conclusion may have to be reassessed.

The computer program for our model is included on a diskette along with an instruction manual (also found in the Appendix). We hope the examples we have chosen have provided some insight into the utility of computer approaches, and that the readers will take the opportunity to familiarize themselves with the program and use it as both a didactic and experimental tool.

ACKNOWLEDGMENTS

These studies were supported, in part, by Helopharm, and by USPHS grants HL20558 and HL28958.

Appendix: User Manual for the Computer Model of Purkinje Action Potential

INTRODUCTION

purkinje is a computer program that can be used to synthesize (compute numerically) cardiac action potentials derived from a mathematical model describing the different ionic currents in mammalian Purkinje fibers. This appendix contains detailed instructions for running the program. The mathematical model is described in Chapter 8, which also shows examples of using the program to simulate several different experimental scenarios. The equations comprising the model are shown below. All model adjustable parameters, as well as their default values, are shown in Table 1. The quantities that are computed by the program are listed in Table 2.

COMPUTATIONAL REQUIREMENTS

purkinje.exe is an executable program that is run from the command prompt on a IBM-based PC running under the Microsoft Windows 95 or Windows NT operating systems (purkinje will *not* run under MS-DOS or Windows 3.*x*). The program is a so-called console application: a text-based application that provides no graphical user interface. Model calculations are written to an ASCII (text) output file for subsequent importing into a spreadsheet (e.g., Excel) or graphics program (e.g., SigmaPlot) for graphical representation of results.

RUNNING THE PROGRAM

To run the program, first copy purkinje.exe to a suitable directory and invoke an MS-DOS command prompt. Since some of the program commands result in the display of more than 24 lines of text (the default window size), the "properties" of the MS-DOS window should be set to display 40 (or more) lines. Then simply enter the program name. For example:

```
c: \mydir>copy a:\purkinje.exe
c: \mydir>purkinje
Model: purkinje (ver. 10-Jan-98)
purkinje>
```

Table 1 Default parameter values and their position (indices) in variable arrays*. Superscript numbers in parentheses refer to footnotes (see legend)

Indices (position of variable in list):

	1	2	3	4	5	6	7	8	9	10	11	12	13
Membrane currents:	i_{Na}	i_{Ca}	i_p	i_{K_2}	i_{Kr}	i_{Ks}	i_{to}	i_{K_1}	$i_{Na,b}$	$i_{Cl,b}$	$i_{Na,p}$	i_f	i_{leak}

Equation values (e.g., gating variables, membrane potential) and their derivatives:

	1	2	3	4	5	6	7	8	9	10	11
	m	h	d	f	q	r	s	X_1	X_2	y	V_m

$\bar{\alpha}$ values that can be changed with the set alphabar command:

	1	2	3	4	5	6	7	8	9	10
	$\bar{\alpha}_m^{(1)}$	–	$\bar{\alpha}_d^{(3)}$	–	$\bar{\alpha}_q^{(4)}$	$\bar{\alpha}_r^{(4)}$	$\bar{\alpha}_s^{(4)}$	$\bar{\alpha}_{X_1}^{(4)}$	$\bar{\alpha}_{X_2}^{(4)}$	$\bar{\alpha}_y^{(5)}$
	0.32	–	0.5	–	0.008	2.08×10^{-5}	0.001	5×10^{-4}	1.27×10^{-4}	7.29×10^{-6}

$\bar{\beta}$ values that can be changed with the set betabar command:

	1	2	3	4	5	6	7	8	9	10
	$\bar{\beta}_m^{(1)}$	–	$\bar{\beta}_d^{(3)}$	–	$\bar{\beta}_q^{(4)}$	$\bar{\beta}_r^{(4)}$	$\bar{\beta}_s^{(4)}$	$\bar{\beta}_{X_1}^{(4)}$	$\bar{\beta}_{X_2}^{(4)}$	$\bar{\beta}_y^{(5)}$
	5.806	–	0.5	–	0.08	0.02	5×10^{-5}	0.0013	3×10^{-4}	2.913×10^{-3}

$\bar{E}$ values that can be changed with the set ebar command:

	1	2	3	4	5	6	7	8	9	10
	$\bar{E}_m^{(1)}$	–	$\bar{E}_d^{(3)}$	–	$\bar{E}_q^{(4)}$	$\bar{E}_r^{(4)}$	$\bar{E}_s^{(4)}$	–	–	$\bar{E}_y^{(5)}$
	–47.13	–	–6.6	–	0	–26	–52	–	–	–52

Maximum conductances, currents, etc., that can be changed with the set gbar command:

	1	2	3	4	5	6	7	8	9	10	11	12	13
	$\bar{g}_{Na}^{(6)}$	$\bar{g}_{Ca}^{(4)}$	$\bar{g}_{qr}^{(4)}$	$\bar{g}_{Na,b}^{(4)}$	$\bar{g}_{Cl,b}^{(4)}$	$\bar{g}_{K_1}^{(7)}$	$\bar{i}_{K_2}^{(4)}$	$\bar{i}_{X_1}^{(4)}$	$\bar{i}_{X_2}^{(4)}$	$\bar{g}_{X_2}^{(4)}$	$\bar{i}_p^{(8)}$	$\tau_{f,fact}^{(9)}$	$\bar{g}_{Na,p}^{(10)}$
	500	0.8	5	0.105	0.01	2.43	2.8	2.2	25	0.385	5	5	0.075
	$\bar{g}_f^{(5)}$	$\bar{g}_{leak}^{(4)}$											
	0.40	0											

h-kinetics parameters that can be changed with set hkinetics command:

$V_{shift}^{(11)}$	$a_h^{(2)}$	$k_\alpha^{(2)}$	$E_\alpha^{(2)}$	$b_h^{(2)}$	$k_\beta^{(2)}$	$E_\beta^{(2)}$	$C_1^{(2)}$	$C_2^{(2)}$
−7	0.0294	−0.1395	−68.94	0.004898	0.1393	−73.34	0.1876	−0.009857

Reversal (equilibrium) potential values that can be changed with the set erev command:

$E_{Na}^{(4)}$	$E_{Ca}^{(4)}$	$E_{Cl}^{(4)}$	$E_K^{(4)}$	$E_f^{(5)}$	$E_{leak}^{(4)}$	$E_{qr}^{(4)}$
40	70	−70	−100	−41	0	−70

Membrane capacitance that can be changed with the set capacitance command:

$C_m^{(4)}$
10

* See Appendix 1 for definition of symbols. In general, parameters are set within a factor of two of values found in the literature. (1) From Ebihara and Johnson (1980). (2) From re-analysis of data from Ebihara and Johnson (1980) to substitute a continuous function for a piece-wise continuous function in their study. (3) From Wilders *et al.* (1991). (4) From the model of McAllister *et al.* (1975). Given the wide variation in the properties of measured membrane currents in isolated Purkinje myocytes and fibers (I.S. Cohen, *personal observations*), peak conductance parameters were varied up to 100% from ther original values in McAllister *et al.* (1975). In some cases, reversal potentials were adjusted slightly to facilitate model predictions with the earlier study. (5) Derived from analysis of data obtained from Yu *et al.* (1995). (6) Set to generate a maximum upstroke velocity of ≈ 500 V/sec. (7) From Shah *et al.* (1987). (8) Scaled to that obtained in Purkinje myocytes by Cohen *et al.* (1987). (10) Obtained by estimating peak current density of steady-state TTX-sensitive currents from Colatsky (1982) using the cm^2/μF ratio obtained by Colatsky and Tsien (1979). (11) Added to account for difference in the half-inactivation valued of Ebihara and Johnson (1980) in cultured myocytes and the value reported by Weidman (1955).

Table 2*   Output-file contents

Index	Variable	Description (*units*)
–	t	Integration time (msec)

Equation values

1	m	Sodium activation (transient and persistent channels)
2	h	Sodium inactivation (transient channels)
3	d	Calcium activation
4	f	Calcium inactivation
5	q	Transient-outward current activation
6	r	Transient-outward current inactivation
7	s	Potassium pacemaker activation
8	X_1	Plateau-potassium (delayed rectifier) current activation (fast phase)
9	X_2	Plateau-potassium (delayed rectifier) current activation (slow phase)
10	y	Hyperpolarized-activated (pacemaker) current activation
11	V_m	Membrane potential (mV)

Time derivatives (note: $' = \mathrm{d}/\mathrm{d}t$*)*

12	m'	Sodium activation (transient and persistent channels) (msec^{-1})
13	h'	Sodium inactivation (transient channels) (msec^{-1})
14	d'	Calcium activation (msec^{-1})
15	f'	Calcium inactivation (msec^{-1})
16	q'	Transient-outward current activation (msec^{-1})
17	r'	Transient-outward current inactivation (msec^{-1})
18	s'	Potassium pacemaker activation (msec^{-1})
19	X_1'	Plateau-potassium (delayed rectifier) current activation (fast phase) (msec^{-1})
20	X_2'	Plateau-potassium (delayed rectifier) current activation (slow phase) (msec^{-1})
21	y'	Hyperpolarized-activated (pacemaker) current activation (msec^{-1})
22	V_m'	Membrane potential (mV/msec)

Ionic currents:

23	i_{Na}	Fast transient sodium current ($\mu A/cm^2$)
24	i_{Ca}	Calcium current (L-type channel) ($\mu A/cm^2$)
25	i_p	Sodium-pump current ($\mu A/cm^2$)
26	i_{K_2}	Potassium pacemaker current ($\mu A/cm^2$)
27	i_{K_r}	Plateau-potassium (delayed rectifier) current (fast phase) ($\mu A/cm^2$)
28	i_{K_s}	Plateau-potassium (delayed rectifier) current (slow phase) ($\mu A/cm^2$)
29	i_{to}	Transient outward current ($\mu A/cm^2$)
30	i_{K_1}	Potassium background current (inward rectifier) ($\mu A/cm^2$)
31	$i_{Na,b}$	Sodium background current ($\mu A/cm^2$)
32	$i_{Cl,b}$	Chloride background current ($\mu A/cm^2$)
33	$i_{Na,p}$	Persistent sodium current ($\mu A/cm^2$)
34	i_f	Hyperpolarization-activated inward current ($\mu A/cm^2$)
35	i_{leak}	Nonspecific leak current ($\mu A/cm^2$)

* Under default conditions, 36 values are written to the output and snapshot files: time, and all 35 variables listed above. Each line consist of 432-character (byte) records, with each numerical value occupying 12 characters. Values are delimited by spaces (n.b., when importing data into spreadsheets, specify "white space" as the delimiter). The values are written using Fortran "G" format, which switches between fixed (decimal point) format and exponential-notation depending on the amplitude of the value. The `outrec` command can be used to limit output to only those quantities of interest; use the indices (above) to select which quantities to save when using this command.

When the program starts, it identifies itself, displays a prompt (`purkinje >`), and awaits a command from the user.

COMMAND SYNTAX

All commands consist of a command name, *followed by a space*, and then an optional list of arguments (delimited with spaces or commas). For example, the command to open an output file can be entered as follows:

```
purkinje>file test1.txt
```

Alternatively, if the argument is not specified with the command, then the user will be prompted for it:

```
purkinje>file
Output file: test1.dat
```

Only the *first four characters* of a command are significant, so most can be abbreviated if desired.

List Directed Input for Numerical Arguments

A number of commands expect arguments consisting of a list of numeric values. Fortran list-directed input is used in reading the values and permits the entry of all the values, only some of the values (leaving the missing values unchanged), and permits repeating of a single value. The rules for list-directed input are as follows:

- A leading comma skips over the first value, and successive commas (,,) in the input list skip over their respective values, leaving them unchanged;
- A slash (/) terminates the list leaving the following values unchanged;
- A value can be repeated using the asterisk (*) as a repeat indicator (e.g., "4 * 5"is equivalent to entering "5 5 5 5");
- If entered with a command, the list of values terminates with the last entry; if the command is entered alone with the program prompting for the arguments, then the values can be entered on multiple lines (or the list can be terminated with a slash).

An example will help clarify these rules. The set erev command expects seven values as its argument: E_{Na}, E_{Ca}, E_{Cl}, E_K, E_f, E_{leak} and E_{qr} (in that order). Suppose one only wants to change E_{Na} and E_{Cl}, leaving the other values unchanged. This could be done as follows:

```
purkinje>set erev 50,,−100
```

or alternatively,

```
purkinje>set erev
ENa, ECa ECl, EK, Ef, Eleak, Eqr: 50,, −100/
```

Note that if the user omitted the slash on the line above, the program would have waited for entry of the remaining four potentials (E_K, E_f, E_{leak} and E_{qr}) on a second line; the user could at that point enter the slash, thereby leaving their values unchanged.

Parameter Indices

Related lists of variables and parameters are grouped together in lists of numbers called arrays. For example, the `set erev` command (above) modifies an array containing 7 different model parameters. When changing these values, one *must be careful* to specify them in the correct order, as well as the correct position in the list. The position of a given variable or parameter in its associated array is termed its *index*. For example, in the `set erev` command, E_{Cl} corresponds to index number 3 in the array containing the reversal potentials.

Table 1 shows all model parameters that can be changed during execution of the model, as well as their corresponding indices in the respective arrays. Note also that when viewing model parameters using the `show` command, the parameter arrays are labeled, but the individual parameters are *not* labeled. Again, you should refer to Table 1 to find the array position of the parameter in question.

STARTING VERSUS CONTINUING AN INTEGRATION

Two program commands (discussed below) control the actual numerical itegration of the differential equations comparising the model. The `start` command initializes time (t) to 0 msec, and integrates the equations up to a specified ending time. The `continue` command can subsequently be used to extend the integration to future times; it does *not* reinitialize time to 0 msec. These two commands differ in how they initially invoke the numerical integration algorithm, and as such, the user needs to be aware of some of the details regarding numerical integration.

When using the `start` and `continue` commands, apart from specifying an ending time, one also specifies a time interval (Δt) to use when approaching the ending time. For example, the command `start 2 0.1` directs the program to integrate the equations from 0 to 2 msec using 0.1 msec intervals; at each interval, results are written to an output file thereby producing a 20-row table of equation values, currents, etc. When performing numerical integration in general, the accuracy of the results depends on Δt, yet there is no *a priori* reason to believe that the interval specified (in this example, 0.1 msec) is sufficient for the desired accuracy. As such, the algorithm automatically subdivies Δt into smaller subintervals until the specified accuracy (six significant digits, or a relative local error of 10^{-6}) is achieved. During phase 0 of the action potential, when the transient sodium channels are rapidly activating, very small subintervals ($\ll 0.1$ msec) are required in order to resolve this fast event accurately. However, in subsequent phases of the action potential, small subintervals are not required since gating kinetics is much slower. During these phases, the integration algorithm automatically increases the size of the subintervals in order to minimize the number of numerical computations, thereby speeding up running of the program. Integration algorithms that act in this fashion are called adaptive algorithms and, in general, are highly desirable since the user does not have to be concerned the accuracy of the results – the program maintains a specified accuracy automatically.

A major difference between the start and continue commands is as follows: the start command *always* starts with a small time subinterval (0.05 msec), whereas the continue command initially uses the last time subinterval determined at the ending time from the previous start (or continue) command. As such, the continue command can sometimes cause the algorithm to "skip over" or miss abrupt changes resulting from changes made to the model parameters (or equation values) *just prior* to continuing the previously started integration. This most commonly occurs when one integrates the equations for a period of time, abruptly imposes a brief current pulse, and then continues the integration. One should, therefore, avoid changing model parameters prior to continuing an integration: use the continue command solely to extend the period of time, possibly after changing the time interval.

If one wants to integrate the equations to a certain time and *then* impose an abrupt change in a model parameter, equation value, or impose a current pulse, then the integration should be continued by using the start command once again, using the equation values at the ending time of the first start command as the initial conditions for the second. This will reinitialize time to zero, but later (e.g., when plotting the response) one can add an offset to the time values thereby creating a continuous time history.

AN EXAMPLE OF RUNNING THE PROGRAM

All program commands and their arguments are discussed in detail below. In the outset, a straightforward example will illustrate operation of the program. Also see Chapter 8 in the accompanying volume for additional example.

Using the default parameter set, the following example computes an action potential after initializing the gating variables to their equilibrium valus at -80 mV. The initial membrane potential is set at -50 mV, a process that subsequently activates the fast transient sodium channels and initiates an action potential. The equations are initially integrated using brief (0.05 msec) time intervals in order to resolve the maximum upstroke velocity of the action potential. Then, the integration continues to 600 msec using larger (2 msec) intervals. This is accomplished using the following commands, with the computed membrane potential (in this example, the only variable saved) being stored in file test.txt.

Console Input and Output:	Comments:
C: \mydir>purkinje	Start the program
Model: purkinje (ver. 10-Jan-98)	
purkinje>set current 3 ∗ 0	Inhibit a default current pulse
purkinje>init −80	Initialize gating variables
purkinje>setv −50	Initialize membrane potential
purkinje>file test.txt	Open an output file
purkinje>outrec 11 0	Only V_m will be written to file

```
purkinje>print                          Disable console printing
Console print disabled.
purkinje>start 2 0.05                   Integrate to 2 msec
dVm/dt-max of 459.4 at t = .3500
purkinje>cont 600 2                     Continue integrating to 600 msec
dVm/dt-max of 459.4 at t = .3500
purkinje>close                          Close the output file
purkinje>exit                           End the program
c: \mydir>
```

After the program ended (above), a graphics spreadsheet program (e.g., Microsoft Excel) was started, and the results (V_m as a function of time) saved in file `test.txt` were imported into the spreadsheet. These results are plotted in the following graph:

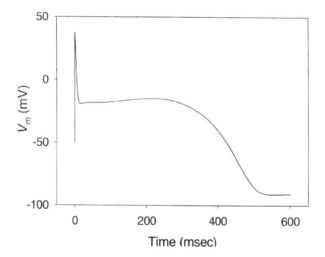

PROGRAM COMMANDS AND THEIR ARGUMENTS

In the description of the commands that follow, the following syntax is used: the program command itself is denoted by courier type font, and optional arguments are denoted by *courier italic* type font. Commands are not case sensitive and can be entered in either UPPER or lower case. Recall that only the first four characters are significant (e.g., "continue", "cont", "contest" and "control" are all equivalent to the actual continue command, see below).

Commands that Display Information on the Console

check
    The check command displays all equation values, derivatives, and membrane currents. See Table 1 for association between equation indices and variable names.

`help`
　　The `help` command displays a concise list of all program commands, with brief descriptions of their function.

`indices`
　　The `indices` command displays the indices of all quantities that can be saved in an output file. These include 11 equation values (gating variables and membrane potential), their time derivatives, and 13 membrane currents (see also the `outrec` command).

`show` *category*
　　The `show` command displays model parameters that can be altered with the `set` command (see below). *category* is one of the following: `alphabar`, `betabar`, `ebar`, `gbar`, `hkinetics`, `erev`, `cap` or `current`. If the user enters `show all`, then all adustable model parameters are displayed. See Table 1 for the correspondence between the lists of values displayed and their associated model-parameter names.

`print`
　　The `print` command is used to enable or disable console printing during integration of the equations. By default, console printing is initially enabled.

Commands that Change Model Parameters

`ic` *numeric_list*
　　The `ic` command is used to specify initial conditions for the 10 gating variables (see Table 1), as well as the membrane potential, V_m (the eleventh element in the list). This command provides the only way to enter initial conditions manually for the gating variables. See also the `initialize` and `rest` commands.

`initialize` *membrane_potential*
　　The `initialize` command is used to initialize all the gating variables (see Table 1) to their equilibrium values at the specified *membrane_potential*; the `initialize` command *does not* set V_m (see the `setv` and `ic` commands). To initialize gating variables to their equilibrium values at the current membrane potential, execute the initialize command supplying the current potential by specifying a slash in lieu of *membrane_potential* (i.e., `initialize /`).

`rest` *membrane_potential_estimate, absolute_error, relative_error*
　　The `rest` command computes the resting membrane potential using an iterative algorithm that determines the membrane potential resulting in zero net membrane current. V_m is then initialized to this resting potential (to view the potential, use the `check` command). One should supply an estimate of the potential, followed by two error criteria to determine the accuracy in computing the true potential. The iterative procedure will stop when successive iterations result in changes in V_m that are less than *absolute_error* (default 0.001 mV) or when the *relative* difference is less than *relative_error* (default 10^{-5}, implying five significant digits accuracy). To accept the defaults, supply only *membrane_potential_estimate* with the

command (i.e., `rest -80`), or use the current membrane potential (default) as the estimate (i.e., `rest /`).

`set alphabar` *numeric_list*
The `set alphabar` command change $\bar{\alpha}$ parameters (see Table 1).

`set betabar` *numeric_list*
The `set betabar` command changes $\bar{\beta}$ parameters (see Table 1).

`see cap` *membrane_capacitance*
The `set cap` command changes the membrane capacitance (C_m) to *membrane_capacitance* (initially, C_m is $10 \,\mu\text{F}/\text{cm}^2$).

`set current` *start_time, end_time, amplitude*
The `set current` command is used to specify the starting time, ending time, and amplitude of a membrane current pulse. Specifying 0 for *amplitude* effectively disables the pulse. The current pulse starts when $t \geq$ *start_time*, and ends when $t >$ *end_time*, By default, the model parameters are set to produce a $0.5\,\text{msec}$ depolarizing current pulse of amplitude $-800 \,\mu\text{A}/\text{cm}^2$ starting at $t = 0$ (i.e., `set current 0 0.5 -800`).

`set ebar` *numeric_list*
The `set ebar` command changes $\bar{E}$ parameters (see Table 1).

`set erev` *numeric_list*
The `set erev` command changes the reversal potentials (equilibrium potentials) for the different ionic species (see Table 1).

`set gbar` *numeric_list*
The `set gbar` command changes $\bar{g}$ and $\bar{i}$ parameters (maximum channel conductances, currents, etc., see Table 1).

`set hkinetics` *numeric_list*
The `set hkinetics` command changes parameters related to fast (transient) sodium-channel inactivation (gating variable h, see Table 1).

`setv` *membrane_potential*
The `setv` command is used to initialize V_m to any potential (see also the `ic` and `rest` commands).

Input-output Commands

`close`
The `close` command closes the ASCII (text) output file. An output file must be closed prior to importing model results into a spreadsheet or graphics program. An output file is automatically closed when a new output file is specified (see the `file` command) or when the program exits (see the `exit` command).

file *file_name*
> The file command opens the ASCII (text) file *file_name* to receive results of model computations. If the file already exists prior to being opened, output will overwrite the existing contents. See Table 2 for a description of the file format.

iv *v_min, v_max, delta_v*
> The iv command computes the instantaneous current-voltage relationship (i.e., I/V curve), and writes the voltage and current values to the output file. The coordinates are computed at V_m values ranging from *v_min* to *v_max*, with voltage increments of *delta_v*. Accepting default values for the arguments (i.e., executing iv /) computes the I/V curve going from -100 to $+50\,\text{mV}$, in $1\,\text{mV}$ increments.

load *file_name*
> The load command loads all model parameters and equation values from a previously-saved parameter file *file_name*. The command effectively restores all model equation and parameter values to their state following a prior execution of the program. See also the save command. Note: Upon restoring all model parameters following a load command, the user must perform the next subsequent integration by *initially* using the start command; one *cannot* simply continue an integration (see the continue command) immediately following a load command.

outrec *numeric_list*, 0
> The outrec command specifies which output fields (numerical quantities) are to be written to the ASCII output file during integration of the equations, or following execution of the snapshot command. The user specifies the numeric indices corresponding to the variables of interest (see Table 2, or the indices command). By default, all 35 values (equaton values, derivatives and currents) are written to an open output file. *numeric_list* can consist of single indices or a specified range of indices, *and should end with 0 (zero)*. To specify a range, enter three numbers consisting of the starting, $-$ending (ending as a negative number), and increment for the index. For example, outrec 1 5 20 $-$30 2 11 0 directs the program to output values corresponding to the following indices: 1, 5, 20, 22, 24, 26, 28, 30 and 11 (in that order). Note: outrec 1 $-$35 1 0 restores the default condition by specifying output of all 35 values.

save *file_name*
> The save command saves all model parameters and variable values in the specified ASCII parameter file *file_name*. This command is useful for saving all values (equation values, derivatives and parameter values) prior to exiting the program, and for restoring the values (with the load command) the next time the model is run.

sclose
> The sclose command closes a snapshot output file (see the sfile and snapshot commands). A snapshot file must be closed prior to importing its data into spreadsheets or graphics programs.

sfile *file_name*

> The sfile command opens the ASCII (text) snapshort file *file_name*. A snap-shot file is an alternate output file (see the file command) that receives results (specified by the outrec command) whenever the snapshot command is executed. If the specified snapshot file already exiss prior to being opened, output will overwrite the existing contents. See Table 2 for a description of the file format.

snapshot

> The snapshot writes one line of output (specified by the outrec command) to an open snapshot output file (see the sfile and sclose commands). The command is useful for saving model results at any arbitrary time (while integration is sus-pended and the program is waiting for a command). A snapshot file is distinct from a normal output file (see the file command), which receives all output at the time intervals specified during integration of the model equations (see the start and continue commands).

Integration Commands

continue *end_time, delta_t*

> The continue command continues a previously started integration (see the start command) by integrating from the current time (see check command) to *end_time*, using time intervals of *delta_t*. If an output file is open, results (specified by the outrec command) are written to the file after each time interval.

start *end_time, delta_t*

> The start command is used to start an integration from $t = 0$ to *end_time*, using *delta_t* time increments. The start command *always* initializes t to 0. If an output file is open, results (specified by the outrec command) are written to the file after each time interval. *delta_t* can equal *end_time* (e.g., start 600 600). To con-tinue an integration from the current time to a new end time, use the continue command. Note: during integration, time, V_m and dV_m/dt are displayed on the console if console printing is enabled (see the print command). When the integ-ration reaches *end_time*, the program also displays the maximum upstoke velocity [$\dot{V}_{max}$ or $(dV_m/dt)_{max}$] and the time at which it occurred. One should initially use short time intervals for *delta_t* (e.g., start 2 0.05) to resolve the maximum velocity accurately.

Commands for Suspending the Program and Automating Processing of Commands

command *file_name*

> The command command provides a means to automate execution of the program by executing a sequence of commands previously stored in a so-called command file. The command opens the ASCII (text) file *file_name*, which contains a list of valid program commands, *one command per line*. If the commands include their respective arguments, the commands are automatically executed one by one until the end of the file is reached. If the commands lack their arguments, then as each command is executed the user is prompted to supply the argument. When the end

of the file is reached, control of the program returns to the keyboard (unless the last command is exit, in which case the program terminates). Note: a command file *can* contain a command command, in which case program input is directed to a second command file. One cannot, however, "branch back" to the first command file in order to execute any commands following the line containing the command command.

exit
  The exit command closes all files, ends the program, and returns the user to the command-window prompt (or closes the window). If one wishes to save the state of the program prior to exiting, then a save command should be executed prior to the exit command (see also the load command).

pause
  The pause command suspends execution of the program, displays the standard command-line prompt (e.g., C: \mydir >) and permits execution of a *single* system command or program. After the command is executed, the model resumes execution.If one wishes to execute multiple system commands while the program is suspended, then a new command interpreter should be invoked (e.g., the system command command on a Windows 95 system). Pausing the program does *not* close output or snapshot files; if one wants to access these files while the program is in a pause state, they should be closed (close or sclose commands) *prior* to executing the pause command. Note: if one reopens an existing output file (after the program resumes), the original contents will be overwritten.

Commands that Control the Internal Operation of the Numerical Integration Algorithm

The following four commands display and change internal values that control the operation of the subprogram that performs the numerical integration. Under normal operating conditions, the user *should not alter* these values, since testing has been done to ascertain the "optimal" operation of the program producing default values that should be more than adequate.

  For more information, consult the documentation (not supplied) for subroutine IVPAG/DIVPAG in the IMSL Math and Statistical Library (see Chapter 8 for further details).

error *error_severity, print_action, stop_action*
  The error command alters the behavior of the numerical integration algorithm by changing how internal errors are reported, and how the algorithm reacts to them. By default, the program displays error messages on the console, and attempts to recover from errors, thereby permitting the user to take corrective action.

setpar *numeric_list*
  The setpar command changes a list of values that controls the numerical integration algorithm (e.g., its accuracy, mode of operation, etc.). The values can be displayed by the showpar command. Under normal operational of the program,

the values *should not be changed*, since improperly set values can results in erratic behavior and inaccurate results.

shopar

The shopar command displays a list of values that controls the numerical integration algorithm (e.g., its accuracy, mode of operation, etc.). The values are useful for debugging purposes only.

tolerance *relative_tolerance*

The tolerance command changes the relative (local) error to accept during integration of the equations. Under default conditions, *relative_tolerance* is set to 10^{-6}, corresponding to six significant digits of accurancy.

MODEL EQUATIONS (see Table 1 for Parameter Values)

Differential equations

For an arbitrary gating variable a (where $a = m, h, d, f, q, r, s, X_1, X_2$ or y),

$$\frac{da}{dt} = \alpha_a(1-a) - \beta_a a. \tag{A1}$$

If i_m is total membrane current (sum of all ionic currents plus applied current) and C_m is membrane capacitacitance,

$$\frac{dV_m}{dt} = -\frac{i_m}{C_m}. \tag{A2}$$

Fast (transient) sodium current

$$i_{Na} = m^3 h \bar{g}_{Na}(V_m - E_{Na}) \tag{A3}$$

$$\alpha_m = \bar{\alpha}_m \frac{\bar{E}_m - V_m}{\exp[0.1(\bar{E}_m - V_m)] - 1} \tag{A4}$$

$$\beta_m = \bar{\beta}_m \exp[(\bar{E}_m - V_m)/11] \tag{A5}$$

$$\alpha_h = \frac{h_\infty}{\tau_h} \tag{A6}$$

$$\beta_h = \frac{1 - h_\infty}{\tau_h} \tag{A7}$$

$$h_\infty = \frac{\alpha'_h}{\alpha'_h + \beta'_h} \tag{A8}$$

$$\tau_h = \frac{1}{\alpha'_h + \beta'_h} + C_1 \exp[C_2(V_m - V_{\text{shift}})] \tag{A9}$$

$$\alpha'_h = a_h \exp[k_\alpha(V_m - V_{\text{shift}} - E_\alpha)] \tag{A10}$$

$$\beta'_h = b_h \exp[k_b(V_m - V_{\text{shift}} - E_\beta)] \tag{A11}$$

Persistent sodium current

$$i_{\text{Na,p}} = m^3 \bar{g}_{\text{Na,p}}(V_m - E_{\text{Na}}) \tag{A12}$$

Calcium current

$$i_{\text{Ca}} = df \bar{g}_{\text{Ca}}(V_m - E_{\text{Ca}}) \tag{A13}$$

$$\alpha_d = \frac{\bar{\alpha}_d}{1 + \exp[(\bar{E}_d - V_m)/6.6]} \tag{A14}$$

$$\beta_d = \bar{\beta}_d \frac{\exp[(\bar{E}_d - V_m)/6.6]}{1 + \exp[(\bar{E}_d - V_m)/6.6]} \tag{A15}$$

$$\alpha_f = \frac{f_\infty}{\tau_f} \tag{A16}$$

$$\beta_f = \frac{1 - f_\infty}{\tau_f} \tag{A17}$$

$$f_\infty = \frac{1}{1 + \exp[(V_m + 25)/6]} \tag{A18}$$

$$\tau_f = \tau_{f,fact} \left[2.21 \left(\frac{1-f}{0.1+f} \right)^2 + 4 \right] \tag{A19}$$

Transient outward current

$$i_{\text{to}} = qr \bar{g}_{qr}(V_m - E_{qr}) \tag{A20}$$

$$\alpha_q = \bar{\alpha}_q \frac{\bar{E}_q - V_m}{\exp[(\bar{E}_q - V_m)/10] - 1} \tag{A21}$$

$$\beta_q = \bar{\beta}_q \exp[(\bar{E}_q - V_m)/11.26] \tag{A22}$$

$$\alpha_r = \bar{\alpha}_r \exp[(\bar{E}_q - V_m)/25] \tag{A23}$$

$$\beta_r = \frac{\bar{\beta}_r}{1 + \exp[(\bar{E}_r - V_m)/11.49]} \tag{A24}$$

Potassium background current

$$i_{K_1} = \bar{g}_{K_1}(V_m - E_K)\frac{P_g p}{P_g + p^3(1 - P_g)} \tag{A25}$$

$$P_g = \frac{1}{1 + \exp[(V_m - E_K + 5)/5]} \tag{A26}$$

$$p = \frac{1}{1 + \exp[(V_m - E_K)/8]} \tag{A27}$$

Plateau potassium (delayed rectifier) currents

$$i_{K_r} = X_1 \bar{i}_{X_1} \frac{\exp[0.04(V_m - E_K - 5)] - 1}{\exp[0.04(V_m - E_K - 55)]} \tag{A28}$$

$$\alpha_{X_1} = \bar{\alpha}_{X_1} \frac{\exp[(V_m + 50)/12.1]}{1 + \exp[(V_m + 50)/17.5]} \tag{A29}$$

$$\beta_{K_s} = \bar{\beta}_{X_1} \frac{\exp[-(V_m + 20)/16.67]}{1 + \exp[-(V_m + 20)/25]} \tag{A30}$$

$$i_{X_2} = X_2[\bar{i}_{X_2} + \bar{g}_{X_2}(V_m - E_K - 100)] \tag{A31}$$

$$\alpha_{X_2} = \frac{\bar{\alpha}_{X_2}}{1 + \exp[-(V_m + 19)/5]} \tag{A32}$$

$$\beta_{X_2} = \bar{\beta}_{X_2} \frac{\exp[-(V_m + 20)/16.67]}{1 + \exp[-(V_m + 20)/25]} \tag{A33}$$

Potassium pacemaker current

$$i_{K_2} = s\bar{i}_{K_2} \frac{\exp[0.04(V_m - E_K + 10)] - 1}{\exp[0.08(V_m - E_K - 40)] + \exp[0.04(V_m - E_K - 40)]} \tag{A34}$$

$$\alpha_s = \bar{\alpha}_s \frac{\bar{E}_s - V_m}{\exp[(\bar{E}_s - V_m)/5] - 1} \tag{A35}$$

$$\beta_s = \bar{\beta}_s \exp[(\bar{E}_s - V_m)/14.93] \tag{A36}$$

Hyperpolarization-activated current

$$i_f = y\bar{g}_f(V_m - E_f) \tag{A37}$$

$$\alpha_y = \bar{\alpha}_y \exp[-0.0554(V_m - \bar{E}_y)] \tag{A38}$$

$$\beta_y = \bar{\beta}_y \frac{\exp[0.0585(V_m - \bar{E}_y)]}{1 + \exp[0.0585(V_m - \bar{E}_y)]} \tag{A39}$$

Sodium-pump current

$$i_p = \frac{\bar{i}_p}{1 + \exp[-0.0368(V_m + 80)]} \tag{A40}$$

Sodium and chloride background currents, and the "leak" current

$$i_{Na,b} = \bar{g}_{Na,b}(V_m - E_{Na}) \tag{A41}$$

$$i_{Cl,b} = \bar{g}_{Cl,b}(V_m - E_{Cl}) \tag{A42}$$

$$i_{leak} = \bar{g}_{leak}(V_m - E_{leak}) \tag{A43}$$

References

Adelman J.P. (1995). Proteins that interact with the pore-forming subunits of voltage-gated ion channels. *Current Opinion in Neurobiology*, 5:286–295.

Advani S.V., Singh B.N. (1995). Pharmacodynamic, pharmacokinetic and antiarrhythmic properties of d-sotalol, the dextro-isomer of sotalol. *Drugs*, 49:664–679.

Aggarwal R., Boyden P.A. (1995). Diminished calcium and barium currents in myocytes surviving in the epicardial border zone of the 5 day infarcted canine heart *Circ. Res.*, 77:1180–1191.

Aggarwal R., Boyden P.A. (1996). Altered pharmacologic responsiveness of reduced L-type calcium currents in myocytes surviving in the infarcted heart. *J. Cardiovasc. Electrophysiol.*, 7:20–35.

Akahane K., Furukawa Y., Ogiwara Y., Haniuda M., Chiba S. (1989). β_2 adrenoceptor-mediated effects on sinus rate and atrial and ventricular contractility on isolated, blood-perfused dog heart preparations. *J. Pharmacol. Exp. Ther.*, 248:1276–1282.

Akiyama T., Pawitan Y., Greenberg H., Kuo C.S., Reynolds-Haertle R.A. (1991). The CAST investigators. Increased risk of death and cardiac arrest from encainide and flecainide in patients after non-Q-wave acute myocardial infarction in the Cardiac Arrhythmia Suppression Trial. *Am. J. Cardiol.*, 68:1551–1558.

Allen J.M., Bircham P.M.M., Edwards A.V., Tatemoto K., Bloom S.R. (1983). Neuropeptide Y (NPY) reduces myocardial perfusion and inhibits the force of contraction of the isolated perfused rabbit heart. *Regul. Peptides*, 6:247–253.

Allen J.M., Goerstrup P., Bjoerkman J-A., Ek L., Abrahamsson T., Bloom S.R. (1986). Studies on cardiac distribution and function of neuropeptide Y. *Acta. Physiol. Scand.*, 126:405–411.

Alter W.A., Weiss G.K., Priola D.V. (1973). Vagally-induced tachycardia in atropinized dogs: effect of β-adrenergic blockade. *Eur. J. Pharmacol.*, 24:329–333.

Altschuld R.A., Starling R.C., Hamlin R.L., Billman G.E., Hensley J., Castillo L., Fertel R.H., Hohl C.M., Robitaille P.M.L., Jones L.R., Xiao R.P., Lakatta E.G. (1995). Response of failing canine and human heart cells to β_2-adrenergic stimulation. *Circulation*, 92:1612–1618.

Alvarez J.L., Vassort G. (1992). Properties of the low threshold Ca^{2+} current in single frog atrial cardiomyocytes. A comparison with the high threshold Ca^{2+} current. *J. Gen. Physiol.*, 100:519–545.

Amiodarone Trials Meta-Analysis Investigators (1977). Effects of prophylactic amiodarone on mortality after acute myocardial infarction and congestive heart failure: meta-analysis of individual data from 6500 patients in randomized trials. *Lancet*, 350:1417–1424.

Anderson J.L. (1990). Clinical implication of new studies in the treatment of benign, potentially malignant and malignant ventricular arrhythmias. *Am. J. Cardiol.*, 65:36B–42B.

Antzelevitch C., Jalife J., Moe G.K. (1980). Characteristics of reflection as a mechanism of reentrant arrhythmias and its relationship to parasystole. *Circulation*, 61:182–191.

Antzelevitch C., Sun Z.Q., Zhang Z.Q., Yan G.X. (1996). Cellular and ionic mechanisms underlying erythromycin-induced long QT intervals and torsade de pointes. *Journal of the American College of Cardiology*, 28:1836–1848.

Anyukhovsky E.P., Guo S.-D., Danilo P. Jr., Rosen M.R. (1997). Responses to norepinephrine of normal and "ischemic" canine Purkinje fibers are consistent with activation of different β_1-receptor subtypes. *J. Cardiovasc. Electrophysiol.*, 8:658–666.

Anyukhovsky E.P., Rybin V.O., Nikashin A.V., Budanova O.P., Rosen M.R. (1992). Positive chronotropic responses induced by α_1-adrenergic stimulation of normal and "ischemic" Purkinje fibers have different receptor-effector coupling mechanisms. *Circ. Res.*, 71:526–534.

Anyukhovsky E.P., Sosunov E.A., Rosen M.R. (1996). Regional differences in electrophysiological properties of epicardium, midmyocardium, and endocardium. *In vitro* and *in vivo* correlations. *Circulation*, 94:1981–1988.

Apkon M., Nerbonne J.M. (1988). α_1-adrenergic agonists selectively suppress voltage-dependent K^+ currents in rat ventricular myocytes. *Proc. Natl. Acad. Sci. USA*, 85:8756–8760.

Ardell J.L., Randall W.C. (1986). Selective vagal innervation of sinoatrial and atrioventricular nodes in canine heart. *Am. J. Physiol.*, 251:H764–H773.

Argentieri T.M., Frame L.H., Colatsky T.J. (1990). Electrical properties of canine subendocardial Purkinje fibers surviving in one-day old experimental myocardial infarction *Circ. Res.*, 66:123–134.

Armstrong C.M. (1971). Interactions of tetraethylammonium ion derivatives with the potassium channels of giant axons. *J. Gen. Physiol.*, 58:413–437.

Armstrong C.M. (1975). Ionic pores, gates, and gating currents. *Q. Rev. Biophys.*, 7:179–210.

Armstrong C.M., Bezanilla F. (1974). Charge movement associated with the opening and closing of the activation gates of the Na channels. *J. Gen. Physiol.*, 63:533–552.

Armstrong C.M., Bezanilla F.M., Rojas E. (1974). Destruction of sodium conductance inactivation in squid axons perfused with pronase. *J. Gen. Physiol.*, 62:375–391.

Armstrong C.M., Bezanilla F. (1977). Inactivation of the sodium channel. II. Gating current experiments. *J. Gen. Physiol.*, 70:567–590.

Armstrong C.M. (1981). Sodium channels and gating currents. *Physiol. Rev.*, 61:644–683.

Armstrong C.M. (1992). Voltage-dependent ion channels and their gating. *Physiological Reviews*, 72:S5–13.

Aronson R.S. (1980). Characteristics of action potentials of hypertrophied myocardium from rats with renal hypertension. *Circ. Res.*, 47:443–454.

Attwell D., Cohen I.S., Eisner D.A., Ohba M., Ojeda C. (1979). The steady state TTX-sensitive ("window") sodium current in cardiac Purkinje fibres. *Pflügers Archives*, 379:137–142.

Auld V.J., Goldin A.L., Krafte D.S., Catterall W.A., Lester H.A., Davidson N., Dunn R.J. (1990). A neutral amino acid change in segment IIS4 dramatically alters the gating properties of the voltage-dependent sodium channel. *Proc. Natl. Acad. Sci. USA*, 87:323–327.

Babila T., Moscucci A., Wang H., Weaver F.E., Koren G. (1994). Assembly of mammalian voltage-gated potassium channels: evidence for an important role of the first transmembrane segment. *Neuron*, 12:615–626.

Backx P.H., Yue D.T., Lawrence J.H., Marban E., Tomaselli G.F. (1992). Molecular localization of an ion-binding site within the pore of mammalian sodium channels. *Science*, 257:248–251.

Bahniski A., Nairn A.C., Greengard P., Gadsby D.C. (1989). Chloride conductance regulated by c-AMP-dependent protein kinase in cardiac myocytes. *Nature*, 340:718–721.

Balasubramaniam A., Sheriff S., Rigel D.F., Fischer J.E. (1990). Characterization of neuropeptide Y binding sites in rat cardiac ventricular membranes. *Peptides*, 11:545–550.

Balser J.R., Bennett P.B., Roden D.M. (1990). Time-dependent outward current in guinea pig ventricular myocytes. Gating kinetics of the delayed rectifier. *Journal of General Physiology*, 96:835–863.

Barbieri M., Varani K., Cerbai E., Guerra L., Li Q., Borea A., Mugelli A. (1994). Electrophysiological basis for the enhanced cardiac arrhythmogenic effect of isoprenaline in aged spontaneously hypertensive rats. *Cardiovas. Res.*, 26:849–860.

Barchi R.L. (1995). Molecular pathology of the skeletal muscle sodium channel. *Annu. Rev. Physiol.*, 57:355–385.

Bargheer K., Bode F., Klein H.U., Trappe H.J., Franz M.R., Lichtlen P.R. (1994). Prolongation of monophasic action potential duration and refractory period in the human heart by tedisamil, a new potassium blocking agent. *Eur. Heart. J.*, 15:1409–1414.

Barhanin J., Lesage F., Guillemare E., Fink M., Lazdunski M., Romey G. (1996). K(V)LQT1 and 1sK (minK) proteins associate to form the I(Ks) cardiac potassium current. *Nature*, 384:78–80.

Barr L., Dewey M.M., Berger W. (1965). Propagation of action potentials and the structure of the nexus in cardiac muscle. *J. Gen. Physiol.*, 48:797–823.

Barr R.C., Plonsey R. (1984). Propagation of excitation in idealized anisotropic two dimensional tissue. *Biophys. J.*, 45:1191–1202.

Barrington P.L., Harvey R.D., Mogul D.J., Bassett A.L., TenEick R.E. (1988). Na$^+$ current and inward rectifying K$^+$ current in cardiocytes from normal and hypertrophic right ventricles of cat. *Biophys. J.*, 53:426.

Bassett A.L., Gelband H. (1973). Chronic partial occlusion of the pulmonary artery in cats. Change in ventricular action potential configuration during early hypertrophy. *Circ. Res.*, 32:15–26.

Beeler G.W., Reuter H. (1977). Reconstruction of the action potential of ventricular myocardial fibers. *J. Physiol.*, 268:177–210.

Benitah J.P., Baily P., D'Agrosa M.C., DaPonte J.P., Delgado C., Lorente P. (1992a). Slow inward current in single cells isolated from adult human ventricles. *Pflügers Arch.*, 421:176–187.

Benitah J.P., Baily P., DaPonte J.P., DeRiberolles C., Lorente P. (1992b). Outward currents in isolated myocytes from human hypertrophied left ventricles. *Circulation*, 86:I-697.

Benitah J.P., Gomez A.M., Bailly P., DaPonte J.P., Berson G., Delgado C., Lorente P. (1993). Heterogeneity of the early outward current in ventricular cells isolated from normal and hypertrophied rat hearts. *J. Physiol.*, 469:111–138.

Benitah J.-P., Gomez A.M., Delgado C., Lorente P., Lederer W.J. (1997). A chloride current component induced by hypertrophy in rat ventricular myocytes. *Am. J. Physiol.*, 272:H2500–H2506.

Bennett P.B. Jr., Makita N., George A.L. Jr. (1993). A molecular basis for gating mode transitions in human skeletal muscle Na$^+$ channels. *FEBS Letters*, 326:21–24.

Bennett P.B., Valenzuela C., Chen L.Q., Kallen R.G. (1995a). On the molecular nature of the lidocaine receptor of cardiac Na$^+$ channels. Modification of block by alterations in the α-subunit III–IV interdomain. *Circulation Research*, 77:584–592.

Bennett P.B., Yazawa K., Makita N., George A.L. Jr. (1995b). Molecular mechanism for an inherited cardiac arrhythmia. *Nature*, 376:683–685.

Berman M.F., Camardo J.S., Robinson R.B., Siegelbaum S.A. (1989). Single sodium channels from canine ventricular myocytes: voltage dependence and relative rates of activation and inactivation. *Journal of Physiology*, 415:503–531.

Bers D.M. (1993). *Excitation-contraction coupling and cardiac contractile force*, Boston: Kluwer Academic Publishers.

Beuckelmann D.J., Nabauer M., Erdmann E. (1991). Characteristics of calcium currents in isolated human ventricular myocytes from patients with terminal heart failure. *J. Mol. Cell. Cardiol.*, 23:929–937.

Beuckelmann D.J., Nabauer M., Erdmann E. (1992). Intracellular calcium handling in isolated ventricular myocytes from patients with terminal heart failure. *Circulation*, 85:1046–1055.

Beuckelmann D.J., Nabauer M., Erdmann E. (1993). Alterations of K^+ currents in isolated human ventricular myocytes from patients with terminal heart failure. *Circ. Res.*, 73:379–385.

Beyer E.C., Veenstra R.D., Kanter H.L., Saffitz J.E. (1995). Molecular sturcture and patterns of expression of cardiac gap junction proteins. In: D.P. Zipes and J. Jalife (eds.), *Cardiac Electrocphysiology: From Cell to Bedside* (2nd edition), W.B. Saunders, Co., Phildelphia, pp. 31–38.

Billette J., Shrier A. (1995). Atrioventricular nodal activation and functional properties. In: D.P. Zipes and J. Jalife, (eds.), *Cardiac Electrophysiology: From Cell to Bedside* (2nd edition), W.B. Saunders Co., Philadelphia, Pa., pp. 216–228.

Black S.C., Chi L., Mu D.X., Lucchesi B.R. (1991). The antifibrillatory actions of UK-68798, a class III antiarrhythmic agent. *J. Pharmacol. Exp. Ther.*, 258:416–423.

Bohm M., Pieske B., Ungerer M., Erdmann E. (1989). Characterization of α_1 adenosine receptors in atrial and ventricular myocardium from diseased human hearts. *Circ. Res.*, 65:1201–1211.

Borea P.A., Amerini S., Masini I., Cerbai E., Ledda F., Mantelli L., Varani K., Mugelli A. (1992). β_1- and β_2-adrenoceptors in sheep cardiac ventricular muscle. *J. Mol. Cell. Cardiol.*, 24:753–764.

Boyden P.A., Pinto J.M.B. (1994). Reduced calcium currents in subendocardial Purkinje myocytes that survive in the 24 and 48 hour infarcted heart. *Circulation*, 89:2747–2759.

Boyden P.A., Albala A., Dresdner K. (1989). Electrophysiology and ultrastructure of canine subendocardial Purkinje cells isolated from control and 24 hour infarcted hearts. *Circ. Res.*, 65:955–970.

Boyden P.A., Tilley L.P., Albala A., Liu S.K., Fenoglio J.J.Jr., Wit A.L. (1984). Mechanisms for atrial arrhythmias associated with cardiomyopathy: a study of feline hearts with primary myocardial disease. *Circulation*, 69:1036–1047.

Boyden P.A., Jeck C.D. (1995). Ion channel function in disease. *Cardiovascular Research*, 29:312–318.

Boyden P.A., Gardner P.I., Wit A.L. (1988). Action potentials of cardiac muscle in healing infarcts: response to norepinephrine and caffeine. *J. Mol. Cell. Cardiol.*, 20:525–537.

Boyett M.R., Jewell B.R. (1980). Analysis of the effects of changes in rate and rhythm upon electrical activity in the heart. *Progress in Biophysics and Molecular Biology*, 36:1–52.

Breithardt G. (1995). Amiodarone in patients with heart failure. *N. Engl. J. Med.*, 333:121–122.

Bridal T.R., Rees S.A., Spinelli W., Colatsky T.J. (1996). Terikalant (RP 62719) is not a selective blocker of inward rectifier current in cat ventricular myocytes. *Circulation*, 94:I-529.

Bril A., Faivre J.F., Forest M.C., Cheval B., Gout B., Linee P., Ruffolo R.R. Jr., Poyser R.H. (1995). Electrophysiological effects of BRL-32872, a novel antiarrhythmic agent with potassium and calcium channel blocking properties, in guinea pig cardiac isolated preparations. *J. Pharmacol. Exp. Ther.*, 273:1264–1272.

Bristow M.R., Ginsburg R., Umans V., Fowler M., Minobe W., Rasmussen R., Zera P., Menlove R., Shah P., Jamison S., Stinson E.B. (1986). β_1- and β_2-adrenergic receptor subpopulations in nonfailing and failing human ventricular myocardium: Coupling of both receptor subtypes to muscle contraction and selective β_1-receptor down-regulation in heart failure. *Circ. Res.*, 59:297–309.

Bristow M.R., Hershberger R.E., Port J.D., Gilbert E.M., Sandoval A., Rasmussen R., Cates A.E., Feldman A.M. (1990). β-adrenergic pathways in nonfailing and failing human ventricular myocardium. *Circulation*, 82:112–125.

Bristow M.R., Hershberger R.E., Port J.D., Rasmussen R. (1989). β_1 and β_2-adrenergic receptor mediated adenylate cyclase stimulation in nonfailing and failing human ventricular myocardium. *Mol. Pharmacol.*, 35:295–303.

Brodde O.E., Khamssi M., Zerkowski H.R. (1991). β-adrenoceptors in the transplanted human heart: unaltered β_1-adrenoceptor density, but increased proportion of β_2-adrenoceptors with posttransplant time. *Naunyn-Schmiedeberg's Arch. Pharmacol.*, 344:430–436.

Brodde O.-E. (1991). β_1- and β_2-adrenoceptors in the human heart: properties, function, and alterations in chronic heart failure. *Pharmacol. Rev.*, 43:203–242.

Brooksby P., Levi A.J., Jones J.V. (1993a). Investigation of the mechanisms underlying the increased contraction of hypertrophied ventricular myocytes isolated from the spontaneously hypertensive rat. *Cardiovasc. Res.*, 27:1268–1277.

Brooksby P., Levi A.J., Jones J.V. (1993b). The electrophysiological characteristics of hypertrophied ventricular myocytes isolated from the spontaneously hypertensive rat. *J. Hypertension*, 11:611–622.

Brown A.M., Birnbaumer L. (1988). Direct G protein gating of ion channels. *Am. J. Physiol.*, 254:H401–H410.

Brown H.F. (1982). Electrophysiology of the sinoatrial node. *Physiol. Rev.*, 62:505–530.

Bryant S.M., Ryder K.O., Hart G. (1991). Effects of neuropeptide Y on cell length and membrane currents in isolated guinea pig ventricular myocytes. *Circ. Res.*, 69:1106–1113.

Buddish D., Isemberg G., Ravens U., Scholtysik G. (1985). The role of sodium channel in the effect of the cardiotonic compound DPI-206–106 on contractility and membrane potentials in isolated mammalian heart preparations. *Eur. J. Pharmacol.*, 118:303–311.

Burgen A.S.V., Terroux K.G. (1953). On the negative inotropic effect in the cat's auricle. *J. Physiol.* (Lond.), 120:449–464.

Busch A.E., Malloy K., Groh W.J., Varnum M.D., Adelman J.P., Mylie J. (1994). The novel class III antiarrhythmic NE-10064 and NE-10133 inhibit I_{Ks} channels expressed in *Xenopus* oocytes and I_{Ks} in guinea pig cardiac myocytes. *Biochem. Biophys. Res. Commun.*, 202:265–270.

Bylund D.B., Eikenberg D.C., Hieble J.P., Langer S.Z., Lefkowitz R.J., Minneman K.P., Molinoff P.B., Ruffolo R.R. Jr., Trendelenburg U. (1994). International Union of Pharmacology IV. Nomenclature of adrenoceptors. *Pharmacol. Rev.*, 46:121–136.

Cabo C., Pertsov A.M., Baxter W.T., Davidenko J.M., Gray R.A., Jalife J. (1994). Wavefront curvature as a cause of slow conduction and block in isolated cardiac muiscle. *Circ. Res.*, 75:1014–1028.

Cabo C., Pertsov A.M., Davidenko J.M., Baxter W.T., Gray R.A., Jalife J. (1996). Vortex shedding as a precursor of turbulent cardiac electrical activity in cardiac muscle. *Biophys. J.*, 70:1105–1111.

Cameron J.S., Myerburg R.J., Wong S.S., Gaide M.S., Epstein K., Alvarez T.R., Gelband H, Guse P.A., Bassett A.L. (1983). Electrophysiologic consequences of chronic experimentally induced left ventricular pressure overload. *Am. J. Cardiol.*, 2:481–487.

Capasso J.M., Strobeck J.E., Sonnenblick E.H. (1981). Myocardial mechanical alterations during the gradual onset long term hypertension in rats. *Am. J. Physiol.*, 10:H435–H441.

Carmeliet E. (1992). Voltage- and time-dependent block of the delayed K$^+$ current in cardiac myocytes by dofetilide. *J. Pharmacol. Ex. Ther.*, 262:809–817.

Carmeliet E. (1993). Use-dependent block and use-dependent unblock of the delayed rectifier K$^+$ current by almokalant in rabbit ventricular myocytes. *Circ. Res.*, 73:857–858.

CAST Investigators (1989). Preliminary report: effect of encainide and flecainide on mortality in a randomized trial of arrhythmia suppression after myocardial infarction. *N. Engl. J. Med.*, 321:406–412.

CAST Investigators (1992). Effect of the antiarrhythmic agent moricizine on survival after myocardial infarction. *N. Engl. J. Med.*, 327:227–333.

Catterall W.A. (1988a). Structure and function of voltage-sensitive sodium channels. *Science*, 242:50–61.

Catterall W.A. (1988b). Molecular pharmacology of voltage-sensitive sodium channels. *ISI Atlas of Science: Pharmacol.*, 2:190–195.

Catterall W.A. (1991). Structure and function of voltage-gated sodium and calcium channels. *Current Opinion in Neurobiology*, 1:5–13.

Catterall W.A. (1993). Structure and modulation of Na$^+$ and Ca^{2+} channels. *Ann. N.Y. Acad. Sci.*, 707:1–19.

Catterall W.A. (1995). Structure and function of voltage-gated ion channels. *Annual Review of Biochemistry*, 64:493–531.

Cerbai E., Barbieri M. Mugelli A. (1996). Occurrence and properties of the hyperpolarization activated current I_f in ventricular myocytes from normotensive and hypertensive rats with aging *Circulation*, 94:1674–1681.

Cerbai E., Barbieri M., Li Q., Mugelli A. (1994). Ionic basis of action potential prolongation of hypertrophied cardiac myocytes isolated from hypertensive rats of different ages *Cardiovasc. Res.*, 28:1180–1187.

Cerbai E., Pino R., Porciatti F., Sani G., Toscano M., Maccherini M., Giunti G., Mugelli A. (1997). Characterization of the hyperpolarization activated current I_f in ventricular myocytes from human failing heart. *Circulation*, 95:568–571.

Chang F., Yu H., Cohen I.S. (1994). Actions of vasoactive intestinal peptide neuropeptide Y on the pacemaker current in canine Purkinje fibers. *Circ. Res.*, 74:157–162.

Chen P.S., Wolf P.D., Dixon E.G., Danieley N.D., Frazier D.W., Smith W.M., Ideker R.E. (1988). Mechanism of ventricular vulnerability to single premature stimuli in open chest dogs. *Circ. Res.*, 62:1191–1209.

Chevalier P., Ruffy F., Danilo P. Jr., Rosen M.R. (1998). Interaction between α_1 adrenergic and vagal effects on cardiac rate and repolarization. *J. Pharmacol Exp. Ther.*, 284:832–837.

Chi L., Uprichard A.C.G., Lucchesi B.R. (1990). Profibrillatory actions of pinacidil in a conscious canine model of sudden coronary death. *J. cardiovasc. Pharmacol.*, 15:452–456.

Chialvo D.R., Jalife J. (1987). Non-linear dynamics of cardiac excitation and impulse propagation. *Nature*, 330:749–752.

Chialvo D.R., Gilmour R.F., Jalife J. (1990a). Low dimensional chaos in cardiac tissue. *Nature*, 343:653–657.

Chialvo D.R., Michaels D.C., Jalife J. (1990b). Supernormal excitability as a mechanism of chaotic dynamics of activation in cardiac Purkinje fibres. *Circ. Res.*, 66:525–545.

Chiamvimonvat N., Kargacin M.E., Clark R.B., Duff H.J. (1995). Effects of intracellular calcium on sodium current density in cultured neonatal rat cardiac myocytes. *J. Physiol.*, 483:307–318.

Choi K.L., Aldrich R.W., Yellen G. (1991). Tetraethylammonium blockade distinguishes two inactivation mechanisms in voltage-activated K^+ channels. *Proc. Natl. Acad. Sci. USA*, 88:5092–5095.

Choi K.L., Mossman C., Aube J., Yellen G. (1993). The internal quaternary ammonium receptor site of shaker potassium channels. *Neuron*, 10:533–541.

Chouinard S.W., Wilson G.F., Schlimgen A.K., Ganetzky B. (1995). A potassium channel β-subunit related to the aldo-keto reductase superfamily is encoded by the Drosophila hyperkinetic locus. *Proc. Natl. Acad. Sci. USA*, 92:6763–6767.

Christophe J., Waelbroeck M., Chatelain P., Robberecht P. (1984). Heart receptors for VIP, PHI and secretin are able to activate adenylate cyclase and to mediate inotropic and chronotropic effects. Species variations and physiopathology. *Peptides*, 5:341–353.

Clerc L. (1976). Directional differences of impulse spread in trabecular muscle from mammalian heart. *J. Physiol.*, (Lond.), 255:335–346.

Cohen N.M., Lederer W.J. (1993). Calcium current in single human cardiac myocytes *J. Cardiovasc. Electrophysiol.*, 4:422–437.

Cohen I.S., Datyner N.B., Gintant G.A., Kline R.P. (1986). Time-dependent outward currents in the heart. In: Fozzard H.A., Haber E., Jennings R.B., Katz A.M., Morgan H.E. (eds.), *The heart and cardiovascular system*, New York: Raven Press, pp. 637–669.

Colatsky T.J. (1982). Mechanisms of action of lidocaine and quinidine on action potential duration in rabbit cardiac Purkinje fibers. An effect on steady state sodium currents? *Circ. Res.*, 50:17–27.

Colatsky T.J., Argentieri T.M. (1994). Potassium channel blockers as antiarrhythmic drugs. *Drug Development Research*, 33:235–249.

Colatsky T.J. (1995). Antiarrhythmic drugs: where are we going? *Pharmaceutical News*, 2:17–23.

Colli Franzone P., Guerri L., Taccardi B. (1993a). Spread of excitation in a myocardial volume: Simulation studies in a model of anisotropic ventricular muscle activated by point stimulation. *C. Cardiovasc. Electrophysiol.*, 4:144–160.

Colli Franzone P., Guerri L., Taccardi B. (1993b). Potential distributions generated by point stimulation in a myocardial volume. Simulation studies in a model of anisotropic ventricular muscle. *J. Cardiovasc. Electrophysiol.*, 4:438–458.

Conforti L., Millhorn D.E. (1997). Selective inhibition of a slow-inactivating voltage-dependent K^+ channel in rat PC12 cells by hypoxia *J. Physiol.*, 502.2:293–305.

Coraboeuf E., Deroubaix E., Coulombe A. (1979). Effect of tetrodotoxin on action potentials of the conducting system in the dog heart. *Am. J. Physiol.*, 236:H561–H567.

Coulombe A., Momtaz A., Richer P., Swynghedauw B., Coraboeuf E. (1994). Reduction of calcium independent outward potassium current density in DOCA salt hypertrophied rat ventricular myocytes *Pflugers Arch.*, 427:47–55.

Coumel P., Attuel P., Lavellée J.P., Flammang D., Leclerc J.F., Slama R. (1978). Syndrome d'arythmie auriculaire d'origine vagale. *Arch. Mal. Coeur.*, 71:645–656.

Courtney K.R. (1980). Interval-dependent effects of small antiarrhythmic drugs on the excitability of guinea pig myocardium. *J. Mol. Cell Cardiol.*, 12:1273–1286.

Courtney K.R. (1987). Review: Quantitative structure/activity relations based on use-dependent block and repriming kinetics in myocardium. *J. Mol. Cell. Cardiol.*, 19:319–330.

Cox M.M., Berman I., Myerburg R.J., Smets M.J.D., Kozlovskis P.L. (1991). Morphometric mapping of regional myocyte diameters after healing of myocardial infarction in cats. *J. Mol. Cell. Cardiol.*, 23:127–135.

Cranefield P.F., Klein H.O., Hoffman B.F. (1971). Conduction of the cardiac impulse. I. Delay, block, and one-way block in depressed Purkinje fibers. *Circ. Res.*, 28:199–219.

Cranefield P.F., Wit A.L., Hoffman B.F. (1972). Conduction of the cardiac impuse. III. Characteristics of very slow conduction. *J. Gen. Physiol.*, 59:227–246.

Curran M.E., Splawski I., Timothy K.W., Vincent G.M., Green E.D., Keating M.T. (1995). A molecular basis for cardiac arrhythmia: HERG mutations cause long QT syndrome. *Cell*, 80:795–804.

Damiano B.P., Rosen M.R. (1984). Effects of pacing on triggered activity induced by early afterdepolarizations. *Circulation*, 69:1013–1025.

Dangman K.H., Hoffman B.F. (1981). In vivo and in vitro antiarrhythmic and arrhythmogenic effects of N-acetylprocainamide. *J. Pharmacol. Exp. Ther.*, 217:851–862.

Danilo P., Rosen M., Hordof A. (1978). Effects of acetylcholine on the ventricular specialized conducting system of neonatal and adult dogs. *Circ. Res.*, 43:777–784.

Datyner N., Cohen I.S. (1993). Slow inactivation and the measurement of L- and T-type calcium current in Purkinje myocytes. *J. Gen. Physiol.*, 102:859–869.

Daut J. (1982). The passive ellectrical properties of guinea-pig ventricular muscle as examined with a voltage-clamp technique. *Journal of Physiology*, 330:221–242.

Daut J., Marier-Rudolph W., von Beckerath N., Mehrke G., Günther K., Goedel-Meinen L. (1990). Hypoxic dilation of coronary arteries is mediated by ATP-sensitive potassium channels. *Science*, 247:1341–1344.

Davidenko J.M. (1993). Spiral wave activity as a common mechanism for polymorphic and monomorphic ventricular tachycardias. *J. Cardiovasc. Electrophysiol.*, 4:730–746.

Davidenko M.J., Pertsov A.M., Salomonsz R., Baxter W., Jalife J. (1991). Stationary and drifting spiral waves of excitation in isolated cardiac muscle. *Nature*, 355:349–351.

Davis L. Jr., Lorento de Nó R. (1947). Contribution to the mathematical theory of the electrotonus. In: Lorento de Nó (ed.), *A study of Nerve Physiology*, Srud Rockefeller Inst. Med. Res., pp. 442–496.

De Bakker J.M.T., vanCapelle F.J.L., Janse M.J., Wilde A.A., Coronel R., Becker A.E., Dingemans K.P., van Hemel N.M., Hauer R.N.W. (1988): Reentry as a cause of ventricular tachycardia in patients with chronic ischemic heart disease: electrophysiologic and anatomic correlations. *Circulation*, 77:589–606.

de la Fuente D., Sasyniuk B., Moe G.K. (1971). Conductance through a narrow isthmus in isolated canine atrial tissue: a model of the W-P-W syndrome. *Circulation*, 44:803–809.

Del Balzo U., Rosen M.R., Malfatto G., Kaplan L.M., Steinberg S.F. (1990). Specific α_1-adrenergic receptor subtypes modulate catecholamine-induced increases and decreases in ventricular automaticity. *Circ. Res.*, 67:1535–1551.

Delgado C., Steinhaus B., Delmar M., Chialvo M., Jalife J. (1990). Directional differences in excitability and margin of safety for propagation in sheep ventricular epicardial muscle. *Circ. Res.*, 67:97–110.

Delmar M., Jalife J. (1990). Wenckebach periodicity: From deductive electrocardiographic analysis to ionic mechanisms. In: D.P. Zipes and J. Jalife (eds.), *Cardiac Electrophysiology. From Cell to Bedside*, W.B. Saunders Co., Philadelphia, In Press. pp. 128–138.

Delmar M., Glass L., Michaels D.C., Jalife J. (1989a). Ionic bases and analytical solution of the Wenckebach phenomenon in guinea pig ventricular myocytes. *Circ. Res.*, 65:775–788.

Delmar M., Michaels D.C., Jalife J. (1989b). Slow recovery of excitability and the Wenckebach phenomenon in the single guinea pig ventricular myocyte. *Circ. Res.*, 65:761–774.

Delmar M., Ibarra J., Davidenko J., Lorente P., Jalife J. (1991). Dynamics of the background outward current in single guinea pig ventricular myocytes. Ionic mechanisms of hysteris in cardiac cells. *Circ. Res.*, 69:1316–1326.

Delmar M., Michaels D.C., Jalife J. (1988). The single ventricular myocyte as a model for Wenckebach periodicity. In: W.A. Clark, R.S. Decker, T.K. Borg (eds.), *Biology of Isolated Adult Cardiac Myocytes*, Elsevier, New York, pp. 426–429.

Delmar M., Michaels D.C., Johnson T., Jalife J. (1987). Effects of increasing intercellular resistance on transverse and longitudinal propagagtion in sheep epicardial muscle. *Circ. Res.*, 60:780–785.

DeMello W.C. (1977). Passive electrical properties of the atrio-ventricular node. *Pflügers Arch.*, 371:135–139.

Demo S.D., Yellen G.(1991). The inactivation gate of the Shaker K^+ channel behaves like an openchannel blocker. *Neuron*, 7:743–753.

Denyer J.C., Brown H.F. (1990). Pacemaking in rabbit isolated sino-atrial node cells during Cs^+ block of the hyperpolarization activated current. If *Journal of Physiology*, 429:401–409.

DiFrancesco D. (1985). The cardiac hyperpolarizing current I_f. Origin and developments. *Prog. Biophys. Molec. Biol.*, 46:163–183.

Difrancesco D. (1981a). A study of the ionic nature of the pace-maker current in calf Purkinje fibres. *Journal of Physiology*, 314:377–393.

DiFrancesco D. (1981b). A new interpretation of the pace-maker current in calf Purkinje fibres. *J. Physiol.*, (London). 314:359–76.

Difrancesco D. (1993). Pacemaker mechanisms in cardiac tissue. *Annu. Rev. Physiol.*, 55:451–467.

DiFrancesco D., Ducouret P., Robinson R.B. (1989). Muscarinic modulation of cardiac rate at low acetylcholine concentrations. *Science*, 243:699–671.

Dillon S.M. (1991). Optical recordings of the rabbit heart show that defibrillation strength shocks prolong the duration of depolarization and the refractory period. *Circ. Res.*, 69:842–856.

Dirksen R.T., Sheu S.S. (1990). Modulation of ventricular action potential by α_1-adrenoceptors and protein kinase C. *Am. J. Physiol.*, 258:H907–H911.

Dixon J.E., Shi W., Wang H.S., McDonald C., Yu H., Wymore R.S., Cohen I.S., Mckinnon D. (1996). Role of the Kv4.3 K^+ channel in ventricular muscle. A molecular correlate for the transient outward current [published erratum appears in *Circ. Res.*, 1997, Jan; 80(1):147]. *Circ. Res.*, 79:659–668.

Dolly J.O., Rettig J., Scott V.E., Parcej D.N., Wittkat R., Sewing S., Pongs O. (1994). Oligomeric and subunit structures of neuronal voltage-sensitive K^+ channels [Review][36 refs]. *Biochemical Society Transactions*, 22:473–478.

Dominguez G., Fozzard H.A. (1970). Influence of extracellular K^+ concentration on cable properties and excitability of sheep cardiac Purkinje fibres. *Circ. Res.*, 26:565–574.

Donald D.E., Samueloff S.I., Ferguson D. (1967). Mechanism of tachycardia caused by atropine in conscious dogs. *Am. J. Physiol.*, 212:901–910.

Dresdner K.P., Kline R.P., Wit A.L. (1987). Intracellular K^+ activity, intracellular Na^+ activity and maximum diastolic potential of canine subendocardial Purkinje cells from one-day-old infarcts *Circ. Res.*, 60:122–132.

Drugge E., Robinson R. (1987). Trophic influence of sympathetic neurons on the cardiac α-adrenergic response requires close nerve-muscle association. *Dev. Pharmacol. Ther.*, 10:47–59.

Dukes I.D., Vaughan-Williams E.M. (1984). Effects of selective α_1, α_2, β_1, and β_2-adrenoceptor stimulation on potentials and contractions in the rabbit heart. *J. Physiol.* (Lond.), 355:523–546.

Dukes I.D., Cleeman L., Morad M. (1990). Tedisamil blocks the transient and delayed rectifier K^+ current in mammalian cardiac and glial cells. *J. Pharm. Exp. Ther.*, 254:560–569.

Eaholtz G., Scheuer T., Catterall W.A. (1994). Restoration of inactivation and block of open sodium channels by an inactivation gate peptide. *Neuron*, 12:1041–1048.

Ebihara L., Johnson E.A. (1980). Fast sodium current in cardiac muscle: a quantitative description. *Biophys. J.*, 32:79–790.

Echt D.S., Liebson P.R., Mitchell L.B., Peter R.W., Obias-Manno D., Barker A.H., Arensberg D., Baker A., Friedman L., Greene H.L., Huther M.L., Richardson D.W., the CAST investigators (1991). Mortality and morbidity in patients receiving encainide, flecainide, or placebo. *N. Engl. J. Med.*, 324:781–788.

Echt D.S., Back J.N., Barbey J.T., Coxe D.R., Cato E. (1989). Evaluation of antiarrhythmic drugs on defibrillation energy requirements in dogs: sodium channels block and action potential prolongation. *Circulation*, 79:1106–1117.

Editorial. Third and long (QT) (1996). *Nature Genetics*, 12:1–2.

Edvinsson L., Hakanson R., Wahlestedt C., Uddman R. (1987). Effects of neuropeptide Y on the cardiovascular system. *Trends in Physiol Sci.*, 8:231–235.

Ek-Vitorin J.F., Calero G., Morley G.E., Coombs W., Taffet S.M., Delmar M. (1996). pH Regulation of connexin43: molecular analysis of the gating particle. *Biophys. J.*, 71:1273–1284.

Elharrar V., Surawicz B. (1983). Cycle length effect on restitution of action potential duration in dog cardiac fibers. *Am. J. Physiol.*, 244:H782–H792.

El-Sherif N., Scherlag B.J., Lazzara R., Samet P. (1974). Pathophysiology of tachycardia-and bradycardia-dependent block in the canine proximal His-Purkinje system after acute myocardial ischemia. *Am. J. Cardiol.*, 33:529–540.

Engelman T.W. (1896). Expériences sur la propagation irréciproque des excitations dans les fibres musculaires. *Arch. néerl.*, 30:165–183.

England S.K., Uebele V.N., Kodali J., Bennett P.B., Tamkun M.M. (1995a). A novel K^+ channel β-subunit (hKv β 1.3) is produced via alternative mRNA splicing. *Journal of Biological Chemistry*, 270:28531–28534.

England S.K., Uebele V.N., Shear H., Kodali J., Bennett P.B., Tamkun M.M. (1995b). Characterization of a voltage-gated K^+ channel β subunit expressed in human heart. *Proceedings of the National Academy of Sciences of the United States of America*, 92:6309–6313.

Erlanger J. (1908). Irregularities of the heart resulting from disturbed conductivity. *Am. J. Med. Sci.*, 135:797–811.

Ertl R., Jahnel U., Nawrath H., Carmeliet E., Vereecke J. (1991). Differntial electrophysiological and inotropic effects of phenylephrine in atrial and ventricular heart muscle preparations from rats. *Naunyn-schmied Arch. Pharmacol.*, 344:574–581.

Escande D., Coulombe A., Faivre J.F., Coraboeuf E. (1986). Characteristics of the time dependent slow inward current in adult human atrial single myocytes *J. Mol. Cell. Cardiol.*, 18:547–551.

Escande D., Coulombe A., Faivre J.F., Deroubaix E., Coraboeuf E. (1987). Two types of transient outward currents in adult human atrial cells. *American Journal of Physiology*, 252:H142–H148.

Escande D., Loisance D., Planche C., Caraboeuf E. (1985). Age-related changes of action potential plateau shape in isolated human atrial fibers. *Am. J. Physiol.*, 249:H843–H850.

Escande D., Mestre M., Cavero I., Brugada J., Kirchof C. (1992). RP 58866 and its active enantiomer RP 62719 (Terikalan): Blockers of the inward rectifier K^+ current acting as pure class III antiarrhythmic. *J. Cardiovasc. Pharmacol.*, 20:S106–S113.

Faivre J.F., Findlay I. (1990). Action potential duration and activation of ATP-sensitive potassium current in isolated guinea pig myocytes. *Biochim. Biophys. Acta.*, 1029:167–172.

References

Faivre J.F., Foest M.C., Cheval B., Gout B., Linee P., Ruffolo R.R. Jr., Poyser R.H., Bril A. (1994). Electrophysiological activity of BRL-32872, a new class III antiarrhythmic agent with calcium antaonist propeties. *FASEB J.*, 8:I-A74.

Farrukh H.M., White M., Port J.D., Handwerger D., Larrabee P., Klein J., Roden R.A., Skerl L., Renlund D.G., Feldman A.M., Bristow M.R. (1993). Up-regulation of β_2-adrenergic receptors in previously transplanted, denervated nonfailing human hearts. *J. Am. Coll. Cardiol.*, 22:1902–1908.

Fast V.G., Kléber A.G. (1995a). Cardiac tissue geometry as a determinant of unidirectional conduction block: assessment of microscopic excitation spread by optical mapping in patterned cell cultures and in a computer model. *Cardiovasc. Res.*, 29:697–707.

Fast V.G., Kléber A.G. (1995a). Block of impulse propagation at an abrupt tissue expansion: evaluation of the critical strand diameter in 2- and 3- dimensional computer models. *Cardiovasc. Res.*, 30:449–459.

Fast V.G., Kléber A.G. (1997). Role of wavefront curvature in propagation of cardiac impulse. *Cardiovasc. Res.*, 33:258–271.

Fast V.G., Darrow B.J., Saffitz J.E., Kléber A.G. (1996). Anisotropic activation spread in heart cell monolayers assessed by high-resolution optical mapping. Role of tissue discontinuities. *Circ. Res.*, 79:115–127.

Fedida D., Shimoni Y., Giles W.R. (1990). α-adrenergic modulation of the transient outward current in rabbit atrial myocytes. *J. Physiol. (Lond).*, 423:257–277.

Feldman A.M., Cates A.E., Bristow M.R., Van Dop C. (1988). Expression of the α G_i gene in the failing heart. *J. Mol. Cell. Cardiol.*, 20:17.

Fenoglio J.J. Pham T.D., Harken A.H., Horowitz L.N., Josephson M.E., Wit A.L. (1983). Recurrent sustained ventricular tachycardia: structure and ultrastructure of subendocardial regions in which tachycardia originates. *Circulation*, 68:518–533.

Fields J.Z., Roeske W.R., Morkin E., Yamamura H.I. (1978). Cardiac muscarinic cholinergic receptors: Biochemical identification and characterization. *J. Biol. Chem.*, 253:3251–3258.

Fischmeister R., Hartzell H.C. (1986). Mechanism of action of acetylcholine on calcium current in single cells from frog ventricle. *J. Physiol.*, 376:183–202.

Fleig A., Fitch J.M., Goldin A.L., Rayner M.D., Starkus J.G., Ruben P.C. (1994). Point mutations in IIS4 alter activation and inactivation of rat brain IIA Na channels in Xenopus oocyte macropatches. *Pflugers archiv.-European Journal of Physiology*, 427:406–413.

Fleming J.W., Strawbridge R.A., Watanabe A.M. (1987). Muscarinic receptor regulation of cardiac adenylate cyclase activity *J. Mol. Cell. Cardiol.*, 19:47–61.

Folander K., Smith J.S., Antanavage J., Bennett C., Stein R.B., Swanson R. (1990). Cloning and expression of the delayed-rectifier IsK channel from neonatal rat heart and diethylstilbestrol-primed rat uterus. *Proc. Natl. Acad. Sci. USA*, 87:2975–2979.

Follmer C.H., Colatsky T.J. (1990). Block of the delayed rectifier potassium current, I_K, by flecainide and E-4031 in cat ventricular myocytes. *Circulation*, 82:289–293.

Follmer C.H., Lodge N.J., Cullinam C.A., Colatsky T.J. (1992). Modulation of the delayed rectifier, I_K, by cadmium in cat ventricular myocytes. *Am. J. Physiol.*, 262:C75–C83.

Fowler M.B., Laser J.A., Hopkins G.L., Minobe W., Bristow M.R. (1986). Assessment of the β-adrenergic receptor pathway in the intact failing human heart: Progressive receptor downregulation and subsensitivity to agonist response. *Circulation*, 74:1290–1302.

Fozzard H.A. (1979). Conduction of the action potential. In: R.M. Berne, N. Sperelakis, and S.R. Geiger (eds.), *Handbook of Physiology. Section 2, The Cardiovascular System*, Vol 1. Bethesda, MD, American Physiological Society, pp. 335–336.

Fozzard H.A., Levin D.N., Walton M. (1982). Control of conduction velocity in cardiac Purkinje fibers. In: Paes de Carvalho A., Hoffman B.F. and Lieberman M. (eds.), *Normal and abnormal Conduction in the Heart*, Futura Publishing Co., New York, pp. 105–116.

Frase L., Gaffney A., Lane L., Buckey J., Said S., Blomqvist G., Krejs G. (1987). Cardiovascular effects of vasoactive intestinal peptide in healthy subjects. *Am. J. Cardiol.*, 60:1356–1361.

Frazier D.W., Krassowska W., Chen P.S., Wolf P.D., Danieley N.D., Smith W.M., Ideker R.E. (1988). Transmural activations and stimulus potentials in three-dimensional anisotropic canine myocardium. *Circ. Res.*, 63:135–146.

Frazier D.W., Wolf P.D., Wharton J.M., Tang A.S.L., Smith W.M., Ideker R.E. (1989). Stimulus-induced critical point: Mechanism for the electrical initiation of reentry in normal canine myocardium. *J. Clin. Invest.*, 83:1039–1052.

Freedman J.C. (1995). Biophysical chemistry of cellular electrolytes. In: Sperelakis N. (ed.), *Cell Physiology. Source book*, Academic Press, San Diego, pp. 3–17.

Friedrichs G.S., Abreu J.N., Driscol E.M., Borlak J., Lucchesi B.R. (1998). Antifibrillatory efficacy of long-term tedisamil administration in a postinfarcted canine model of ischemic ventricular fibrillation. *J. Cardiovasc. Pharmacol.*, 31:56–66.

Furokawa T., Tsujimura Y., Kitamura K., Tanaka H., Habuchi Y. (1989). Time- and voltage-dependent block of the delayed K^+ current in rabbit sinoatrial and atrioventricular nodes. *J. Pharmacol. Exp. Ther.*, 251:756–763.

Furukawa T., Ito H., Nitta J., Tsujino M., Adachi S., Hiroe M., Marumo F., Sawanobori T., Hiraoka M. (1992). Endothelin-1 enhances calcium entry through T type Ca channels in cultured rat ventricular myocytes. *Circ. Res.*, 71:1242–1253.

Furukawa T., Myerburg R.J., Furukawa N., Kimura S., Bassett A.L. (1994). Metabolic inhibition of $I_{Ca, L}$ and I_K differs in feline left ventricular hypertrophy *Am. J. Physiol.*, 266:H1121–H1131.

Gadsby D.C. (1983). β-adrenoceptor agonists increase membrane K conductance in cardiac Purkinje fibres. *Nature Lond.*, 306:691–693.

Gaide M.S., Myerburg R.J., Kozlovskis P.L., Bassett A.L. (1983). Elevated sympathetic response of epicardial proximal to healed myocardial infarction. *Am. J. Physiol.*, 245:H646–H652.

Gao J., Mathias R.T., Cohen I.S., Shi J., Baldo G.J. (1996). The effects of ?-stimulation on the $Na^+ - K^+$ pump current-voltage relationship in guinea-pig ventricular myocytes. *J. Physiol.* (London), 494: 697–708.

Garfinkel A., Spano M.L., Ditto W.L., Weiss J.N. (1992). Controlling cardiac chaos. *Science*, 257:1230–1235.

Gauthier C., Tavernier G., Charpentier F., Langin D., Le Marec H. (1996). Functional β_3-adrenoceptor in human heart. *J. Clin. Invest.*, 98:556–562.

Gengo P.J., Sabbah H.N., Steffen R.P., Sharpe J.K., Kono T., Stein P.D., Goldstein S. (1992). Myocardial β adrenoceptor and voltage sensitive calcium channel changes in a canine model of chronic heart failure. *J. Mol. Cell. Cardiol.*, 24:1361–1369.

Gerisch G. (1965). Standienpezifische Aggregationsmuster bei Distyostelium Discoideum. *Wilhelm Roux Archiv Entwick Org*, 156:127–144.

Gidh-Jain M., Huang B., Jain P., El-Sherif N. (1996). Differential expression of voltage gated K channel genes in left ventricular remodeled myocardium after experimental myocardial infarction *Circ. Res.*, 79:669–675.

Gidh-Jain M., Huang B., Jain P., Battula V., El-Sherif N. (1995). Reemergence of the fetal pattern of L-type calcium channel gene expression in non infarcted myocardium during left ventricular remodeling. *Biochem. Biophys. Res. Comm.*, 216(3):892–897.

Gilmour R.F.J., Zipes D.P. (1986). Abnormal automaticity and related phenomena. In: Fozzard H.A., Haber E., Jennings R.B., Katz A.M., Morgan H.E. (eds.), *The heart and cardiovascular system. Scientific foundations*, New York: Raven Press, Ltd., pp. 1239–1257.

Gintant G.A. (1996). Two components of delayed rectifier current in canine atrium and ventricle: Does I_{Ks} play a role in the reverse rate dependence of class III agents? *Circ. Res.*, 78:26–37.

Gintant G.A., Datyner N.B., Cohen I.S. (1984). Slow inactivation of a tetrodotoxin-sensitive current in canine Purkinje fibers. *Biophysical Journal*, 45:509–512.

Gintant G.A., Datyner N.B., Cohen I.S. (1985). Gating of delayed rectification in acutely isolated canine cardiac Purkinje myocytes. Evidence for a single voltage-gated conductance. *Biophys. J.*, 48:1059–1064.

Glossman H., Ferry D.R., Rombusch M. (1984). Molecular pharmacology of the calcium channel: evidence for subtypes, multiple drug-receptor sites, channel subunits, and the development of a radioiodinated 1,4 dhydropyridine calcium channel label, $[I^{125}]$ iodipine. *J. Cardiovasc. Pharmacol.*, 6:608–621.

Goldman D.E. (1943). Potential, impedance and rectification in membranes. *J. Gen. Physiol.*, 27:37–60.

Gomez A.M., Valdivia H.H., Cheng H., Lederer M.R., Santana L.F., Cannell M.B., McCune S.A., Altschuld R.A., Lederer W.J. (1997). Defective excitation-contraction coupling in experimental cardiac hypertrophy and heart failure. *Science*, 276:800–806.

Gorelova N.A., Bures J. (1983). Spiral waves of spreading depression in the isolated chicken retina. *Neurobiology*, 14:353–363.

Grant A.O., Starmer F., Strauss H.C. (1984). Antiarrhythmic drug action: Blockade of the inward sodium channel. *Circ. Res.*, 55:427–439.

Gray R.A., Jalife J., Panfilov A., Baxter W.T., Cabo C., Davidenko J.M., Pertsov A.M. (1995a). Nonstationary vortexlike reentrant activity as a mechanism of polymorphic ventricular tachycardia in the isolated rabbit heart. *Circulation*, 91:2454–2469.

Gray R.A., Jalife J., Panflilov A.V., Baxter W.T., Cabo C., Davidenko J., Pertsov A.M. (1995b). Mechanisms of cardiac fibrillation. *Science*, 270:1222–1225.

Gray R.A., Pertsov A.M., Jalife J. (1996). Incomplete reentry and epicardial breakthrough patterns during atrial fibrillation in the sheep heart. *Circulation*, 94:2649–2661.

Greenbaum R.A., Ho S.Y., Gibson D.G., Becker A.E., Anderson R.H. (1981). Left ventricular fiber architecture in man. *Br. Heart. J.*, 45:248–263.

Gross A., Abramson T., MacKinnon R. (1994). Transfer of the scorpion toxin receptor to an insensitive potassium channel. *Neuron*, 13:961–966.

Grover G.J., McCullogh Jr., Henry D.E., Conder M.L., Sleph P.G. (1989). Anti-ischemic effects of the potassium channel activators pinacidil and cromakalim and the reversal of these effects with the potassium channel blocker glyburide. *J. Pharmacol. Exp. Ther.*, 251:98–104.

Grover G.J., Sleph P.G., Dzwonczyk S. (1990). Pharmacologic profile of cromakalim in the treatment of myocardial ischemia in isolated rat hearts and anesthetized dogs. *J. Cardiovasc. Pharmacol.*, 16:853–864.

Gruver E.J., Glass M.G., Marsh J.D., Gwathmey J.K. (1993). An animal model of dilated cardiomyopathy: characterization of dihydropyridine receptors and contractile performance. *Am. J. Physiol.*, 265:H1704–H1711.

Gu J., Polak J.M., Allen J.M., Huang W.M., Sheppard M.N., Tatemoto K., Bloom S.R. (1984). High concentrations of a novel peptide, neuropeptide Y, in the innervation of mouse and rat heart. *J. Histochem. Cytochem.*, 32:467–472.

Guevara M.R., Glass L., Shrier A. (1981). Phase locking, period doubling bifurcations and irregular dynamics in periodically stimulated cardiac cells. *Science*, 214:1350–1351.

Gul'ko F.B., Petrov A.A. (1972). Mechanism of the formation of closed pathways of conduction in excitable media. *Biophysics*, 17:271–281.

Gulch R.W., Baumann R., Jacob R. (1979). Analysis of myocardial action potentials in left ventricular hypertrophy of the Goldblatt rat. *Basic Res. Cardiol.*, 74:69–82.

Guo J., Ono K., Noma A. (1995). A sustained inward current activated at the diastolic range in rabbit sino-atrial node cells. *Journal of Physiology*, 483:1–13.

Haas M., Cheng B., Richardt G., Lang R.E., Schomig A. (1989). Characterization and presynaptic modulation of stimulation-evoked exocytotic co-release of noradrenaline and neuropeptide Y in guinea-pig heart. *Naunyn-Schmiedeberg's Arch. Pharmacol.*, 339:71–78.

Hagiwara N., Irisawa H., Kameyama M. (1988). Contribution of two types of calcium currents to the pacemaker potentials of rabbit sino-atrial node cells. *Journal of Physiology*, 395:233–253.

Hagiwara N., Irisawa H., Kasanuki H., Hosoda S. (1992). Background current in sino-atrial node cells of the rabbit heart. *Journal of Physiology*, 448:53–72.

Hall J.A., Petch M.C., Brown M.J. (1989). Intracoronary injections of salbutamol demonstrate the presence of functional β_2 receptors in the human heart. *Circ. Res.*, 65:546–553.

Hamrell B.B., Alpert N.R. (1977). The mechanical characteristics of hypertrophied rabbit cardiac muscle in the absence of congestive heart failure: The contractile and series elastic elements. *Circ. Res.*, 40:20–25.

Hart G. (1994). Cellular electrophysiology in cardiac hypertrophy and failure. *Cardiovasc. Res.*, 28:933–946.

Hartmann H.A., Tiedeman A.A., Chen S.F., Brown A.M., Kirsch G.E. (1994). Effects of III–IV linker mutations on human heart Na^+ channel inactivation gating. *Circulation Research*, 75:114–122.

Hartshorne R.P., Catterall W.A. (1984). The sodium channel from rat brain. Purification and subunit composition. *J. Biol. Chem.*, 259:1667–1675.

Hartzell H.C. (1988). Regulation of cardiac ion channels by catecholamines, acetylcholine and second messenger systems. *Prog. Biophys. Mol. Biol.*, 52:165–247.

Hartzell H.C., Simmons M.A. (1987). Comparison of effects of acetylcholine on calcium and potassium currents in frog atrium and ventricle. *J. Physiol.*, 389:411–422.

Harvey R.D., Hume J.R. (1989). Autonomic regulation of a chloride current in heart. *Science*, 244:983–985.

Hauswirth O., Noble D., Tsien R.W. (1972). The dependence of plateau currents in sheep Purkinje fibers on the interval between action potentials. *J. Physiol. (Lond.)*, 222:27–49.

Hayashi H., Shibata S. (1974). Electrical properties of cardiac cell membrane of spontaneously hypertensive rat. *Eur. J. Pharmacol.*, 27:355–359.

Heginbotham L., MacKinnon R. (1992). The aromatic binding site for tetraethylammonium ion on potassium channels. *Neuron*, 8:483–491.

Heinemann S.H., Rettig J., Wunder F., Pongs O. (1995). Molecular and functional characterization of a rat brain Kv β_3 potassium channel subunit. *FEBS Lett.*, 377:383–389.

Heinemann S.H., Schlief T., Mori Y., Imoto K. (1994). Molecular pore structure of voltage-gated sodium and calcium channels. [54 refs]. *Brazilian Journal of Medical Biological Research*, 27:2781–2802.

Heinemann S.H., Terlau H., Stuhmer W., Imoto K., Numa S. (1992). Calcium channel characteristics conferred on the sodium channel by single mutations. *Nature*, 356:441–443.

Henning R.J. (1992). Vagal stimulation during muscarinic and adrenergic blockade increased atrial contractility and heart rate. *J. Auton. Nerv. Syst.*, 40:121–130.

Hershman K.M., Levitan E.S. (1997). Cardiac myocyte Kvl.5 K^+ channel mRNA expression is influenced by cell-cell interactions. *Biophys. J.*, 72:A-265. (Abstract)

Hescheler J., Kameyama M., Trautwein W.(1986). On the mechanism of muscarinic inhibition of the cardiac Ca current. *Pflügers. Arch.*, 407:182–189.

Hescheler J., Kameyama M., Trautwein W., Mieshes G., Soling H.D. (1987). Regulation of the cardiac calcium channel by protein phosphatases. *Eur. J. Biochem.*, 165:261–266.

Hescheler J., Mieskes G., Ruegg J.C., Takai A., Trautwein W. (1988). Effects of a protein phosphatase inhibitor, okadaic acid, on membrane currents of isolated guinea-pig cardiac myocytes. *Pflügers Arch.*, 412:248–252.

Hess P., Lansman J.B., Tsien R.W. (1984). Different modes of Ca channel gating behaviour favored by dihydropyridine Ca agonist and antagonist. *Nature* (Lond.), 311:538–544.

Hidalgo P., MacKinnon R. (1995). Revealing the architecture of a K^+ channel pore through mutant cycles with a peptide inhibitor. *Science*, 268:307–310.

Hieble J.P., Bylund D.B., Clark D.E., Eikenburg D.C., Langer S.Z., Lefkowitz R.J., Minneman K.P., Ruffolo R.R. Jr. (1995). International Union of Pharmacology. X. Recommendation for nomenclature of α_1-adrenoreceptors: Consensus update. *Pharmacol. Rev.*, 47:267–270.

Hille B. (1977). Local anesthetics: hydrophilic and hydrophobic pathways for the drug-receptor interaction. *J. Gen. Physiol.*, 69:469–515.

Hille B. (1984). *Ionic Channels of excitable Membranes*, 1st ed. Sinauer Associates Inc. Publishers, Sunderland, Massachusetts.

Hille B. (1992). *Ionic Channels of Excitable Membranes*, 2nd ed. Sinauer Associates, Sunderland, MA.

Hirano Y., Fozzard H.A., January C.T. (1989). Characteristics of L- and T-type Ca^{2+} currents in canine cardiac Purkinje cells. *American Journal of Physiology*, 256:H1478–H1492.

Hirano Y., Moscucci A., January C.T. (1992). Direct measurement of L-type Ca^{++} window current in heart cells. *Circulation Research*, 70:445–455.

Hiraoka M., Kawano S. (1989). Calcium-sensitive and insensitive transient outward current in rabbit ventricular myocytes. *Journal of Physiology*, 410:187–212.

Hirschberg B., Rovner A., Lieberman M., Patlak J. (1995). Transfer of twelve charges is needed to open skeletal muscle Na^+ channels. *J. Gen. Physiol.*, 106:1053–1068.

His W. (1899). Ein fall von Adams-Stokes'scher Krankeit mit ungleichzeitigem schlagen der vorhofe U. Herzkammern (Herzblock). *Deutsch Archiv. f. klin. Med.*, 64:316–331.

Ho K.K., Pinsky J.L., Kannel W.B., Levy D. (1993). The epidemiology of heart failure: The Framingham Study. *JACC*, 22:6A–13A.

Hockerman G.H., Johnson B.D., Scheuer T., Catterall W.A. (1995). Molecular determinants of high affinity block of L-type calcium channels by phenylalkylamines. *J. Biol. Chem.*, 270:22119–22122.

Hockerman G.H., Peterson B.Z., Johnson B.D., Catterall W.A. (1997). Molecular determinants of drug binding and actions on L-type calcium channels. *Ann. Rev. Pharmacol. Toxicol.*, 37:361–398.

Hodgkin A.L. (1937a). Evidence for electrical transmission in nerve. Part I. *J. Physiol.*, (Lond.), 90:183–210.

Hodgkin A.L. (1937b). Evidence for electrical transmission in nerve. Part II. *J. Physiol.* (Lond.), 90: 211–232.

Hodgkin A.L., Huxley A.F. (1952a). A quantitative description of membrane current and its application to conduction and excitation in nerve. *J. Physiol.* (Lond.), 117:500–544.

Hodgkin A.L., Huxley A.F. (1952b). Currents carried by sodium and potassium ions through the membrane of the giant axon of *Loligo. J. Journal of Physiology*, 116:449–472.

Hodgkin A.L., Katz B. (1949). The effect of sodium ions on the electrical activity of the giant axon of the squid. *J. Physiol.*, 108:37–77.

Hodgkin A.L., Rushton W.A.H. (1946). The electrical constants of a crustacean nerve fiber. *Proc. R. Soc. Lond. B.*, 133:444–479.

Hoffman B.F., Cranefield P.F. (1960). *Electrophysiology of the Heart*. New York, NY, McGraw-Hill.

Hoffman B.F., Cranefield P.F. (1976). *Electrophysiology of the Heart*. Futura Publishing Company, Inc. Mount Kisko, New York.

Hoffman B.F., Paes de Carvalho A., DeMello W.C. (1958). Transmembrane potentials of single fibers of the atrio-ventricular node. *Nature*, 181:66–67.

Hondeghem L.M. (1987). Antiarrhythmic agents: modulated receptor applications. *Circulation*, 75:514–520.

Hondeghem L.M., Katzung B.G. (1984). Antiarrhythmic agents: The modulated receptor mechanism of action of sodium and calcium channel-blocking drugs. *Ann. Rev. Pharmacol. Toxicol.*, 24:387–423.

Hondeghem L.M., Snyders D.J. (1990). Class III antiarrhythmic agents have a lot of potential but a long way to go: Reduced effectiveness and dangers of reverse use-dependence. *Circulation*, 81:686–690.

Hoppe U.C., Jansen E., Sudkamp M., Beuckelmann D.J. (1998). Hyperpolarization activated inward current in ventricular myocytes from normal and failing human hearts. *Circulation*, 97:55–65.

Hoshi T., Zagotta W.N., Aldrich R.W. (1990). Biophysical and molecular mechanisms of Shaker potassium channel inactivation. *Science*, 250:533–538.

Hoshi T., Zagotta W.N., Aldrich R.W. (1991). Two types of inactivation in Shaker K^+ channels: effects of alterations in the carboxy-terminal region. *Neuron*, 7:547–556.

Hoshi T., Zagotta W.N., Aldrich R.W. (1994). Shaker potassium channel gating. I: Transitions near the open state. *J. Gen. Physiol.*, 103:249–278.

Hoshino K., Anumonwo J., Delmar M., Jalife J. (1990). Wenckebach periodicity in single atrioventricular nodal cells from the rabbit heart. *Circulation*, 82:2201–2216.

Hume J.R., Harvey R.D. (1991). Chloride conductance pathways in the heart. *Am. J. Physiol.*, 261: C399–C412.

Hunter P.J., Smail B.H. (1988). The analysis of cardiac function: a continuum approach. *Prog. Biophys. Mol. Biol.*, 52:101–164.

Imaizumi S., Mazgalev T., Dreifus L.S., Michelson E.L., Miyugawa A., Bharati S., Lev M. (1990). Morphological and electrophysiological correlates of atrioventricular nodal response to increased vagal activity. *Circulation*, 82:951–964.

Imanishi S., Surawicz B. (1976). Automatic activity in depolarized guinea pig ventricular myocardium. Characteristics and mechanisms. *Circulation Research*, 39:751–759.

Inoue H., Zipes D.P. (1987). Results of sympathetic denervation in the canine heart; Supersensitivity that may be arrhythmogenic. *Circulation*, 75:877–887.

Isom L.L., DeJongh K.S., Catterall W.A. (1994). Auxillary subunits of voltage gated ion channels. *Neuron*, 12:1183–1194.

Isom L.L., DeJongh K.S., Patton D.E., Reber B.F., Offord J., Charbonneau H., Walsh K., Goldin A.L., Catterall W.A. (1992). Primary structure and functional expression of the β_1 subunit of the rat brain sodium channel. *Science*, 256:839–842.

Itaya T., Hashimoto H., Uematsu T., Nakashima M. (1990). Alteration of responsiveness to adrenoceptor agonists and calcium of non-infarcted hypertrophied muscles from rats with chronic myocardial infarction. *Br. J. Pharmacol.*, 99:572–576.

Ito H., Tung R.T., Sugimoto T., Kobayashi I., Takahashi K., Katada T., Ui M., Kurachi Y. (1992). On the mechanism of G protein $\beta\gamma$ subunit activation of the muscarinic K^+ channel in guinea pig atrial cell membrane. *J. Gen. Physiol.*, 99:961–983.

Jack J.J.B., Noble D., Tsien R.W. (1975). *Electric Current Flow in Excitable Cells*, Oxford University Press, Oxford.

Jalife J. (1983). The sucrose gap preparation as a model of AV nodal transmission: Are dual pathways necessary for reciprocation and AV nodal echoes? *PACE*, 6:1106–1122.

Jalife J., Antzelevitch C., Lamanna V., Moe G.K. (1983). Rate-dependent changes in excitability of depressed cardiac Purkinje fibers as a mechanism of intermittent bundle branch block. *Circulation*, 67:912–922.

Jalife J. (1993a). Chaos theory and the study of arrhythmogenesis: Part I. *ACC Current Journal Review*, May/June. pp. 13–16.

Jalife J. (1993b). Chaos theory and the study of arrhythmogenesis: Part II. *ACC Current Journal Review*, July/August. pp. 13–16.

Jalife J., Delmar M. (1991). Ionic basis of the Wenckebach phenomenon. In: L. Glass, P. Hunter A. McCulloch (eds.), *Theory of Heart*, Springer Verlag, New York, NY, pp. 359–376.

Jalife J., Gray R. (1996). Drifting vortices of electrical waves underline ventricular fibrillation in the rabbit heart. *Acta Physiol. Scand.*, 157:123–131.

Jalife J., Moe G.K. (1981). Excitation, conduction and reflection of impulses in isolated bovine and canine cardiac Purkinje fibers. *Circ. Res.*, 49:233–247.

Jalife J., Sicouri S., Delmar M., Michaels D.C. (1989). Electrical uncoupling and impulse propagation in isolated sheep Purkinje fibers. *Am. J. Physiol.*, 257:H179–H189.

Janes R.D., Brandys J.C., Hopkins D.A., Johnstone D.E., Murphy D.A., Armour J.A. (1986). Anatomy of human extrinsic cardiac nerves and ganglia. *Am. J. Cardiol.*, 57:299–309.

January C.T., Riddle J.M. (1989). Early afterdepolarizations: Mechanism of induction and block. A role for L-type Ca^{2+} current. *Circulation Research*, 64:977–990.

Jeck D., Lindmar R., Löffelholz K., Wanke M. (1988). Subtypes of muscarinic receptor on cholinergic nerves and atrial cells of chicken and guinea pig hearts. *Br. J. Pharmacol.*, 93:357–366.

Josephson I.R., Sanchez-Chapula A.M., Brown A.M. (1984). Early outward current in rat single ventricular cells. *Circulation Research*, 54:157–162.

Joyner R.W., Westerfeld M., Moore J.W. (1980). Effects of cellular geometry on current flow during a propagated action potential. *Biophys. J.*, 31:183–194.

Jurevicius J., Fischmeister R. (1996). cAMP compartmentation is responsible for a local activation of cardiac Ca^{2+} channels by β-adrenergic agonists. *Proc. Natl. Acad. Sci. USA*, 93:295–299.

Jurkiewicz N.K., Sanguinetti M.C. (1993). Rate-dependent prolongation of cardiac action potentials by a methanesulfonanilide class III antiarrhythmic agent. Specific block of rapidly activating delayed rectifier current by dofetilide. *Circulation Research*, 72:75–83.

Jurkiewicz N.K., Wang J., Fermini B., Sanguinetti M.C., Salata J.J. (1996). Mechanism of action potential prolongation by RP 58866 and its active enantiomer, terikalant: Block of the rapidly activating delayed rectifier K^+ current, I_{Kr}. *Circulation*, 94:2938–2946.

Kaab S., Nuss H.B., Chiamvimonvat N., O'Rourke B., Pak P.H., Kass D.A., Marban E., Tomaselli G.F. (1996a). Ionic mechanism of action potential prolongation in ventricular myocytes from dogs with pacing-induced heart failure. *Circ. Res.*, 78:262–273.

Kaab S.H., Duc J., Ashen D., Nabauer M., Beuckelmann D.J., Dixon J., McKinnon D., Tomaselli G.F. (1996b). Quantitative analysis of K^+ channel mRNA expression in normal and failing human ventricle reveals the molecular identity of I_{to} *Circulation*, 94:I-592. (Abstract)

Kavanaugh M.P., Hurst R.S., Yakel J., Varnum M.D., Adelman J.P., North R.A. (1992). Multiple subunits of a voltage-dependent potassium channel contribute to the binding site for tetraethylammonium. *Neuron*, 8:493–497.

Keener J.P. (1981). On cardiac arrhythmias: AV conduction block. *J. Math. Biol.*, 12:215–225.

Keener J.P. (1991). An eikonal-curvature equation for action potential propagation in myocardium. *J. Math. Biol.*, 29:629–651.

Keener J.P., Panfilov A.V. (1995). Three-dimensional propagation in the heart: The effects of geometry and fiber orientation on propagation in myocardium. In: D.P. Zipes and J. Jalife, (eds.), *Cardiac Electrophysiology: From Cell to Bedside*, W.B. Saunders Co., Philadelphia, pp. 335–347.

Kellenberger S., Scheuer T., Catterall W.A. (1996). Movement of the Na^+ channel inactivation gate during inactivation. *J. Biol. Chem.*, 271:30971–30979.

Kellenberger S., West J.W., Catterall W.A., Scheuer T. (1997a). Molecular analysis of potential hinge residues in the inactivation gate of brain type IIA Na^+ channels. *J. Gen. Physiol.*, 109:607–617.

Kellenberger S., West J.W., Scheuer T., Catterall W.A. (1997b). Molecular analysis of the putative inactivation particle in the inactivation gate of brain type IIA Na^+ channels. *J. Gen. Physiol.*, 109: 589–605.

Kenyon J.L., Gibbons W.R. (1979). 4-aminopyridine and the early outward current in sheep Purkinje fibers. *Journal of General Physiology*, 73:139–157.

Keung E.C. (1989). Calcium current is increased in isolated adult myocytes from hypertrophied rat myocardium. *Circulation Research*, 64:753–763.

Kimura S., Bassett A.L., Gaide M.S., Kozlovskis P.L., Myerburg R.J. (1986). Regional changes in intracellular potassium and sodium activity after healing of experimental myocardial infarction in cats. *Circ. Res.*, 58:202–208.

Kirchhof C.J.H.J., Boersma L.V.A., Allessie M.A. (1994). Atrial fibrillation begets atrial fibrillation. In: S.B. Olsson, M.A. Allessie, R.W.F. Campbell (eds.), *Atrial Fibrillation: Mechanisms and Therapeutic Strategies*, Futura Publishing Co., Inc., Armonk, N.Y., pp. 195–201.

Kisselev O., Gautam N. (1993). Specific interaction with rhodopsin is dependent on the γ subunit type in a G protein. *J. Biol. Chem.*, 268:24519–24522.

Kitzen J., McCallum J., Harvey C., Morin M.E., Oshiro G., Colatsky T.J. (1992). Potassium channel activators cromakalim (WAY-120, 491) fail to decrease myocardial infarct size in the anesthetized canine. *Pharmacology*, 45:71–82.

Kiyosue T., Arita M. (1989). Late sodium current and its contribution to action potential configuration in guinea pig ventricular myocytes. *Circulation Research*, 64:389–397.

Kleiman R.B., Houser S.R. (1988). Calcium currents in normal and hypertrophied isolated feline ventricular myocytes. *Am. J. Physiol.*, 255:H1434–H1442.

Kleiman R.B., Houser S.R. (1989). Outward currents in normal and hypertrophied feline ventricular myocytes. *Am. J. Physiol.*, 256:H1450–H1461.

Kleuss C., Scherubl H., Herschler J., Schultz G., Wittig B. (1993). Selectivity in signal transduction determined by γ subunits of heterotrimeric G proteins. *Science*, 259:832–834.

Kou W.H., Nelson S.D., Lynch J.J., Montgomery D.G., DiCarlo L., Lucchesi B.R. (1987). Effect of flecainide acetate on prevention of electrical induction of ventricular tachycardia and occurrence of ischemic ventricular fibrillation during the early postmyocardial infarction period: Evaluation in a conscious canine model of sudden death. *J. Am. Coll. Cardiol.*, 9:359–365.

Koumi S.I., Arentzen C.E., Backer C.L., Wasserstrom J.A. (1994). Alterations in muscarinic potassium channel response to acetylcholine and to G protein-mediated activation in atrial myocytes isolated from failing human hearts. *Circulation*, 90:2213–2224.

Koumi S.I., Backer C.L., Arentzen C.E., Sato R. (1995). β-adrenergic modulation of the inwardly rectifying potassium channel in isolated human ventricular myocytes. *J. Clin. Invest.*, 96:2870–2881.

Koumi S.I., Sato R., Nagasawa K., Hayakawa H. (1997). Activation of inwardly rectifying potassium channels by muscarinic receptor-linked G protein in isolated human ventricular myocytes. *J. Membr. Biol.*, 157:71–81.

Kowey P.R., Frielling T.D., Sewter J., Wu Y., Sokil A., Paul J., Nocella J. (1991). Electrophysiological effects of left ventricular hypertrophy. Effects of calcium and potassium channel blockade. *Circulation*, 83:2067–2075.

Kozlovskis P.L., Gerdes A.M., Smets M., Moore J.A., Bassett A.L., Myerburg R.J. (1991). Regional increase in isolated myocyte volume in chronic myocardial infarction in cats. *J. Mol. Cell. Cardiol.*, 23:1459–1466.

Krezel A.M., Kasibhatla C., Hidalgo P., MacKinnon R., Wagner (1995). Solution structure of the potassium channel inhibitor agitoxin 2: caliper for probing channel geometry. *Protein Science*, 4:1478–1489.

Krinsky V.I., (1978). Mathematical models of cardiac arrhythmias (spiral waves). *Pharmac. Ther. B.*, 3: 539–555.

Kuffler S.W., Nicholls J.G. (1976). *From Neuron to Brain*. Sinauer Associates, Inc. Publishers, Sunderland, Massachusetts.

Laider K.J., Meiser J.H. (1982). *Physical Chemistry*, The Benjamin/Cummings Publishing Company, Inc.

Latham K.R., Sellitti D.F., Goldstein R.E. (1987). Interaction of amiodarone and desethylamiodarone with solubilized nuclear thyroyd hormone receptors. *J. Am. Coll. Cardiol.*, 9:872–876.

Lazzara R., Scherlag B.J. (1984). Electrophysiologic basis for arrhythmias in ischemic heart disease. *Am. J. Cardiol.*, 53:1B–7B.

Le Grande B., Deroubaix E., Coulombe A., Coraboeuf E. (1990). Stimulatory effect of ouabain on T- and L-type calcium currents in guinea pig cardiac myocytes *Am. J. Physiol.*, 258:H1620–H1623.

Lechleiter J., Girard S., Peralta E., Clapham D. (1991). Spiral calcium wave propagation and annihilation in *Xenopus laevis*, oocytes. *Science*, 252:123–126.

Ledda F., Marchetti P., Manni A. (1971). Influence of phenylephrine on transmembrane potentials and effective refractory period of single Purkinje fibers of sheep heart. *Pharmacol. Res. Commun.*, 3: 195–206.

Lee J.H., Rosen M.R. (1994). α_1-adrenergic receptor modulation of repolarization in canine Purkinje fibers. *J. Cardiovasc. Electrophysiol.*, 5:232–240.

Lee J.H., Steinberg S.F., Rosen M.R. (1991). A WB 4101-sensitive α_1-adrenergic receptor subtype modulates repolarization in canine Purkinje fibers. *J. Pharmacol. Exp. Ther.*, 258:681–687.

Lee K.S. (1992). Ibutilide, a new compound with potent class III antiarrhythmic activity, activates a slow inward Na^+ current in guinea pig ventricular cells. *J. Pharmacol. Exp. Ther.*, 262:99–108.

Lee K.S., Marban E., Tsien R.W. (1985). Inactivation of calcium channels in mammalian heart cells: joint dependence on membrane potential and intracellular calcium. *Journal of Physiology*, 364:395–411.

Lee K.S., Tsai T.D., Lee E.W. (1993). Membrane activity of class III antiarrhythmic compounds: a comparison between ibutilide, d-sotalol, E-4031, sematilide and dofetilide. *Eur. J. Pharmacol.*, 234:43–53.

Legssyer A., Hove-Madsen L., Hoerter J., Fischmeister R. (1997). Sympathetic modulation of the effect of nifedipine on myocardial contraction and Ca current in the rat. *J. Mol. Cell. Cardiol.*, 29:579–591.

Levy F.O., Zhu X., Kaumann A.J., Birnbaumer L. (1993). Efficacy of β_1-adrenergic receptors is lower than that of β_2-adrenergic receptors. *Proc. Natl. Acad. Sci. USA*, 90:10798–10802.

Levy M.N. (1971). Sympathetic-parasympathetic interactions in the heart. *Circ. Res.*, 29:437–445.

Levy M.N., Martin P.J. (1995). Autonomic neural control of cardiac function. In: N. Sperelakis (ed.), *Physiology and Pathophysiology of the Heart*, (3rd edition), Kluwer Academic Publishers, Norwell, MA, pp. 413–430.

Levy M.N., Martin P.J., Zieske H., Adler D. (1974). Role of positive feedback in the atrioventricular nodal Wenckebach phenomenon. *Circ. Res.*, 24:697–710.

Lewis T. (1925). *The Mechanism and Graphic Registration of the Heart Beat*, Shaw and Sons Ltd., London.

Li G.-R., Feng J., Yue L., Carrier M., Nattel S. (1996). Evidence for two components of delayed rectifier K^+ current in human ventricular myocytes. *Circulation Research*, 78:689–696.

Litovsky S.H., Antzelevitch C. (1988). Transient outward current prominent in canine ventricular epicardium but not endocardium. *Circulation Research*, 62:116–126.

Litwin S.E., Bridge J.H.B. (1997). Enhanced NaCa exchange in the infarcted heart. Implications for excitation contraction coupling. *Circ. Res.*, 81:1083–1093.

Litwin S.E., Morgan J.P. (1992). Captopril enhances intracellular calcium handling and β-adrenergic responsiveness of myocardium from rats with postinfarction failure. *Circ. Res.*, 71:797–807.

Liu D.W., Gintant G.A., Antzelevitch C. (1993). Ionic bases for electrophysiological distinctions among epicardial, midmyocardial, and endocardial myocytes from the free wall of the canine left ventricle. *Circ. Res.*, 72:671–687.

Liu D.-W., Antzelevitch C. (1995). Characteristics of the delayed rectifier current (IKr and IKs) in canine ventricular epicardial, midmyocardial, and endocardial myocytes. A weaker IKs contributes to the longer action potential of the M cell. *Circulation Research*, 76:351–365.

Liu D.-W., Gintant G.A., Antzelevitch C. (1990). Ionic bases for electrophysiologic distinctions among epicardial, midmyocardial and endocardial myocytes from the free wall of the canine left ventricle. *Circulation Research*, 67:1287–1291.

Liu Q.-Y., Rosen M.R., Robinson R.B. (1997). Alpha-adrenergic agonists modulate I_{to} in rat epicardial but not endocardial myocytes. *Circulation*, 96:I-296.

Liu S., Taffet S., Stoner L., Delmar M., Vallano M.L. and Jalife J. (1993). A structural basis for the unequal sensitivity of the major cardiac and liver gap junctions to intercellular acidification: the carboxyl tail length. *Biophys. J.*, 64:1422–1433.

Löffelholz K., Pappano A.J. (1985). The parasympathetic neuroeffector junction of the heart. *Pharmacol. Rev.*, 37:1–24.

Logothetis D.E., Kim D., Northup J.K., Neer E.J., Clapham D.E. (1988). Specificity of action of guanine nucleotide-binding regulatory protein subunits on the cardiac muscarinic K^+ channel. *Proc. Natl. Acad. Sci. USA.*, 85:5814–5818.

London B., Trudeau M.C., Newton K.P., Beyer A.K., Copeland N.G., Gilbert D.J., Jenkins N.A., Satler C.A., Robertson G.A. (1997). Two isoforms of the mouse ether-a-go-go-related gene coassemble to form channels with properties similar to the rapidly activating component of the cardiac delayed rectifier K^+ current. *Circ. Res.*, 81:870–878.

Lopatin A.N., Makhina E.N., Nichols C.G. (1994). Potassium channel block by cytoplasmic polyamines as the mechanism of intrinsic rectification. *Nature*, 372:366–369.

Lue W.-M., Boyden P.A. (1992). Abnormal electrical properties of myocytes from chronically infarcted canine heart. Alterations in V_{max} and the transient outward current. *Circulation*, 85:1175–1188.

Lumma W.C. Jr., Wohol R.A., Davey D.D., Argentieri T.M., DeVita R.J., Jain V.K., Marisca A.J., Morgan T.K., Reiser H.J., Wiggins J., Wong S.S. (1987). Rational design of 4-[(methylsulfonyl)amino] benzamides as Class III antiarrhythmic agents. *J. Med. Chem.*, 30:755–758.

Lundberg J.M., Hökfelt T. (1983). Co-existence of peptides and classical neurotransmitters. *Trends Neurosci.*, 6:325–333.

Lundberg J.M., Hökfelt T. (1986). Multiple co-existence of peptides and classical transmitters in peripheral autonomic and sensory neurons – functional and pharmacological implications. *Progress in Brain Research*, 68:241–262.

Lundberg J.M., Martinsson A., Theodorsson-Norheim E., Svedenhag E., Ekblom B., Hjemdahl P. (1985). Co-release of neuropeptide Y and catecholamines during physical exercise in man. *Biochem. Biophys. Res. Commun.*, 133:30–36.

Luo C.-H., Rudy Y. (1994). A dynamic model of the cardiac ventricular action potential. I. Simulation of ionic currents and concentration changes. *Circulation Research*, 74:1071–1096.

Machado B.H., Brody M.J. (1988). Role of the nucleus ambiguous in the regulation of heart rate and arterial pressure. *Hypertension*, 11:602–607.

Mackaay A.J.C., Opthof T., Bleeker W.K., Jongsma H.J., Bouman L.N. (1980). Interaction of adrenaline and acetylcholine on cardiac pacemaker function. *Journal of Pharmacology and Experimental Therapeutics*, 214:417–422.

Mackaay A.J.C., Opthof T., Bleeker W.K., Jongsma H.J., Bouman L.N., (1982). Interaction of adrenaline and acetylcholine on rabbit sinoatrial node function. In: Bouman L.N., Jongsma H.J. (eds.), *Cardiac rate and rhythm*, The Hague: Martinus Nijhoff, pp. 507–523.

MacKinnon R., Yellen G. (1990). Mutations affecting TEA blockade and ion permeation in voltage-activated K^+ channels. *Science*, 250:276–279.

Maki T., Gruver E.J., Toupin D., Marks A.R., Davidoff A., Marsh J.D. (1993). Catecholamines regulate calcium channel expression in rat cardiomyocytes: distinct α and β adrenergic regulatory mechanisms. *Circulation*, 88:I-276.

Malfatto G., Zaza A., Schwartz P.J. (1993). Parasympathetic control of cycle length dependence of endocardial ventricular repolarisation in the intact feline heart during steady state conditions. *Cardiovascular Research*, 27:823–827.

Maltsev V.A., Wobus A.M., Rohwedel J., Bader M., Hescheler J. (1994). Cardiomyocytes differentiated in vitro from embryonic stem cells developmentally express cardiac-specific genes and ionic currents. *Circulation Research*, 75:233–244.

Manning A., Thisse V., Hodeige D., Richard J., Heynrickx Chatelain P. (1995). SR 33589, a new amiodarone-like antiarrhythmic agent: electrophysiological effects in anesthetized dogs. *J. Cardiovasc. Pharmacol.*, 25:252–261.

Marzo K.P., Frey M.J., Wilson J.R., Lian B.T., Manning D.R., Lanoce V., Molinoff P.B. (1991). β-adrenergic receptor-G protein-adenylate cyclase complex in experimental canine congestive heart failure produced by rapid ventricular pacing. *Circ. Res.*, 69:1546–1556.

Masini I., Porciatti F., Borea P.A., Barbieri M., Cerbai E., Mugelli A. (1991). Cardiac β-adrenoceptors in the normal and failing heart: electrophysiological aspects. *Pharmacol. Res.*, 24:21–27.

Matsubara H., Suzuki J., Inada M. (1993a). Shaker-related potassium channel, Kv1.4, mRNA regulation in cultured rat heart myocytes and differential expression of Kv1.4 and Kv1.5 genes in myocardial development and hypertrophy. *J. Clin. Invest.*, 92:1659–1666.

Matsubara H., Suzuki J., Murasawa S., Inada M. (1993b). Kv1.4 mRNA regulation in cultured rat heart myocytes and differential expression of Kv1.4 and Kv1.5 genes in myocardial development and hypertrophy *Circulation*, 88:I86.

Matsuda H., Saigusa A., Irisawa H. (1987). Ohmic conductance through the inwardly rectifying K channel and blocking by internal Mg^{++}. *Nature*, 325:156–159.

Mazzanti M., Difrancesco D. (1989). Intracellular Ca modulates K-inward rectification in cardiac myocytes. *Pflügers Archives*, 413:322–324.

McAllister R.E., Noble D., Tsien R.W. (1975). Reconstruction of the electrical activity of cardiac Purkinje fibres. *J. Physiol.* (London), 251:1–59.

McCormack K., Lin L., Sigworth F.J. (1993). Substitution of a hydrophobic residue alters the conformational stability of Shaker K^+ channels during gating and assembly. *Biophys. J.*, 65:1740–1748.

McDermott B.J., Millar B.C., Piper H.M. (1993). Cardiovascular effects of neuropeptide Y: Receptor interactions and cellular mechanisms. *Cardiovasc. Res.*, 27:893–905.

McPhee J.C., Ragsdale D.S., Scheuer T., Catterall W.A. (1994). A mutation in segment IVS6 disrupts fast inactivation of sodium channels. *Proc. Natl. Acad. Sci. USA*, 91:12346–12350.

McPhee J.C., Ragsdale D.S., Scheuer T., Catterall W.A. (1995). A critical role for transmembrane segment IVS6 of the sodium channel alpha subunit in fast inactivation. *J. Biol. Chem.*, 270:12025–12034.

Mendez C., Mueller W.J., Urquiaga X. (1970). Propagation of impulses across the Purkinje fiber-muscle junctions in the dog heart. *Circ. Res.*, 26:135–150.

Merideth J., Mendez C., Mueller W.J., Moe G.K. (1968). Electrical excitability of atrioventricular nodal cells. *Circ. Res.*, 23:69–85.

Meszaros J., Levai G. (1992). Catecholamine-induced cardiac hypertrophy uncouples β-adrenoceptors from slow calcium channel. *Eur. J. Pharmacol.*, 210:333–338.

Mewes T., Ravens V. (1994). L-type calcium currents of human myocytes from ventricle of non-failing and failing hearts and from atrium. *J. Mol. Cell. Cardiol.*, 26:1307–1320.

Millar B.C., Weis T., Piper H.M., Weber M., Borchard U., McDermott B.J., Balasubramaniam A. (1991). Positive and negative contractile effects of neuropeptide Y on ventricular cardiomyocytes. *Am. J. Physiol.*, 261:H1727–H1733.

Mines G.R. (1914). On circulating excitation on heart muscles and their possible relation to tachycardia and fibrillation. *Trans. R. Soc. Can.*, 4:43–53.

Mizeres M.J. (1958). The origin and course of the cardioaccelerator fibers in the dog. *Anat. Record.*, 132:261–279.

Mobitz W. (1924). Uber die unvollstandige Storung der Erregungsuberleitung zwischen Vorhof und Kammer des menschlichen Herzens. *Zeitschr. f. d. ges. exper. Med.*, 41:180–237.

Moe G.K., Childers R.W., Merideth J. (1968). An appraisal of "supernormal" A-V conduction. *Circulation*, 38:5–28.

Molenaar P., Smolich J.J., Russel F.D., Mc Martin L.R., Summers R.J. (1990). Differential regulation of β_1 and β_2 adrenoceptors in guinea pig atrioventricular conducting system after chronic (-)-isoproterenol infusion. *J. Pharmacol. Exp. Ther.*, 255:393–400.

Molina-Viamonte V., Steinberg S.F., Chow Y.K., Legato M.J., Robinson R.B., Rosen M.R. (1990). Phospholipase C modulates automaticity of canine cardiac Purkinje fibers. *J. Pharmacol. Exp. Ther.*, 252:886–893.

Moorman J.R., Kirsch G.E., Brown A.M., Joho R.H. (1990). Changes in sodium channel gating produced by point mutations in a cytoplasmic linker. *Science*, 250:688–691.

Morales M.J., Castellino R.C., Crews A.L., Rasmusson R.L., Strauss H.C. (1995). A novel beta subunit increases rate of inactivation of specific voltage-gated potassium channel alpha subunits. *J. Biol. Chem.*, 270:6272–6277.

Mori Y., Matsubara H., Folco E., Siegel A., Koren G. (1993). The transcription of a mammalian voltage-gated potassium channel is regulated by cAMP in a cell-specific manner *J. Biol. Chem.*, 268(35):26482–26493.

Motomura S., Hashimoto K. (1992). β_2-adrenoceptor-mediated positive dromotropic effects on atrioventricular node of dogs. *Am. J. Physiol.*, 262:H123–H129.

Mubagwa K., Flameng W., Carmeliet E. (1994). Resting and action potentials of nonischemic and chronically ischemic human ventricular muscle. *J. Cardiovasc. Electrophysiol.*, 5:659–671.

Myerburg R.J., Gelband H., Nilsson K., Sung R.J., Thurer R.J., Morales A.R., Bassett A.L. (1977). Long-term electrophysiological abnormalities resulting from experimental myocardial infarction in cats *Circ. Res.*, 41:73–84.

Nair L.A., Grant A.O. (1997). Emerging class III antiarrhythmic agents: mechanism of action and proarrhythmic potential. *Cardiovasc. Drugs. Ther.*, 11:149–157.

Nakayama T., Kurachi Y., Noma A., Irisawa H. (1984). Action potentials and membrane currents of single pacemaker cells of the rabbit heart. *Pflügers Arch.*, 402:248–257.

Narahashi T., Frazier D.T. (1971). Site of action and active form of local anesthetics. *Neurosci. Res.*, 4: 65–99.

Nattel S. (1991). Antiarrhythmic drug classifications: a critical appraisal of their history, present status and clinical relevance. *Drugs*, 41:672–701.

Nattel S., Pedersen D.H., Zipes D.P. (1981). Alterations in regional myocardial distribution and arrhythmogenic effects of apridine produced by coronary artery occlusion in the dog. *Cardiovasc. Res.*, 15:80–85.

Nielsen P.M.F., Le Grice I.J., Smaill B.H., Hunter P.J. (1991). Mathematical model of geometry and fibrous structure of the heart. *Am. J. Physiol.*, 260:H1365–H1378.

Nishimura M., Habuchi Y., Hiromasa S., Watanabe Y. (1988). Ionic basis of depressed automaticity and conduction by acetylcholine in rabbit AV node. *Am. J. Physiol.*, 255:H7.

Nitta J.-I., Furukawa T., Marumo F., Sawanobori T., Hiraoka M. (1994). Subcellular mechanism for Ca^{2+}-dependent enhancement of delayed rectifier K^+ current in isolated membrane patches of guinea pig ventricular myocytes. *Circulation Research*, 74:96–104.

Noble D. (1975). *The Initiation of the Heart Beat*, Oxford University Press, Oxford.

Noble D., Tsien R.W. (1968). The kinetics and rectifier properties of the slow potassium current in cardiac Purkinje fibres. *J. Physiol.* (London), 195:185–214.

Noda M., Shimizu S., Tanabe T., Takai T., Kayano T., Ikeda T., Takahashi H., Nakayama H., Kanaoka Y., Minamino N. *et al.*, (1984). Primary structure of Electrophorus electricus sodium channel deduced from cDNA sequence. *Nature*, 312:121–127.

Noda M., Suzuki H., Numa S., Stühmer W. (1989). A single point mutation confers tetrodotoxin and saxotoxin insensitivity on the sodium channel II. *FEBS Lett.*, 259:213–216.

Noma A. (1983). ATP-regulated K^+ channels in cardiac muscle. *Nature*, 305:147–148.

Noma A., Irisawa H. (1976). Membrane currents in the rabbit sinoatrial node cell studied by the double microelectrode method. *Pflügers Arch.*, 366:45–52.

Noma A., Nakayama T., Kurachi Y., Irisawa H. (1984). Resting K conductances in pacemaker and non-pacemaker heart cells of the rabbit. *Japanese Journal of Physiology*, 34:245–254.

Nuss H.B., Houser S.R. (1993). T type Ca current is expressed in hypertrophied adult feline left ventricular myocytes *Circ. Res.*, 73:777–782.

O'Hara G., Villemarie C., Talajic M., Nattel S. (1992). Effects of flecainide on atrial refractoriness, atrial repolarization and atrioventricular nodal conduction in anesthetized dogs. *J. Am. Coll. Cardiol.*, 19:1335–1342.

Ogawa S., Barnett J.V., Sen L., Galper J.B., Smith T.W., Marsh J.D. (1992). Direct contact between sympathetic neurons and rat cardiac myocytes in vitro increases expression of functional calcium channels. *J. Clin. Invest.*, 89:1085–1093.

Ohler A., Amos G.J., Wettwer E., Ravens U. (1994). Frequency-dependent effects of E-4031, almokalant, dofetilide and tedisamil on action potential duration: No evidence for "reverse use-dependent block". *Naunyn Schmiedeberg's Arch. Pharmacol.*, 349:62–61.

Oiunuma H., Miyake K., Yamanaka M., Nomoto K.I., Sawada K., Shino M., Hamano S. (1990). 4'[(4-Piperidyl (carbonyl)] methanesulfonalides as potent, selective, bioavailable Class III antiarrhythmic agents. *J. Med. Chem.*, 22:903–905.

Olgin J.E., Kalman J.M., Fitzpatrick A.P., Lesh M.D. (1995): Role of right atrial endocardial structures as barriers to conduction during human type I atrial flutter. Activation and entrainment guided by intracardiac echocardiography. *Circulation*, 92:1839–1848.

Oliva C., Cohen I.S., Pennefather P. (1990). The mechanism of rectification of I_{K1} in canine Purkinje myocytes. *J. Gen. Physiol.*, 96:299–318.

Olivetti G., Capasso J.M., Meggs L.G., Sonnenblick E.H., Anversa P. (1991). Cellular basis of chronic ventricular remodeling after myocardial infarction in rats. *Circ. Res.*, 68:856–869.

Osaka T., Joyner R.W. (1992). Developmental changes in β-adrenergic modulation of calcium currents in rabbit ventricular cells. *Circ. Res.*, 70:104–115.

Ouadid H., Seguin J., Richard S., Chaptal P.A., Nargeot J. (1991). Properties and modulation of Ca channels in adult human atrial cells. *J. Mol. Cell. Cardiol.*, 23:41–54.

Paes de Carvalho A., de Almeida D.F. (1960). Spread of activity through the atrioventricular node. *Circ. Res.*, 8:801–809.

Panfilov A.V., Keener J.P. (1995). Reentry in an anatomical model of the heart. *Chaos, Solitons and Fractals*, 5:681–689.

Pappano A.J. (1971). Propranolol-insensitive effects of epinephrine in action potential repolarization in electrically driven atria of the guinea pig. *J. Pharmacol. Exp. Ther.*, 177:85–95.

Pappano A.J. (1995). Modulation of the heartbeat by the vagus nerve. In: D.P. Zipes and J. Jalife (eds.), *Cardiac Electrophysiology: From Cell to Bedside* (2nd edition), W.B. Saunders Co., Philadelphia, Pa., pp. 411–422.

Parcej D.N., Dolly J.O. (1989). Dendrotoxin acceptor from bovine synaptic plasma membranes. Binding properties, purification and subunit composition of a putative constituent of certain voltage-activated K^+ channels [see comments]. *Biochemical Journal*, 257:899–903.

Parcej D.N., Scott V.E., Dolly J.O. (1992). Oligomeric properties of α-dendrotoxin-sensitive potassium ion channels purified from bovine brain. *Biochem.*, 31:11084–11088.

Park C.S., Miller C. (1992). Mapping function to structure in a channel-blocking peptide: electrostatic mutants of charybdotoxin. *Biochem.*, 31:7749–7755.

Patterson E., Scherlag B.J., Lazzara R. (1993). Rapid inward current in ischemically-injured subepicardial myocytes bordering myocardial infarction. *J. Cardiovasc. Electrophysiol.*, 4:9–22.

Patton D.E., West J.W., Catterall W.A., Goldin A.L. (1992). Amino acid residues required for fast $Na^{(+)}$-channel inactivation: charge neutralizations and deletions in the III–IV linker. *Proceedings. Of the National Academy of Sciences of the United States of America*, 89:10905–10909.

Pernow J.M., Lundberg J.M., Kaijser L., Hjemdahl P., Theodorsson-Norheim E., Martinsson A., Pernow B. (1986). Plasma neuropeptide Y-like immunoreactivity and catecholamines during various degrees of sympathetic activation in man. *Clin. Physiol.*, 6:561–578.

Pertsov A.M., Jalife J. (1995). Three-dimensional vortex-like reentry. In: D.P. Zipes J. Jalife (eds.), *Cardiac Electrophysiology: From Cell to Bedside* (2nd edition), W.B. Saunders Co., Philadelphia, pp. 403–410.

Pertsov A.M., Davidenko J.M., Salomonsz R., Baxter W.T., Jalife J. (1993). Spiral waves of excitation underlie reentrant activity in isolated cardiac muscle. *Circ. Res.*, 72:631–650.

Pinto J.M.B., Boyden P.A. (1998). Reduced inward rectifying and increased E4031 sensitive K^+ channel function in arrhythmogenic subendocardial Purkinje myocytes from the infarcted heart. *J. Cardiovasc. Electrophysiol.*, 9:299–311.

Pinto J.M.B., Yuan F., Wasserlauf B.J., Bassett A.L., Myerburg R.J. (1997). Regional gradation of L-type calcium currents in the feline heart with a healed myocardial infarct. *J. Cardiovasc. Electrophysiol.*, 8:548–560.

Piper H.M., Millar B.C., McDermott B.J. (1989). The negative inotropic effect of neuropeptide Y on the ventricular cardiomyocyte. *Naunyn-Schmiedeberg's Arch. Pharmacol.*, 340:333–337.

Po S., Roberds S., Snyders D.J., Tamkun M.M., Bennett P.B. (1993). Heteromultimeric assembly of human potassium channels. Molecular basis of a transient outward current? *Circulation Research*, 72:1326–1336.

Potter E.K. (1988). Neuropeptide Y as an autonomic neurotransmitter. *Pharmacol. Ther.*, 37:251–273.

Pu J., Boyden P.A. (1997). Alterations of Na^+ currents in myocytes from epicardial border zone of the infarcted heart. A possible ionic mechanism for reduced excitability and postrepolarization refractoriness *Circ. Res.*, 81:110–119.

Qin D., Jain P., Boutjdir M., El-Sherif N. (1995). Expression of T-type calcium current in remodeled hypertrophied left ventricle from adult rat following myocardial infarction. *Circulation*, 92(suppl I): I-587.

Qin D., Zhang Z.-H., Caref E., Boutjdir M., Jain P., El-Sherif N. (1996). Cellular and ionic basis of arrhythmias in postinfarction remodeled ventricular myocardium. *Circ. Res.*, 79:461–473.

Qu Y., Rogers J., Tanada T., Scheuer T., Catterall W.A. (1995). Molecular determinants of drug access to the receptor site for antiarrhythmic drugs in the cardiac Na^+ channel. *Proc. Natl. Acad. Sci. USA*, 92:11839–11843.

Quarmby L.M., Hartzell H.C. (1995). Molecular biology of G proteins and their role in cardiac excitability. In: D.P., Zipes J. Jalife (eds.), *Cardiac Electrophysiology: From Cell to Bedside* (2nd edition), W.B., Saunders Co., Philadelphia Pa., pp. 38–48.

Ragsdale D.S., McPhee J.C., Scheuer T., Catterall W.A. (1996). Common molecular determinants of local anesthetic, antiarrhythmic, and anticonvulsant block of voltage-gated Na^+ channels. *Proc. Natl. Acad. Sci. USA*, 93:9270–9275.

Ragsdale D.S., McPhee J.C., Scheuer T., Catterall W.A. (1994). Molecular determinants of state-dependent block of Na^+ channels by local anesthetics. *Science*, 265:1724–1728.

Rampe D., Wible B., Brown A.M., Dage R.C. (1993). Effects of terfenidine and its metabolites on a delayed rectifier K^+ channel cloned from the human heart. *Mol. Pharmacol.*, 44:124–1245.

Randall W.C. (1984). Selective autonomic innervation of the heart. In: W.C. Randall (ed.), *Nervous Control of Cardiovascular Function*, New York: Oxford University Press, pp. 46–67.

Randall W.C., Armour J.A. (1977). Gross and microscopic anatomy of the cardiac innervation. In: W.C. Randall (ed.), *Neural Regulation of the Heart*, Oxford University Press, NY, pp. 13–41.

Rasmussen H.S., Allen M.J., Blackburn K.J., Butrous G.S., Dalrymple H.W. (1992). Dofetilide, a novel class III antiarrhythmic agent. *J. Cardiovasc. Pharmacol.*, 20:S96–S105.

Rees S.A., Curtis M.J. (1993). Specific I_{K1} blockade: A new antiarrhythmic mechanism? *Circulation*, 87:1979–1989.

Rettig J., Heinemann S.H., Wunder F., Lorra C., Parcej D.N., Dolly J.O., Pongs O. (1994). Inactivation properties of voltage-gated K^+ channels altered by presence of β-subunit. *Nature*, 369:289–294.

Riegel D.F., Lipson D., Katona P.G. (1986). Excess tachycardia: heart rate after antimuscarinic agents in conscious dogs. *J. Pharmacol. Exp. Ther.*, 238:367–371.

Rioux F., Bachelard H., Martel J.-C., St. Pierre S. (1985). The vasoconstrictor effect of neuropeptide Y and related peptides in the guinea pig isolated heart. *Peptides*, 7:27–31.

Ritchie J.M., Greengard P. (1966). On the mode of action of local anesthetics. *Ann. Rev. Pharmacol.*, 6:405–430.

Robertson W., van B., Dunhue F.W. (1954). Water and electrolyte distribution in cardiac muscle. *Am. J. Physiol.*, 177:292–297.

Roden D.M., Hoffman B.F. (1985). Action potential prolongation and induction of abnormal automaticity by low quinidine concentrations in canine Purkinje fibers: relationship to potassium and cycle length. *Circ. Res.*, 56:857–867.

Roden D.M. (1993). Torsade de pointes. *Clinical Cardiology*, 16:683–686.

Roden D.M., George A.L. Jr., Bennett P.B. (1995). Recent advances in understanding the molecular mechanisms of the long QT syndrome. *J. Cardiovasc. Electrophysiol.*, 6:1023–1031.

Rohr S., Kucera J.P. (1997). Involvement of the calcium inward current in cardiac impulse propagation: induction of unidirectional conduction block by nifedipine and reversal by Bay K 8644. *Biophysical Journal*, 72:754–766.

Rohr S., Kucera J.P., Fast V., Kléber A. (1997). Paradoxical improvement of impulse conduction in cardiac tissue by partial cellular uncoupling. *Science*, 275:841–844.

Rojas E., Rudy B. (1976). Destruction of the sodium conductance inactivation by a specific protease in perfused nerve fibres from Loligo. *Journal of Physiology*, 262:501–531.

Rosen M.R., Hordof A.J., Ilvento J.P., Danilo P. Jr. (1977). Effects of adrenergic amines on electro-physiological properties and automaticity of neonatal and adult canine Purkinje fibers. *Circ. Res.*, 40:390–400.

Rosenblueth A. (1958a). Functional refractory period of cardiac tissues. *Am. J. Physiol.*, 194:171–183.

Rosenblueth A. (1958b). Mechanism of the Wenckebach-Luciani cycyles. *Am. J. Physiol.*, 194:491–494.

Rozanski G.J., Jalife J., Moe G.K. (1984). Determinants of post-reppolarization refractoriness in depressed mammalian ventricular muscle. *Circ. Res.*, 55:486–496.

Rushton W.A.H. (1937). Initiation of the propagated disturbance. *Proc. Roy. Soc. B.*, 124:210.

Ryder K.O., Bryant S.M., Hart G. (1993). Membrane current changes in left ventricular myocytes isolated from guinea pigs after abdominal aortic coarctation *Cardiovasc. Res.*, 27:1278–1287.

Sager P.T., Uppal P., Follmer C., Antimisiaris M., Pruitt C., Singh B.N. (1993). Frequency-dependent electrophysiologic effects of amiodarone in humans. *Circulation*, 88:1063–1071.

Saint D.A., Ju Y.K., Gage P.W. (1992). A persistent sodium current in rat ventricular myocytes. *J. Physiol.* (London), 453:219–231.

Sakakibara Y., Furukawa T., Singer D.W., Jia H., Backer C.L., Arentzen C.E., Wasserstrom J.A. (1993). Sodium current in isolated human ventricular myocytes. *Am. J. Physiol.*, 265:H1301–H1309.

Sakakibara Y., Wasserstrom J.A., Furukawa T., Jia H., Arentzen C.E., Hartz R.S., Singer D.H. (1992). Characterization of the sodium current in single human atrial myocytes. *Circ. Res.*, 71:535–546.

Sakmann B., Trube G. (1984). Conductance properties of single inwardly rectifying potassium channels in ventricular cells from the guinea pig heart. *Journal of Physiology*, 347:641–657.

Sakmann B., Neher E. (1995). *Single-Channel Recording*, Plenum, NY and London.

Salama G., Morad M. (1976). Merocyanine 540 as an optical probe of transmembrane electrical activity in the heart. *Science*, 191:485–487.

Salata J.J., Brooks R.R. (1997). Pharmacology of azimilide dihydrochloride (NE-10064), a class III antiarrhythmic agent. *Cardiovascular. Drug. Rev.*, 15:137–156.

Salata J.J., Jurkiewicz N.K., Wang J., Sanguinetti M.C., Siegl P.K., Claremon D.A., Remy D.C., Elliot J.M., Libby B.E. (1996). The novel class III antiarrhythmic agent. L-735, 821 is a potent and selective blocker of I_{Ks} in guinea pig ventricular myocytes. *Circulation*, 94:I-528.

Sanguinetti M.C., Jurkiewicz N.K. (1990a). Two components of cardiac delayed rectifier K^+ current: differential sensitivity to block by class III antiarrhythmic agents. *J. Gen. Physiol.*, 96:195–215.

Sanguinetti M.C., Jurkiewicz N.K. (1990b). Lanthanum blocks a specific component of I_K and screens membrane surface charges in cardiac cells. *Am. J. Physiol.*, 259:H1881–1889.

Sanguinetti M.C., Curran M.E., Spector P.S., Keating M.T. (1996a). Spectrum of Herg K^+-channel dys-function in an inherited cardiac arrhythmia. *Proceedings of the National Academy of Sciences, USA*, 93:2208–2212.

Sanguinetti M.C., Curran M.E., Zou A., Shen J., Spector P.S., Atkinson D.L., Keating M.T. (1996b). Coassembly of K(V)LQTI and minK (IsK) proteins to form cardiac I(Ks) potassium channel [see comments]. *Nature*, 384:80–83.

Sanguinetti M.C., Jiang C., Curran M.E., Keating M.K. (1995). A mechanistic link between an inherited and an acquired cardiac arrhythmia: HERG encodes the I_{Kr} potassium channel. *Cell*, 81:299–307.

Sanguinetti M.C., Jurkiewicz N.K., Scott A., Siegl P.K.S. (1991). Isoproterenol antagonizes prolongation of refractory period by the class III antiarrhythmic agent E-4031 in guinea pig myocytes. Mechanism of action. *Circulation Research*, 68:77–84.

Sanny J., Moebs W. (1996). *University Physics*, Wm. C. Brown Publishers.

Sano T., Takayama N., Shimamoto T. (1959). Directional difference of conduction velocity in cardiac ventricular syncytium studied by microelectrodes. *Circ. Res.*, 7:262–267.

Santos P.E.B., Barcellos L.C., Mill J.G., Masuda M.O. (1995). Ventricular action potential and L-type calcium channel in infarct-induced hypertrophy in rats. *J. Cardiovasc. Electrophysiol.*, 6:1004–1014.

Sasyniuk B.I., Mendez C. (1971). A mechanism for reentry in canine ventricular tissue. *Circ. Res.*, 28:3–15.

Scamps F., Mayoux E., Charlemagne D., Vassort G. (1990). Calcium current in single cells isolated from normal and hypertrophied rat heart. Effects of β-adrenergic stimulation. *Circ. Res.*, 67:199–208.

Scamps F., Undrovinas A., Vassort G. (1989). Inhibition of I_{Ca} by quinidine, flecainide, ethmozin, and ethacizin. *Am. J. Physiol.*, 256:C549–559.

Schlief T., Schonherr R., Imoto K., Heinemann S.H. (1996). Pore properties of rat brain II sodium channels mutated in the selectivity filter domain. *Eur. Biophys. J.*, 25:75–91.

Schmitt F.O., Erlanger J. (1928–29). Directional differences in the conduction of the impulse through heart muscle and their possible relation to extrasystolic and fibrillary contractions. *Am. J. Physiol.*, 87:326–347.

Schoppa N.E., McCormack K., Tanouye M.A., Sigworth F.J. (1992). The size of gating charge in wild-type and mutant Shaker potassium channels. *Science*, 255:1712–1715.

Schroeder M. (1990). *Fractals, Chaos, Power Laws*, W.H. Freeman and Company, New York, NY, pp. 168: 336–339.

Schuessler R.B., Grayson T.M., Bromberg B.I., Cox J.L., Boineau J.P. (1992). Cholinergically mediated tachyarrhythmias induced by a single extrastimulus in the isolated canine right atrium. *Circ. Res.*, 71:1254–1267.

Schuessler R.B., Kawamoto T., Hand D.E., Mitsuno M., Bromberg B.I., Cox J.L., Boineau J.P. (1993). Simultaneous epicardial and endocardial activation sequence mapping in the isolated canine right atrium. *Circulation*, 88:250–263.

Schumacher C., Becker H., Conrads R., Schotten U., Pott S., Kellinghaus M., Sigmund M., Schondube F., Preusse C., Schulte H.D., Hanrath P. (1995). Hypertrophic cardiomyopathy: A desensitized cardiac β-adrenergic system in the presence of normal plasma catecholamine concentrations. *Naunyn-Schmeideberg's Arch. Pharmacol.*, 351:398–407.

Schwartz P.J., Priori S.G., Locati E.H., Napolitano C., Cantu F., Tobin J.A., Keating M.T., Hammoude H., Brown A.M., Chen L.S.K., Colatsky T.J. (1995). Long QT syndrome patients with mutations of the *SCN5A* and *HERG* genes have differential responses to Na[+] channel blockade and to increases in heart rate: Implications for gene-specific therapy. *Circulation*, 95:3381–3386.

Sewing S., Roeper J., Pongs O. (1996). Kv β_1 subunit binding specific for shaker-related potassium channel α-subunits. *Neuron*, 16:455–463.

Shah A., Cohen I.S., Rosen M.R. (1988). Stimulation of cardiac α receptors increases Na/K pump current and decreases gK via a pertussis toxin-sensitive pathway. *Biophys. J.*, 54:219–225.

Sheridan D.J., Penkoske P.A., Sobel B.E., Corr P.B. (1980). Alpha adrenergic contributors to dysrhythmia during myocardial ischemia and reperfusion in cats. *J. Clin. Invest.*, 65:161–171.

Sherman S.J., Catterall W.A. (1984). Electrical activity and cytosolic calcium regulate levels of tetrodotoxin sensitive sodium channels in rat muscle cells. *Proc. Natl. Acad. Sci.*, 81:262–266.

Sherman S.J., Chrivia J., Catterall W.A. (1985). Cyclic adenosine 3′ 5′-monophosphate and cytosolic calcium exert opposing effects on biosynthesis of tetrodotoxin sensitive sodium channels in rat muscle cells. *J. Neurosci.*, 5:1570–1576.

Shi G., Nakahira K., Hammond S., Rhodes K.J., Schechter L.E., Trimmer J.S. (1996). β subunits promote K[+] channel surface expression through effects early in biosynthesis. *Neuron*, 16:843–852.

Shi W.M., Wymore R.S., Wang H.S., Pan Z.M., Cohen I.S., Mckinnon Dixon J.E. (1997). Identification of two nervous system-specific members of the erg potassium channel gene family. *J. Neurosci.*, 17:9423–9432.

Shibata E.F., Drury T., Refsum H., Aldrete V., Giles W. (1989). Contributions of a transient outward current to repolarization in human atrium *Am. J. Physiol.*, 257:H1773–H1781.

Shimoni Y., Giles W.R. (1992). Role of inwardly rectifying potassium current in rabbit ventricular action potential *J. Physiol.*, 448:709–727.

Shimony E., Sun T., Kolmakova-Partensky L., Miller C. (1994). Engineering a uniquely reactive thiol into a cysteine-rich peptide. *Protein Engineering*, 7:503–507.

Shrier A., Adjemian R.A., Munk A.A. (1995). Ionic mechanisms of atrioventricular nodal cell excitability. In: D.P. Zipes J. Jalife (eds.), *Cardiac Electrophysiology: From Cell to Bedside* (2nd ed.), W.B. Saunders Co., Philadelphia, pp. 164–173.

Shrier A., Dubarski H., Rosengarten M., Guevara M.R., Nattel S., Glass L. (1987). Prediction of complex atrioventricular conduction rhythms in humans with use of the atrioventricular nodal recovery curve. *Circulation*, 76:1196–1205.

Shvilkin A., Danilo P. Jr., Chevalier P., Chang F., Cohen I.S., Rosen M.R. (1994). Vagal release of vasoactive intestinal peptide can promote vagotonic tachycardia in the isolated innervated rat heart. *Cardiovasc. Res.*, 28:1769–1773.

Sicouri S., Antzelevitch C. (1991). A subpopulation of cells with unique electrophysiological properties in the deep subepicardium of the canine ventricle. The M cell. *Circulation Research*, 68:1729–1741.

Siegelbaum S.A., Tsien R.W. (1980). Calcium-activated transient outward current in calf cardiac Purkinjie fibers. *J. Physiol.*, (Lond.), 299:485–506.

Smallwood J.K., Ertl P.G., Steinberg M.I. (1990). Modification by glibenclamide of the electrophysiological consequences of myocardial ischemia in dogs and rabbits. *Naunyn-Schmiedeberg's Arch. Pharmacol.*, 342:214–220.

Smith C., Phillips M., Miller C. (1986). Purification of charybdotoxin, a specific inhibitor of the high-conductance Ca^{2+}-activated K^+ channel. *J. Biol. Chem.*, 261:14607–14613.

Smith P.L., Baukrowitz T., Yellen G. (1996). The inward rectification mechanism of the HERG cardiac potassium channel. *Nature*, 379:833–836.

Snyder D.J., Knoth K.M., Roberds S.L., Tamkum M.M. (1992). Time-, voltage- and state-dependent block by quinidine of a cloned human cardiac potassium channel. *Mol. Pharmacol.*, 41:322–330.

Sosunov E.A., Anyukhovsky E.P., Rosen M.R. (1996). Effects of exogenous neuropeptide Y on automaticity of isolated Purkinje fibers and atrium. *J. Mol. Cell. Cardiol.*, 28:967–975.

Spach M.S., Dolber P.C., Heidlage J.F. (1988). Influence of the passive anisotropic properties on directional differences in propagation following modification of sodium conductance in human atrial muscle: a model of reentry based on anisotropic discontinuous propagation. *Circ. Res.*, 62:811–832.

Spach M.S., Dolber P.C., Heidlage J.F. (1989). Interaction of inhomogeneities of repolarization with anisotropic propagation in dog atria. A mechanism for both preventing and initiating reentry. *Circ. Res.*, 65:1612–1631.

Spach M.S., Heidlage J.F. (1992). A multidimensional model of cellular effects on the spread of electrotonic currents and on propagating action potentials. *Crit. Rev. Biomed. Eng.*, 20:141–169.

Spach M.S., Kootsey J.M. (1983). The nature of electrical propagation in cardiac muscle. *Am. J. Physiol.*, 244:H3–H22.

Spach M.S., Kootsey J.M., Sloan J.D. (1982a). Active modulation of electrical coupling between cardiac cells in the dog: A mechanism for transient and steady state variations in conduction velocity. *Circ. Res.*, 51:347–362.

Spach M.S., Miller III W.T., Dolber P.C., Kootsey M., Sommer J.R., Mosher C.E. (1982b). The functional role of structural complexities in the propagation of depolarization in the atrium of the dog. Cardiac conduction disturbances due to discontinuities of effective axial resistivity. *Circ. Res.*, 50:175–191.

Spach M.S., Miller III W.T., Miller-Jones E., Warren R.B., Barr R.C. (1979). Extracellular potentials related to intracellular action potentials during impulse conduction in anisotropic canine cardiac muscle. *Circ. Res.*, 45:188–204.

Spach M.S., Miller W.T., Geselowitz D.B., Barr R.C., Kootsey J.M., Johnson E.A. (1981). The discontinuous pattern of propagation in normal canine cardiac muscle. *Circ. Res.*, 48:39–54.

Spector P.S., Curran M.E., Zou A., Keating M.T., Sanguinetti M.C. (1996). Fast inactivation causes rectification of the IKr channel. *Journal of General Physiology*, 107:611–619.

Sperelakis N. (1994). Cable properties and propagation of action potentials. In: N. Sperelakis (ed.), *Cell Physiology Source book*, Academic press, Inc. San Diego, CA, pp. 245–254.

Sperelakis N. (1995). Gibbs-Donnan equilibrium potentials. In Cell Physiology. Source book (Sperelakis N ed). Academic Press, San Diego; pp. 91–95.

Spinelli W., Hoffman B.F. (1989). Mechanism of termination of reentrant atrial arrhythmias by class I and class III antiarrhythmic agents. *Circ. Res.*, 65:1565–1579.

Spinelli W., Follmer C.H., Parsons R., Colatsky T.J. (1990). Effects of cromakalim, pinacidil, and nicorandil on cardiac refractoriness and arterial pressure in open-chest dog. *Eur. J. Pharmacol.*, 179: 243–252.

Spinelli W., Parsons R.W., Colatsky T.J. (1992). Effects of WAY-123, 398, a new class III antiarrhythmic agent, on cardiac refractoriness and ventricular fibrillation threshold in anesthetized dogs: A comparison with UK-68798, E-4031 and dl-sotalol. *J. Cardiovasc. Pharmacol.*, 20:913–922.

Spinelli W., Sorota S., Siegal M., Hoffman B.F. (1991). Antiarrhythmic actions of the ATP-regulated K^+ current activated by pinacidil. *Circ. Res.*, 68:1127–1137.

Spyer K.M. (1981). Neural organization and control of the baroreceptor reflex. *Rev. Physiol. Biochem. Pharmacol.*, 88:23–124.

Stambler B.S., Wood M.A., Ellenbogen K.A., Perry K.T., Wakefield L.K., Wanderlugt J.T., the Ibutilide Repeat Dose Study Investigators (1996). Efficacy and safety of repeated intravenous doses of ibutilide for rapid conversion of atrial flutter or fibrillation. *Circulation*, 94:1613–1621.

Stampe P., Kolmakova-Partensky L., Miller C. (1994). Intimations of K^+ channel structure from a complete functional map of the molecular surface of charybdotoxin. *Biochem.*, 33:443–450.

Starmer C.F., Grant A.O., Stauss H.C. (1984). Mechanism of use-dependent block of sodium channels in excitable membranes by local anesthetics. *Biophys. J.*, 46:15–27.

Steinberg S.F., Chow Y.K., Robinson R.B., Bilezikian J.P. (1987). A pertussis toxin substrate regulates α_1-adrenergic dependent phosphatidylinositol hydrolysis in cultured rat myocytes. *Endocrinology*, 120:1889–1895.

Steinberg S.F., Drugge E.D., Bilezikian J.P., Robinson R.B. (1985). Acquisition by innervated cardiac myocytes of a pertussis toxin-specific regulatory protein linked to the α_1-receptor. *Science*, 230: 186–188.

Steinberg S.F., Robinson R.B., Rosen M.R. (1998). Molecular and cellular bases of β-adrenergic modulation of cardiac rhythm. In: D.P. Zipes and J. Jalife (eds.), *Cardiac Electrophysiology: From Cell to Bedside* (3rd edition), W.B. Saunders Co., Philadelphia, Pa., in press.

Steinberg S.F., Zhang H., Pak E., Pagnotta G., Boyden P.A. (1995). Characteristics of the β-adrenergic receptor complex in the epicardial border zone of the 5-day infarcted canine heart. *Circulation*, 91:2824–2833.

Stevens C.F. (1978). Interactions between intrinsic membrane protein and electric field. An approach to studying nerve excitability. *Biophys. J.*, 22:295–306.

Stockbridge N. (1988). Differential conduction at axonal bifurcations. II. Theoretical basis. *J. Neurophysiol.*, 59:1286–1295.

Stockbridge N., Stockbridge L.L. (1988). Differential conduction at axonal bifurcations. I. Effect of electrotonic length. *J. Neurophysiol.*, 59:1277–1285.

Stocker M., Miller C. (1994). Electrostatic distance geometry in a K^+ channel vestibule. *Proc. Natl. Acad. Sci. USA*, 91:9509–9513.

Strauss H.C., Bigger J.T., Hoffman B.F. (1970). Electrophysiological and β-receptor blocking effects of MJ 1999 on dog and rabbit cardiac tissue. *Circ. Res.*, 26:661–678.

Streeter D. (1979). Gross morphology and fiber geometry of the heart. In: Berne R.M. (ed.), *Handbook of Physiology Vol. 1: The Heart, Section 2: The Cardiovascular System*, Williams Wilkins, Baltimore, MD, pp. 61–112.

Stuhmer W., Conti F., Suzuki H., Wang X.D., Noda M., Yahagi N., Kubo H., Numa S. (1989). Structural parts involved in activation and inactivation of the sodium channel. *Nature*, 339:597–603.

Sugiura H., Joyner R.W. (1992). Action potential conduction between guinea pig ventricular cells can be modulated by Ca current. *American Journal of Physiology*, 263:H1591–H1604.

Surawicz B. (1992). Role of potassium channels in cycle length dependent regulation of action potential duration in mammalian cardiac Purkinje and ventricular muscle fibres. *Cardiovascular Research*, 26:1021–1029.

Szabo B., Sweidan R., Rajagopalan C.V., Lazzara R. (1994). Role of Na^+-Ca^{2+} current in Cs^+-induced early afterdepolarizations in Purkinje fibers. *J. Cardiovasc. Electrophysiol.*, 5:933–944.

Taccardi B., Macchi E., Lux R.L., Ershler P.R., Spaggiari S., Baruffi S., Vyhmeister Y. (1994). Effect of myocardial fiber direction on epicardial potentials. *Circulation*, 90:3076–3090.

Takei M., Furukawa Y., Narita M., Ren L.-M., Chiba S. (1992). Cardiac electrical responses to catecholamines are differentially mediated by β_2-adrenoceptors in anesthetized dogs. *Eur. J. Pharmacol.*, 219:15–21.

Takimoto K., Li D., Hershman K.M., Li P., Jackson E.K., Levitan E.S. (1997). Decreased expression of Kv4.2 and novel Kv4.3 K^+ channel subunit mRNAs in ventricles of renovascular hypertensive rats. *Circ. Res.*, 81:533–539.

Takumi T., Ohkubo H., Nakanishi S. (1988). Cloning of a membrane protein that induces a slow voltage-gated potassium current. *Science*, 242:1042–1045.

Talajic M., Papadatos D., Villemarie C., Glass L., Nattel S. (1991). A unified model of atrioventricular nodal conduction predicts dynamic changes in Wenckebach periodicity. *Circ. Res.*, 68:1280–1293.

Tang L., Kallen R.G., Horn R. (1996). Role of an S4-S5 linker in sodium channel inactivation probed by mutagenesis and a peptide blocker. *J. Gen. Physiol.*, 108:89–104.

Task Force of the Working Group on Arrhythmias of the European Society of Cardiology: The Sicilian Gambit (1991). A New Approach to the Classification of Antiarrhythmic Drugs Based on their Actions on Arrhythmogenic Mechanisms. *Circulation*, 84:1831–1851.

Taton G., Chatelain P., Delhaye M., Camus J., DeNeef P., Waelbroeck M., Tatemoto K., Robberecht P., Christophe J. (1982). Vasoactive intestinal peptide and peptide having n-terminal histidine and c-terminal isoleucine amide (PHI) stimulate adenylate cyclase in human heart membranes. *Peptides*, 3:897–900.

Taussig R., Gilman A.G. (1995). Mammalian membrane-bound adenylyl cyclases. *J. Biol. Chem.*, 270:1–4.

Tempel B.L., Papazian D., Schwarz T., Jan Y.N., Jan L.Y. (1987). Sequence of a probable potassium channel component encoded at *Shaker* locus of Drosophila. *Science*, 237:770–775.

TenEick R.E., Singer D.H. (1979). Electrophysiological properties of diseased human atria. Low diastolic potential and altered cellular response to potassium. *Circ. Res.*, 44:545–557.

TenEick R.E., Zhang K., Harvey R.D., Bassett A.L. (1993). Enhanced functional expression of transient outward current in hypertrophied feline myocytes. *Cardiovasc. Drugs Ther.*, 7:611–619.

Terlau H., Heinemann S.H., Stuhmer W., Pusch M., Conti F., Imoto K., Numa S. (1991). Mapping the site of block by tetrodotoxin and saxitoxin of sodium channel II. *FEBS Lett.*, 293:93–96.

Terzic A., Puceat M., Vassort G., Vogel S.M. (1993). Cardiac α_1-adrenoceptors: An Overview. *Pharmacol. Rev.*, 45:147–175.

The BEST Steering Committee (1995). Design of the β-blocker evaluation survival trial (BEST). *Am. J. Cardiol.*, 75:1220–1223.

Thomas G., Chung M., Cohen C.J. (1985). A dihydropyridine (Bay K 8644) that enhances calcium currents in guinea pig and calf myocardial cells. A new type of positive inotropic agent. *Circ. Res.*, 56:87–96.

Tomaselli G.F., Beuckelmann D.J., Calkins H.G., Berger R.D., Kessler P.D., Lawrence J.D., Kass D., Feldman A.M., Marban E. (1994). Sudden cardiac death in heart failure. The role of abnormal repolarization. *Circulation*, 90:2534–2539.

Tomita F., Bassett A.L., Myerburg R.J., Kimura S. (1994). Diminished transient outward currents in rat hypertrophied ventricular myocytes. *Circ. Res.*, 75:296–303.

Tourneur Y. (1986). Action potential-like responses due to the inward rectifying potassium channel. *J. Memb. Biol.*, 90:115–122.

Tritthart H., Luedcke H., Bayer R., Stierle H., Kaufmann R. (1975). Right ventricular hypertrophy in the cat. An electrophysiological and anatomical study. *J. Mol. Cell. Cardiol.*, 7:163–174.

Trudeau M.C., Warmke J.W., Ganetzky B., Robertson G.A. (1995). HERG, a human inward rectifier in the voltage-gated potassium channel family. *Science*, 269:92–95.

Trudeau M.C., Warmke J.W., Ganetzky B., Robertson G.A. (1996). HERG sequence correction [letter]. *Science*, 272:1087.

Tseng G-N., Boyden P.A. (1991). Different effects of intracellular Ca^{2+} and a phorbol ester on the T and L types Ca^{2+} currents in ventricular and Purkinje cells. *Am. J. Physiol.*, 261:H364–H379.

Tseng G-N., Hoffman B.F. (1989). Two components of transient outward current in canine ventricular myocytes. *Circ. Res.*, 64:633–647.

Tsuobi N., Kodama I., Takayama J., Yamada K. (1985). Anisotropic conduction properties of canine ventricular muscles. *Jpn. Cir. J.*, 49:487–498.

Unverferth D.V., O'Dorisio T.M., Muir III W.W., White J., Miller M.M., Hamlin R.L., Magorien R.D. (1985). Effect of vasoactive intestinal polypeptide on the canine cardiovascular system. *J. Lab. Clin. Med.*, 106:542–550.

Ursell P.C., Gardner P.I., Albala A., Fenoglio J.J. Jr., Wit A.L. (1985). Structural and electrophysiological changes in the epicardial border zone of canine myocardial infarcts during infarcts healing. *Circ. Res.*, 56:436–451.

Ursell P., Ren C.L., Albala A., Danilo P. Jr. (1991a). Nonadrenergic noncholinergic innervation. *Circ. Res.*, 68:131–140.

Ursell P., Ren C.L., Danilo P. Jr. (1991b). Anatomic distribution of autonomic neural tissue in the developing dog heart. *Anat. Rec.*, 230:531–538.

Valenzuela C., Bennett P.B. Jr. (1994). Gating of cardiac Na^+ channels in excised membrane patches after modification by α-chymotrypsin. *Biophysical Journal*, 67:161–171.

van Capelle F.J.L. (1983). *Slow Conduction and Cardiac Arrhythmias* (thesis), Amsterdam, Netherlands, University of Amsterdam, pp. 118–132.

Vandenberg C.A., Bezanilla F. (1991). Single-channel, macroscopic, and gating currents from sodium channels in the squid giant axon. *Biophys. J.*, 60:1499–1510.

Vassalle M. (1970). Electrogenic suppression of automaticity in sheep and dog Purkinje fibers. *Circulation Research*, 27:361–377.

Vassalle M., Yu H., Cohen I.S. (1995). The pacemaker current in cardiac Purkinje myocytes. *Journal of General Physiology*, 106:559–578.

Vassilev P., Scheuer T., Catterall W.A. (1989). Inhibition of inactivation of single sodium channels by a site-directed antibody. *Proc. Natl. Acad. Sci. USA*, 86:8147–8151.

Vassort G., Alvarez J. (1994). Cardiac T-type calcium current: pharmacology and role in cardiac tissues. *Journal of Cardiovascular Electrophysiology*, 5:376–393.

Waldo A.L., Camm A.J., deRuyter H. *et al.*, for the SWORD investigators (1996). Effects of *d*-sotalol on mortality in patients with left ventricular dysfunction after recent and remote myocardial infarction. *Lancet*, 348:7–12.

Walker P., Grouzmann E., Burnier M., Waeber B. (1991). The role of neuropeptide Y in cardiovascular regulation. *Trends in Physiol. Sci.*, 12:111–115.

Wallace A.A., Stupienski R.F., Baskin E.P. (1995). Cardiac electrophysiologic and antiarrhythmic actions of tedisamil. *J. Pharmacol. Exp. Ther.*, 273:168–175.

Wallace A.A., Stupiensky R.F., Brooks L.M., Selnick H.G., Claremon D.A., Lynch J.J. Jr. (1991). Cardiac electrophysiologic and inotropic actions of new and potent methanesulfonanilide class III anti-arrhythmic agents in anesthetized dogs. *J. Cardiovasc. Pharmacol.*, 18:687–695.

Wang Q., Curran M.E., Splawski I., Burn T.C., Millholland J.M., VanRaay T.J., Shen J., Timothy K.W., Vincent G.M., de Jager T., Schwartz P.J., Toubin J.A., Moss A.J., Atkinson D.L., Landes G.M., Connors T.D., Keating M.T. (1996). Positional cloning of a novel potassium channel gene: KVLQT1 mutations cause cardiac arrhythmias. *Nature Genetics*, 12:17–23.

Wang Q., Shen J., Li Z., Timothy K., Vincent G.M., Priori S.G., Schwartz P.J., Keating M.T. (1995a). Cardiac sodium channel mutations in patients with long QT syndrome, an inherited cardiac arrhythmia. *Human Molecular Genetics*, 4:1603–1607.

Wang Q., Shen J., Splawski I., Atkinson D., Li Z., Robinson J.L., Moss A.J., Towbin J.A., Keating M.T. (1995b). SCN5A mutations associated with an inherited cardiac arrhythmia, long QT syndrome. *Cell*, 80:805–811.

Wang S., Morales M.J., Liu S., Strauss H.C., Rasmusson R.L. (1996). Time, voltage and ionic concentration dependence of rectification of h-erg expressed in Xenopus oocytes. *FEBS Letters*, 389:167–173.

Wang S., Liu S., Morales M.J., Strauss H.C., Rasmusson R.L. (1997). A quantitative analysis of the activation and inactivation kinetics of HERG expressed in Xenopus oocytes. *Journal of Physiology*, 502:45–60.

Wang Z., Fermini B., Nattel S. (1993). Mechanism of flecainide's rate-dependent actions on action potential duration in canine atrial tissue. *J. Pharmacol. Exp. Ther.*, 267:575–581.

Wang Z., Fermini B., Nattel S. (1995). Effects of flecainide, quinidine, and 4-aminopyridine on transient outward and ultrarapid delayed rectifier currents in human atrial myocytes. *J. Pharmacol. Exp. Ther.*, 272:184–196.

Wang Z., Pelletier L.C., Talajic M., Nattel S. (1990). The effects of flecainide and quinidine on human atrial action potential. *Circulation*, 82:274–283.

Warner M.R., Levy M. (1989). Inhibition of cardiac vagal effects by neurally released and exogenous neuropeptide Y. *Circ. Res.*, 65:1536–1546.

Wasserstrom J.A., Schwartz D.J., Fozzard H.A. (1982). Catecholamine effects on intracellular sodium activity and tension in dog heart. *Am. J. Physiol.*, 243 (Heart Circ. Physiol., 12):H670–H675.

Wei J.-W., Sulakhe P. (1978). Regional and subcellular distribution of myocardial muscarinic cholinergic receptors. *Eur. J. Pharmacol.*, 52:235–238.

Weidmann S. (1952). The electrical constants of Purkinje fibers. *J. Physiol.* (Lond.), 118:348–360.

Weidmann S. (1955a). The effect of cardiac membrane potential on the rapid availability of the sodium carrying system. *J. Physiol.* (Lond.), 127:213–224.

Weidmann S. (1955b). The effects of calcium ions and local anesthetics on electrical properties of Purkinje fibers. *J. Physiol.* (Lond.), 129:568–582.

Weidmann S. (1966). The diffusion of radiopotassium across intercalated disks of mammalian cardiac muscle. *J. Physiol.* (Lond.), 187:323–342.

Weidmann S. (1970). Electrical constants of trabecular muscle from mammalian heart. *J. Physiol.*, 210:1041–1054.

Wenckebach K.F. (1899). Zur Analyse des unregelmassigen Pulses. II. Ueber den regelmassig intermittirenden puls. *Zeitschr. Klin. Med.*, 37:475–488.

West J.W., Patton D.E., Scheuer T., Wang Y., Goldin A.L., Catterall W.A. (1992). A cluster of hydrophobic amino acid residues required for fast Na^+-channel inactivation. *Proc. Natl. Acad. Sci. USA*, 89:10910–10914.

Wettwer E., Amos G.J., Posival H., Ravens U. (1994). Transient outward current in human ventricular myocytes of subepicardial and subendocardial origin *Circ. Res.*, 75:473–482.

White M., Roden R., Minobe W., Khan F., Larrabee P., Wollmering M., Port J.D., Anderson F., Campbell D., Feldman A.M., Bristow M.R. (1994). Age-related changes in β-adrenergic neuroeffector systems in the human heart. *Circulation*, 90:1225–1238.

Wickman K., Nemec J., Gendler S.J., Clapham D.E. (1998). Abnormal heart rate regulation in GIRK4 knockout mice. *Neuron*, 20:103–114.

Wilde A.A.M., Escande E., Schumaker C.A., Thuringer D., Mestre M., Fiolet J.W.T., Janse M.J. (1990). Potassium accumulation in the globally ischemic mammalian heart: A role for the ATP-sensitive potassium channel. *Circ. Res.*, 67:835–843.

Wilders R., Jongsma H.J., van Ginneken A.C.G. (1991). Pacemaker activity of the rabbit sinoatrial node: A comparison of mathematical models. *Biophys. J.*, 60:1202–1216.

Winfree A.T. (1972). Spiral waves of chemical activity. *Science*, 175:634–636.

Winfree A.T. (1973). Scroll-shaped waves in chemical activity in three dimensions. *Science*, 181:937–939.

Winfree A.T. (1987). *When Time Breaks Down*, Princeton University Press, Princeton N.J.

Winfree A.T. (1994). Electrical turbulence in three-dimensional heart muscle. *Science*, 266:1003–1006.

Winfree A.T. (1995). Theory of spirals. In: D.P. Zipes and J. Jalife (eds.), *Cardiac Electrophysiology: From Cell to Bedside*, W.B. Saunders, Philadelphia, pp. 379–389.

Wit A.L., Rosen M.R. (1992). Afterdepolarizations and triggered activity: distinction from automaticity as an arrhythmogenic mechanism. In: Fozzard H.A., Haber E., Jennings R.B., Katz A.M., Morgan H.E., (eds.), *The heart and cardiovascular system. Scientific foundations*, New York: Raven Press Ltd., pp. 2113–2163.

Wit A.L., Janse M.J. (1993). *The Ventricular Arrhythmias of Ischemia and Infarction. Electrophysiological Mechanisms*, Mount Kisco, NY: Futura Publishing Co, Inc.

Wong S.S., Bassett A.L., Cameron J.S., Epstein K., Kozlovskis P., Myerburg R.J. (1982). Dissimilarities in the electrophysiological abnormalities of lateral border and central infarct zone cells after healing of myocardial infarction in cats. *Circ. Res.*, 51:486–493.

Xiao R.P., Ji X., Lakatta E.G. (1995). Functional coupling of the β_2-adrenoceptor to a pertussis toxin-sensitive G protein in cardiac myocytes. *Mol. Pharmacol.*, 47:322–329.

Xu X., Best P.M. (1990). Increase in T type calcium current in atrial myocytes from adult rats with growth hormone-secreting tumors. *Proc. Natl. Acad. Sci. USA*, 87:4655–4659.

Yang J., Ellinor P.T., Sather W.A., Zhang J.F., Tsien R.W. (1993). Molecular determinants of Ca^{2+} selectivity and ion permeation in L-type Ca^{2+} channels. *Nature*, 366:158–161.

Yang N., George A.L. Jr., Horn R. (1996). Molecular basis of charge movement in voltage-gated sodium channels. *Neuron*, 16:113–122.

Yang T., Snyders D.J., Roden D.M. (1995). Ibutilide, a methanesulfonanilide antiarryhthmic, is a potent blocker of the rapidly activating delayed rectifier K^+ current in AT-1 cells. *Circulation*, 91:1799–1806.

Yao J.-A., Jang M., Fan J.-S., Zhou Y.-Y., Tseng G.-N. (1997). Differential effects of myocardial infarction on transient outward, delayed rectifier and inward rectifier currents in rat ventricle. *Biophys. J.* 72:A143.

Yee H.F., Weiss J.N., Langer G.A. (1989). Neuraminidase selectively enhances transient Ca current in cardiac myocytes. *Am. J. Physiol.*, 256:C1267–C1272.

Yeola S.W., Rich T.C., Ubele V.N., Tamkum M.M., Snyders D.J. (1996). Molecular analysis of a binding site for quinidine in a human cardiac delayed rectifier K^+ channel: role of S6 in antiarrhythmic drug binding. *Circ. Res.*, 78:1105–1114.

Yool A.J., Schwarz T.L. (1991). Alteration of ionic selectivity of a K^+ channel by mutation of the H5 region. *Nature*, 349:700–704.

Yu H., Chang F., Cohen I.S. (1995). Pacemaker current I_f in adult canine cardiac ventricular myocytes. *Journal of Physiology*, 485:469–483.

Yuan F., Pinto J.M.B., Hong Z., Myerburg R., Bassett A.L. (1995). Abnormal delayed rectifier potassium current (I_K) in feline left ventricular myocytes adjacent to healed myocardial infarct area. *Circulation*, 92:I-158.

Yuan F., Pinto J.M.B., Li Q., Wasserlauf B.J., Bassett A.L., Myerburg R.J. (1999). Characteristics of I_K and its response to quinidine in myocytes from sites of regional hypertrophy in experimental healed infarction. *J. Cardiovasc. Electro. Physiology.*, (in press).

Yue L., Feng J., Li G.R., Nattel S. (1996). Characterization of an ultrarapid delayed rectifier potassium channel involved in canine atrial repolarization. *Journal of Physiology*, 496:647–662.

Zagotta W.N., Aldrich R.W. (1990a). Voltage-dependent gating of Shaker A-type potassium channels in Drosophila muscle. *J. Gen. Physiol.*, 95:29–60.

Zagotta W.N., Hoshi T., Aldrich R.W. (1990b). Restoration of inactivation in mutants of *Shaker* potassium channels by a peptide derived from *ShB. Science*, 250:568–571.

Zagotta W.N., Hoshi T., Aldrich R.W. (1994a). Shaker potassium channel gating. III: Evaluation of kinetic models for activation. *J. Gen. Physiol.*, 103:321–362.

Zagotta W.N., Hoshi T., Dittman J., Aldrich R.W. (1994b). Shaker potassium channel gating. II: Transitions in the activation pathway. *J. Gen. Physiol.*, 103:279–319.

Zaza A., Kline R., Rosen M. (1990). Effects of α-adrenergic stimulation on intracellular sodium activity and automaticity in canine Purkinje fibers. *Circ. Res.*, 66, 416–426.

Zaza A., Malfatto G., Schwartz P.J. (1991). Sympathetic modulation of the relation between ventricular repolarization and cycle length. *Circulation Research*, 68:1191–1203.

Zaza A., Micheletti M., Brioschi A., Rocchetti M. (1997). Ionic currents during sustained pacemaker activity in rabbit sino-atrial myocytes. *Journal of Physiology*, 505:677–688.

Zaza A., Robinson R.B., Difrancesco D. (1996a). Basal responses of the L-type Ca^{2+} and hyperpolarization-activated currents to autonomic agonists in the rabbit sinoatrial node. *Journal of Physiology*, 491:347–355.

Zaza A., Rocchetti M., Difrancesco D. (1996b). Modulation of the hyperpolarization activated current (I_f) by adenosine in rabbit sinoatrial myocytes. *Circulation*, 94:734–741.

Zaza A., Rocchetti M., Brioschi A., Cantadori A., Ferroni A. (1998). Dynamic Ca^{2+}-induced rectification of I_{K1} during the ventricular action potential. *Circulation Research*, 82:947–956.

Zhang K., Harvey R.D., Martin R.L., Bassett A.L., TenEick R.E. (1991). Inward rectifying K current in normal and hypertrophied cat right ventricular myocytes *Biophys. J.*, 59:279a.

Zhou J.Y., Potts J.F., Trimmer J.S., Agnew W.S., Sigworth F.J. (1991). Multiple gating modes and the effect of modulating factors on the microI sodium channel. *Neuron*, 7:775–785.

Zipes D.G., Mendez C. (1973). Actions of manganese ions and tetrodotoxin on atrioventricular nodal transmembrane potentials in isolated rabbit hearts. *Circ. Res.*, 32:447–454.

Zipes D.G., Mendez C., Moe G.K. (1983). Some examples of Wenckebach periodicity in cardiac tissues, with an appraisal of mechanisms. In: M.V. Elizari and M.B. Rosenbaum (eds.), *Frontiers of Cardiac Electrophysiology*, Martinus Nijhoff, Boston, pp. 357–375.

Zygmunt A.C., Gibbons W.R. (1991). Calcium-activated chloride current in rabbit ventricular myocytes. *Circulation Research*, 68:424–437.

Zygmunt A.C., Gibbons W.R. (1992). Properties of the calcium-activated chloride current in heart. *Journal of General Physiology*, 99:391–414.

Zykov V.S. (1980). Analytical evaluation of the dependence of the speed of an excitation wave in two-dimensional excitable medium on the curvature of its front. *Biophizica*, 25:888–892.

Zykov V.S. (1987). *Simulations of Wave Processes in Excitable Media*, Manchester University Press, Manchester, U.K.

Index

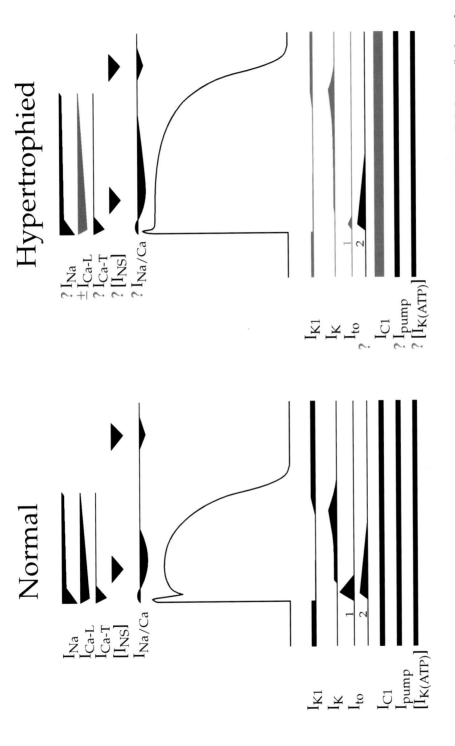

Color Plate 1 Schematic illustrating action potentials of epicardial ventricular myocytes from normal and hypertrophied hearts. Relative contributions of selected ionic currents are shown. Currents in red are those that have been found to be altered in myocytes from hypertrophied hearts. Question marks indicate there is still incomplete knowledge of ion channel function in these types of myocytes. See text for more detail. Modified after The Sicilian Gambit I (1991). *See* Page 180.

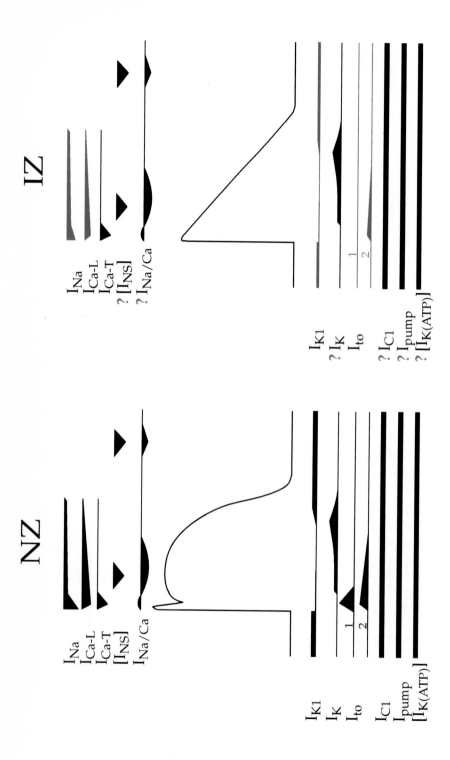

Color Plate 2 Schematic illustrating action potentials of epicardial ventricular myocyte from a normal heart and from the epicardial border zone of a 5 day infarcted heart. Relative contributions of selected ionic currents are shown. Currents in red are those that have been found to be altered in myocytes from the diseased heart. Question marks indicate there is still incomplete knowledge of ion channel function in these types of myocytes. See text for more detail. Modified after Sicilian Gambit I (1991). *See* Page 187.